D0913317

Power, Intimacy, and the Life Story
Personological Inquiries into Identity

Power, Intimacy, and the Life Story

Personological Inquiries into Identity

Dan P. McAdams

Foreword by Lawrence A. Pervin

THE GUILFORD PRESS
New York   London

To Rebecca

Last digit is print number: 9 8 7 6 5 4 3 2

Library of Congress Cataloging-in-Publication Data
McAdams, Dan P.
    Power, intimacy, and the life story.

    Reprint. Originally published: Homewood, Ill.:
Dorsey Press, © 1985. With new foreword and pref.
    Bibliography: p.
    Includes indexes.
    1. Identity (Psychology) 2. Personality.
3. Control (Psychology) 4. Intimacy (Psychology)
I. Title.
BF697.M16 1988   155.2   88-5285
ISBN 0-89862-506-8 (pbk.)

Foreword

For some time the field of personality has been in the doldrums. First the Skinnerian revolution led to an emphasis on determinants of behavior that were external to the person. Then the cognitive revolution led to an emphasis on thoughts, to the neglect of feelings and motives. While regaining its mind, the field of psychology in general, and personality in particular, appeared to have lost its soul. And, in the emphasis on specific pieces of behavior, common to both the Skinnerian and cognitive revolutions, the person as a whole was lost.

There are signs now that the field of personality is emerging from the doldrums, seeking new answers to such old problems as: What is it that motivates people? How do people go about making sense out of themselves and their lives? How can we study aspects of people without losing sight of the importance of the whole? How can we study people scientifically and develop general laws without losing sight of the richness of detail that is part of each individual? These are the questions that Dan McAdams directly addresses in this scholarly and beautifully written book. Following the intellectual tradition of such brilliant psychologists as Erik Erikson and Henry Murray, who played an important role in the development of his thinking, McAdams seeks nothing less than a psychology of personality that emphasizes the whole person—*personology.* As applied by McAdams, personology involves the use of biographical and motivational methods and concepts in the study of whole persons. In particular, McAdams suggests that we understand people in terms of their life stories, the dynamic narrative that we each create to make sense out of the past and orient us toward the future. Beginning in late adolescence we construct stories that form the basis of our identity—identity is a life story. Thus, rather than a mere abstraction or playful work, our life story has the power to provide unity and purpose to our lives. In the words of the author, ''We create stories, and we live according to narrative assumptions.''

While the content of each life story is unique to the individual, McAdams suggests that we can systematically analyze all such stories according to common components—*nuclear episodes* that represent critical scenes and turning points in our lives, *imagoes* that represent images of the self, *ideological settings* that represent the beliefs and values that provide the backdrop for the story, and a *generativity script* that provides a plan for life. In developing these components of the life story, and in illustrating the potential for their systematic study, McAdams ranges over such diverse areas as mythic archetypes, modern literature, and the efforts of such distinguished psychologists as Erikson, Murray, David McClelland, Jane Loevinger, and Sylvan Tomkins. Thus, the breadth of scholarship is of an order that few can match.

In attempting to demonstrate the empirical utility of his proposed framework, McAdams sets forth a number of hypotheses and utilizes a number of important new instruments that warrant the attention of others in the field. The populations studied include not only the readily available college sophomore, but also adults going through midlife crises. Many of the results provide impressive support for the proposed research procedures and theoretical model. For example, fantasy measures of intimacy and power motives are found to be related to spontaneous thought and behavior, patterns of interpersonal relationships, and overall psychological adjustment. Individuals high in intimacy motivation tend to have more close relationships, to be more self-disclosing, and to have a better psychological adjustment than individuals low in such motivation. Thus, the suggestion is made that the desire and capacity to engage in intimate relationships with others is a virtual sine qua non of psychosocial adaptation in the adult years. In contrast with men high on intimacy motivation, men high on power motivation tend to adopt authoritarian leadership strategies and to have problems in love relationships. Thus, the interplay between intimacy and power motives, as assessed through fantasy measures, is seen as accounting for fundamental aspects of human functioning. Along with such supportive results are others that suggest that the complexity of human personalities and human stories is even greater than had originally been recognized. Such is inevitably the case with any first effort, and it is to McAdams's credit that he invites us to join with him in the effort to understand this greater complexity.

While breaking new ground in the study of personality, McAdams would appear to be part of major developments occurring in the field. Three such linkages can be noted. First, there is an emphasis on the importance of motives. A person's power and intimacy motives confer upon his or her identity a predictable thematic emphasis. David McClelland, McAdams's mentor and colleague, has been one of the few psychologists to maintain an interest in, and commitment to, the study of human motivation. The present work follows in McClelland's tradition and stands as a worthy addition to that field of study. I would suspect that an understanding of the role of intimacy motivation in people's lives will be an important challenge for psychologists in the years ahead.

Second, there is an emphasis on images of the self. While interest in the self has waxed and waned in psychology, recently it has increased dramatically. And, in an interesting point of convergence, this is the case within both academic psychology and psychoanalytic object relations theory. The concept of imagoes of the self, with its links to motives, would appear to be similar to Hazel Markus's discussion of possible selves within academic psychology and the concept of internalized object representations in psychoanalytic theory. Thus, McAdams's work may yet serve as a bridge between these two important currents.

Third, there is an emphasis on both cognition and affect. Too often psychologists have studied one to the neglect of the other, as if a person only had thoughts or feelings, or one could only follow from the other. To McAdams's credit, attention is given to both cognition and affect in personality functioning. Motives and goals have both cognitive and affective components to them, and one's life story is a cognitive construction that is derived from, expressive of, and impacts upon powerful emotional experiences.

In sum, McAdams approaches the study of personality with the sensitivity of the clinician and the rigor of the scientist. To whom, then, should the book be of interest? The author aimed his work at social scientists and practitioners in the helping professions whose mission it is to understand the whole person, as well as laypersons concerned with the mystery of their own identity and the identities of others. With a graceful shift between the poetic and the empirical, McAdams has told a story that should be of interest to everyone in his intended audience. Against the backdrop of 20th century discord and malaise, he highlights the adult challenge to be both powerful and intimate, both expanding the self and surrendering it to others in the same self-defining way.

Lawrence A. Pervin

*P*reface

Joan Didion writes, "We tell ourselves stories in order to live." This book is about those stories. So that we may understand who we are and how we fit into our ever-so-complex world, we begin in late adolescence and early adulthood to construct a dynamic narrative of self, a mythological saga of identity complete with gods and goddesses, heroes and villains, tales of power and love, creation, demise, the rise, the fall, the rebirth, and the adventures of the self. Like stories in literature, our life stories embody settings, scenes, characters, plots, and recurrent themes. And like stories in literature, the stories we tell ourselves in order to live bring together diverse elements into an integrated whole, organizing the multiple and conflicting facets of our lives within a narrative framework which connects past, present, and an anticipated future and confers upon our lives a sense of sameness and continuity—indeed, an *identity*. As the story evolves and our identity takes form, we come to *live* the story as we *write* it, assimilating our daily experience to a schema of self that is a product of that experience. Thus, in identity, life gives birth to art and then imitates it. We create stories, and we live according to narrative assumptions.

I have undertaken an exploration of the structure and content of life stories. The inquiry draws upon methods and concepts from within and outside the social sciences, and the tentative synthesis I have forged falls within the domain of what Henry Murray termed *personology*—the scientific study of the whole person. This book is, in part, aimed at those social scientists and practitioners in various helping professions who understand their mission to be that of understanding the whole person, either from the standpoint of research or intervention. The book is also aimed at a broader audience of educated laypersons who find themselves pondering now and again the mysteries of their own identities and the identities of their friends, family, loved ones, and even casual acquaintances. For this broader audience, some familiarity with psychological theory and methods is probably helpful for appreciating what I am doing in this book, but it may not be essential. Rather technical information concerning data collection and analysis is often relegated to the appendixes or footnotes. Thus, I believe that the substance and form of the chapters which follow should be interesting, relevant, and accessible to a wide range of readers, professional and nonprofessional alike.

This paperback edition of *Power, Intimacy, and the Life Story,* published by The Guilford Press, appears at a time when psychologists and many other social scientists are expressing a greater and greater interest in the narrative dimensions of human life. Since the publication of the hardcover edition of this book almost three years ago, we have witnessed an upsurge of research and theorizing about the role of story in persons' lives. For instance, John Kotre's (1985) *Outliving the Self* presents eight fascinating case studies of American adults' attempts to find immortality through their children and other life products, each recast into a concise dramatic narrative to bring out the succession of conflict and resolution and the development of character in the storyteller's life. Kotre believes that the story is the natural vehicle for understanding a life, whether it be somebody else's or one's own. His insight was anticipated by the philosopher Jean Paul Sartre, whose views on narrative and lives have been articulated with clarity and beauty in Stuart Charme's (1984) recent book, *Meaning and Myth in the Study of Lives.* Sartre believed that each person makes sense of his or her own life by constructing and then living a "true novel." As he puts it, "a man is always a teller of tales, he lives surrounded by his stories and the stories of others, he sees everything that happens to him through them; and he tries to live his life as if he were telling a story."

The integrative power of story in human life has been reinforced by two very important books recently written by eminent psychologists who have made wide-ranging contributions to the field over the last 30 years. In *Actual Minds, Possible Worlds*, Jerome Bruner (1986) argues that psychologists have traditionally neglected the narrative mode of human thought, in favor of logical and deductive thinking. Yet the narrative mode seems to be a natural means by which people operate in many different spheres of life, including making sense of their own existence. In *Narrative Psychology*, Ted Sarbin (1986) raises the intriguing possibility that "narrative" might be considered a "root metaphor" for understanding human behavior and experience. Sarbin believes that a focus on story and narrative in human lives may signal a major conceptual shift in the social sciences in the direction of a new and broader paradigm for interpreting individual lives and social systems.

While I am not ready to claim that *Power, Intimacy, and the Life Story* heralds the birth of a new paradigm in psychology, I do believe that the content and the spirit of this book reflect important changes occurring in psychology and the social sciences today. The enthusiastic reception of the hardcover edition of the book reinforces my belief. With the same enthusiasm, I thank Sharon Panulla and The Guilford Press for publishing this new edition.

A book on life stories doubtlessly reflects the life story of the author. This book is no exception. The final product is a culmination of a number of trends in my own intellectual and personal life over the course of the last few years. Though a number of people have had a major influence upon my thinking about life stories over this time, I can presently point to three dominant influences. First and foremost, I would like to thank David McClelland who, more than anyone else, has been an inspiration in my intellectual life. Through my association with him in graduate school and afterwards, I have developed an abiding interest in human motivation and its place in the complicated gamut we call "personality." David taught me, and continues to teach others, that scientists can, in fact, ask the "big questions"—questions about love, power, identity, adaptation—and can design reasonable methodologies and measurement techniques for examining these questions in disciplined empirical ways. Second, I would like to thank another teacher in graduate school—George Goethals—whose influence has been more subtle. Through his legendary classes at Harvard on the psychology of the human life cycle, George has made the work of Freud, Erikson, Sullivan, and a host of others sparkle with an enduring relevance for two generations of students, and in that lucky group I find myself. Third, I would like to extend a belated thank-you to a group of dedicated teachers who shaped my earliest inquiries into human psychology. These are the professors involved in the Christ College honors program in the humanities for undergraduates at Valparaiso University. I would like, therefore, to thank the Christ College program in humanities and in particular Professors Warren Rubel, Bill Olmsted, Arlin Meyer, and Don Affeldt Allen.

I would like to extend a special thank-you to David Winter, whose comments on earlier drafts of the manuscript greatly improved the end product. I am also grateful to all of the following friends and colleagues whose comments and criticisms have been of valuable assistance in putting together this project: Skip Alexander, David Berndt, Fred Bryant, Michael Carney, John Carroll, Robert Casas, Joe Durlak, Jeanne Foley, Carroll Izard, Michael Jeffers, Carol Kirshnit, Michael Klinger, Dick Maier, Mark Mayzner, Dan Perlman, Joe Powers, Joe Rychlak, Abigail Stewart, and Eugene Walker. I would also like to thank all of the following who assisted in data coding and analysis: Don Allen, Erica Bokor, Mirel Castle, Carrie Craven, Kathy Farrell, Sheila Healy, Joan Hong, Marianne Hough, Michele Koslowski, Steven Krause, Nancy Martin, Jim McKay, Dan Rebek, Terri Slaughter, and Steven Wodka. A very special thank-you is extended to Karin Ruetzel who completed the herculean task of collecting most of the data for Sample B.

Maggie Melville and Judy Savage typed most of the manuscript, and to them I am extremely grateful. Finally, I would like to thank my wife, Rebecca Pallmeyer, who has been a companion, a counselor, and the most rigorous of editors throughout the writing of this book.

Part of the research described in this book was funded by a summer research grant from Loyola University of Chicago. The initial investigation into religious ideology reported in Chapter 7 was funded by a grant from the American Lutheran Church.

Dan P. McAdams

REFERENCES

Bruner, J. *Actual minds, possible worlds.* Cambridge, Mass.: Harvard University Press, 1986.

Charme, S.L. *Meaning and myth in the study of lives: A Sartrean perspective.* Philadelphia: University of Pennsylvania Press, 1984.

Kotre, J. *Outliving the self: Generativity and the interpretation of lives.* Baltimore: Johns Hopkins University Press, 1985.

Sarbin, T.R. (Ed.). *Narrative psychology: The storied nature of human conduct.* New York: Praeger, 1986.

Contents

Chapter 1

The Problem of Identity

The integration now taking place in the form of ego identity is, as pointed out, more than the sum of the childhood identifications. It is the accrued experience of the ego's ability to integrate all identifications with the vicissitudes of the libido, with the aptitudes developed out of endowment, and with the opportunities offered in social roles. The sense of ego identity, then, is the accrued confidence that the inner sameness and continuity prepared in the past are matched by the sameness and continuity of one's meaning for others.

(Erik Erikson, 1963, p. 261)

The discord and the malaise of the 20th century are reflected in our images of who we are. The century that has shown us the ultimate brutality and anonymity of Auschwitz and Hiroshima has produced images of identity that are frightening and confusing, fail to affirm life, fail to give us direction, and fail to instill within us the hope that what we feel and believe really matters and what we do really makes a difference. The images inhabit our poetry, drama, fiction, and newspapers. They are implicit in our best offerings from the humanities and the social sciences. And they animate our lives, though we may be aware of them only in our moments of greatest insight.

Consider one of these images—what Robert Langbaum (1982) calls the image of the *walking dead:*

A crowd flowed over London Bridge, so many,
I had not thought death had undone so many.
Sighs, short and infrequent, were exhaled,
And each man fixed his eyes before his feet.

(T. S. Eliot, *The Waste Land*, I. 62–65)

The walking dead trudge anonymously through T. S. Eliot's prophetic verses of *The Waste Land* (1922). Eliot's protagonists wander from place to place without direction for they are incapable of sustaining vital, energizing, direction-giving identities. Cut off from nature, religion, and their own unconscious selves, the walking dead are nameless and faceless, each bereft of a distinctive sense of individual continuity and sameness. The walking dead cannot address the twin questions of identity—"Who am I?" and "How do I fit into an adult world?"—because they fear these questions. As a result, they pass time ruminating over the trivialities of daily existence. The anxious upper-class lady in *The Waste Land* asks,

> *What shall I do now? What shall I do?*
> *What shall we do tomorrow?*
> *What shall we ever do?*
>> (T. S. Eliot, *The Waste Land*, II.
>> 131, 133–34)

And the protagonist of another poem, J. Alfred Prufrock, muses,

> *I grow old . . . I grow old . . .*
> *I shall wear the bottoms of my trousers rolled.*
> *Shall I part my hair behind? Do I dare to eat a peach?*
> *I shall wear white flannel trousers, and walk upon the beach.*
>> (T. S. Eliot, "The Love Song of J. Alfred Prufrock,"
>> 120–23)

Consider another, more haunting, image. In some of the most significant works of contemporary literature, we are confronted with what Langbaum (1982) terms the image of *zero identity*. In the stories and poems of such modern writers as Pynchon, Ionesco, and Beckett, we meet characters who, unlike Eliot's walking dead, do not even walk. The apotheosis of zero identity is identity stripped of even a trace of vitality: the emasculated and solitary identity of Beckett's Krapp or the random and chaotic life stories we hear in Pynchon's *V.* Langbaum writes,

> Beckett's living dead do not even walk—in the novels they hobble and crawl, in the plays they are remarkably stationary. Beckett presents in his plays unindividuated characters with stylized faces, whose single names do not name them, give no clue to family, class, nation (we do not identify Vladimir as Russian or Pozzo as Italian). His characters come from nowhere, belong nowhere, have no occupation or place in society. There is no society. Society appears as the small band that beats Estragon when he sleeps nights in the ditch. Godot beats his messenger's brother; Pozzo beats Lucky. Beating seems the last vestige of the social principle; and for certain pairs (Pozzo-Lucky, Hamm-Clov) the tyrant-victim relation is all that remains of love. Beckett goes farther than early Eliot, who portrays the breaking down of civilization; Beckett portrays the period after the wreck. (1982, p. 120)

Consider an image from an influential social critic. Christopher Lasch (1979) indicts the *narcissistic personality* of our time (p. 71). As prototype of the modern American identity, the narcissist has forfeited a vital engagement of others and world and retreated to an endlessly recursive arena of self. Like Eliot's walking dead, Lasch's narcissist experiences a sense of inner emptiness. But Lasch attributes to the narcissist a host of other character traits drawn from psychoanalytic theory. These include repressed rage, "unconscious oral cravings," Machiavellian seductiveness, "pseudoself insight," and a "dependence upon vicarious warmth provided by others combined with a fear of dependence" (pp. 74–75). For Lasch, the personal identity of the narcissist is a microcosm of contemporary Western culture's corporate identity.

Finally, consider the image of Proteus identified by psychiatrist Robert Lifton (1979). Lifton's *protean man* appears on the surface to be a well-rounded, individuated human being. He or she is actively involved in many life pursuits and has a host of interests and avocations. But in this individual an inner emptiness still prevails. The protean man lacks coherence; no unifying theme binds together his or her disparate interests and activities. The image is scattered identity, with pieces of self thrown together into a patternless mélange.

Unity and Purpose

The problem of identity is the problem of unity and purpose in human lives. These 20th-century images of identity are frightening, partly because they lack unity and purpose. Eliot's walking dead appear to be going nowhere. Lacking a destination, the inhabitants of *The Waste Land* do not know what to do. Alienated from self and world, they do not sense that their lives are integral parts of a superordinate and purposeful whole. At best, they are left to walk through their routines; at worst, they become the faceless and nameless victims of the destruction wrought by tyrannical systems. Beckett's isolated dyads are the survivors of the destruction, but survival is a Pyrrhic victory at best. The elimination of society and nature leaves behind a lunar-like landscape upon which Beckett's characters either crawl or sit. Isolated from others and their environments, Lasch's narcissists have been severed from a purpose to their lives, though Lasch intimates that the severing is their own doing. And Lifton's protean man discovers no underlying purpose for his myriad behaviors and experiences. There are many roles to be played, but no identity to integrate them. The protean man searches for unity to define the self, but, like the Greek god Proteus, his fate is to flip back and forth among the various guises he can so readily adopt. Unity and purpose remain outside his desperate grasp.

Unity and purpose in human lives are products of a complex set of interactions between the individual person and the society in which his or her behavior and experience are embedded. Societies provide occupational, ideological, and relational resources upon which the individual can draw in formulating his or her own identity. The resources are shaped into a personalized life product which, ideally, confers upon the individual a sense of unity and purpose—a feeling/belief that the person is whole and that his or her life is justified by a reason, mission, or goal. If identity is to be vital, the person must in some sense transform the world and, thereby, leave his or her mark upon it. Yet, the world—the sociohistorical environment—is not an object that can be "completely" transformed or transcended. Consequently, forming an identity is not simply a matter of distinguishing oneself from the surround. The counterpoint to separation in formulating a personal identity is reintegration within one's sociohistorical context; that is, establishing connections as well as separations. If identity is like a painting, environmental opportunities are the canvas and colors. Though the final artistic creation is a unique expression, highly personalized, and thus differentiated from all other works of art, the artist is limited by the materials at hand. In art and in living, we cannot transcend our resources.

It has been the belief of many 20th-century observers that the resources at hand for forging individual identities embodying unity and purpose have diminished markedly for Westerners living in the postindustrial age. Though the material and bodily well-being of Westerners has reaped the benefits of unprecedented scientific and technological advancement in the last 200 years, such resources have become scarce. These resources are, for the most part, ideological—they are beliefs and values, affirmed by societies, concerning humankind's appropriate place in the cosmos; they are the questions and answers formulated by persons throughout history in response to issues of ultimate concern.

For hundreds of years before the Enlightenment, Christianity served as a system of beliefs and values which provided Westerners with an agenda for their own identity work. The unity and purpose of one's life on earth was seen in the context of God's plan for the universe. Langbaum (1982) writes, "As long as men believed in a soul created and sustained (continuously *known* and *seen*) by God, there could be no question about the unity of self" (p. 25). With the Enlightenment's attack upon the Christian church and the subsequent erosion of Christianity's synthesizing power as a framework for individual identity in the last 200 years, Westerners have searched for alternative frameworks of meaning, but no all-encompassing substitute has risen to the fore. Depending upon one's view of history, a number of other factors can be implicated, along with the erosion of

Christianity, in the gradual breakdown of an integrative agenda for personal identity in the West. Among these might be the industrial revolution, widespread urbanization, the rise of capitalism, the alienation of worker and work, demystification through science, the discovery of the unconscious, two world wars, and the atom bomb.

The traditional identity agenda has decayed steadily in the West over the past 200 years. In its place, we have experimented with a number of substitutes. Langbaum (1982) argues that these substitutes can be found in the great literature of the last two centuries. For instance, Wordsworth and other Romantic poets of the early 19th century extolled an image of identity which was to serve as an alternative to what was perceived as an effete Christian vision of a God-created self. For the Romantics, identity drew vitality from its organic connection with nature. Wordsworth understood identity as a creative act of imagination in which the self and the natural world come to be seen as intricately woven together. In epiphanies of great joy, Romantic men and women are to apprehend the tapestry of self and nature. To imagine and thereby create the tapestry is to bind oneself to one's environment and past. For Wordsworth, joyful and creative epiphanies in the presence of nature enable the person to travel back in his or her mind to the beginning, to reassess life so as to "bind" one's "days together anew" (Langbaum, 1982, p. 44). Identity is thereby consolidated as one's life comes to be characterized by an inner peace and confidence concerning unity and purpose, what Wordsworth described as "the calm existence which is mine" (*The Prelude.* I, 349).

Unfortunately for the Romantics, the West has failed to embrace this Romantic identity agenda as it has likewise passed over other alternatives which Langbaum (1982) identifies as "secular religions" in literature. And, therefore, identity remains today the "spiritual problem of our time," according to Langbaum (p. 352), as each of us attempts to create, in our own lives, a sense of personal continuity to provide unity and purpose in a world appearing fragmented and without aim.

The urgency of the identity problem is underscored by a number of 20th-century existentialist philosophers who argue that identity is an issue of imperative morality. For not only do modern men and women need to forge personalized identities to attain unity and purpose in a world that provides few easy identity solutions, argue the existentialists, but it is indeed the moral responsibility of men and women to forge identities. For Jean Paul Sartre (1966) and for Gabriel Marcel (1964), human beings must continue to create themselves anew through conscious introspection. Responsible men and women are to confront the angst which results from the seeming purposelessness of human existence through reflection upon "some project of consciousness" (Fingarette, 1969, p. 99). Not to do so is to live in *bad faith* (Sartre, 1966)—to shrink from the moral imperative to create an authentic identity. The individual who lives in bad faith mindlessly plays out the various roles which structure his or her interaction with the world, but in failing to transcend roles he or she continues to deceive self. Like Lifton's protean man, the person living in bad faith is unable to bind together the scattered constituents of his or her life.

The existentialists maintain that to the extent persons can achieve unity and purpose in lives, their achievements are products of concerted introspection or self-examination. Despite major disagreements concerning the process of knowing and the nature of the self to be known, the existentialists agree with the psychoanalysts in asserting that the good (authentic living, psychological health) resides in "knowing thyself." The unexamined life, for the existentialists, means bad faith; for the psychoanalysts, it may mean neurosis. The proliferation, in recent years, of psychological therapies designed to facilitate self-awareness as well as the keen interest expressed by some Westerners in Eastern religions and their attendant practices of meditation and reflection suggests that the Socratic imperative to know thyself has found its way into most contemporary understandings of psychological health and adaptation.

Today, we are encouraged to get in touch with ourselves and with each other. We are asked to reflect upon where the other person "is coming from," and indeed where we ourselves are coming from and to where we may be going. We are urged to maximize our potential, to lead a fulfilling life, and to attain self-actualization. We may even purchase products which enable "me to be me." The 1970s and early 1980s have not promoted the "me generation" simply because we as Westerners have become more egocentric and selfish. The focus upon me has also implied increasing self-reflection—turning inward and questioning the self (Yankelovich, 1981). We as knowers have come to reflect more upon the self as known or what William James (1890) termed "the me or empirical ego."

According to many psychologists, knowing thyself involves being open to change. We are to emancipate ourselves from childhood identifications (Kernberg, 1975), ingrained thought patterns (Beck, 1970; Ellis, 1970), antiquated life "scripts" (Berne, 1972; Steiner, 1974), and worn-out "life structures" (Levinson, 1978). To discover ourselves anew, we must separate from our pasts or at least develop new perspectives from which to view our pasts. In the extreme we may come to view our lives as embodying continual flux and, therefore, to conclude that the only thing unchanging in lives—the sole element of continuity and sameness—is the fact of change. Gould (1980) appears on the verge of this extreme conclusion:

I see transformation as the central concept of adult development. If we are to understand the subtle day-to-day changes as well as the large crises in work and love, we must appeal to these central, ongoing processes whereby each of us is driven by maturational necessity to be more whole, to include within us disenfranchised parts, and to be as internally free as we are capable of being. We do this in steps throughout our life and rarely reach a steady state with either our work or our love life (p. 224).

For Gould, change implies freedom, freedom to be whoever one is able to be. When we are free, we are able to "include within us disenfranchised parts" of the self. When free we are able to attain unity in our lives, though Gould does not mention "purpose." In her popular survey of adult lives, Gail Sheehy (1976) echoes Gould, imploring men and women to emancipate themselves from their pasts and to embrace the continually changing future. We are to welcome the "passages" or "predictable crises" of adulthood and to discover, thereby, continuity in change.

One wonders, however, if a coherent and purposeful identity is likely to emerge amidst relentless flux. Does Gould's ideal eventually commit himself or herself to an identity which provides unity and purpose, or does he or she undertake instead a series of provisional commitments? Is there anything less protean about formulating one identity after another in response to each predictable crisis across the life span than entertaining several at once as does Lifton's protean man? In the former, images of self follow in rapid-fire sequence; in the latter, they abound simultaneously. But both may be examples of Sartre's bad faith. Though Gould argues that the succession of identities across a human life span is progressive such that with each new formulation the person reaches a higher level of unity ("wholeness"), the less sanguine observer might counter that continual transformation in lives implies a *false* freedom from the past. Indeed, Wordsworth wrote that identity binds the past, present, and future. To recapture an earlier metaphor, our personal histories constitute one class of resources upon which we must draw in forging individual identities. Thus, we do *not* achieve unity and purpose by freeing ourselves from our pasts. This critical theme appears again and again in the work of the preeminent observer of contemporary identity— Erik Erikson.

Erikson's Theory of Identity

The Early and the Late

The story of theory and life flowing together in the case of Erik Erikson has been told many times before (Coles, 1970; Erikson, 1975; Goethals, 1976; Hogan, 1976; Monte, 1980; Yankelovich & Barrett,

1971). Erikson, the man who observed significant personality changes in his own life during his adult years, extended the Freudian developmental model to encompass developmental issues of adulthood. Erikson, the poet-turned-analyst who found that answering the questions "Who am I?" and "How do I fit into an adult world?" required a protracted period of "moratorium" in his own life, created a special place in his own theory of personality development for the issue of identity versus role confusion. Erikson, the young adult who was a wanderer and yet appeared to remain optimistic through all his identity journeys, cast psychoanalytic theory in a more positive, life-affirming mold than did the more pessimistic founder who knew from early childhood that his lot in life was "to understand something of the riddles of the world in which we live and perhaps even to contribute something to their solution" (Jones, 1961, p. 22). As a theme of "the early determining the late" is reflected in the life *and* the theory of Sigmund Freud, so a theme of "the late reorganizing the early" appears in the life and theory of one of Freud's most original successors.

For Erikson, identity is a reorganization of the "early" into a pattern which connects the individual's past to the perceived present and anticipated future. The late—adolescence and adulthood—serves to reorganize the early—the individual's history as a child functioning in a child's world. As Erikson (1959) writes, identity formation begins

> where the usefulness of identification ends. It arises from the selective repudiation and mutual assimilation of childhood identifications, and their absorption in a new configuration, which in turn, is dependent on the process by which a *society* (often through subsocieties) *identifies the young individual*, recognizing him as somebody who had to become the way he is, and who, being the way he is, is taken for granted. (p. 113)

In adolescence and young adulthood, the person is confronted for the first time with the twin identity questions of "Who am I?" and "How do I fit into an adult world?" According to Erikson, successfully answering the identity questions presupposes an understanding of "Who have I been in the past?" and "Who am I to be in the future?" This binding together of past, present, and future is beautifully portrayed in the identity sagas of such great men as Gandhi (Erikson, 1969) and Luther (Erikson, 1958), and Erikson adds that "it would be well to trace its development through the life histories or significant life episodes of ordinary individuals" (1959, p. 110).

The binding together of past, present, and future cannot occur in a person's life until he or she has indeed established a past and recognized it as such. The time in the human life cycle which is ripe for this realization is, according to Erikson, late adolescence and young adulthood. The reasons for this are many. Biologically, young girls and boys find themselves the reluctant inhabitants (in adolescence) of suddenly adult-like bodies. Psychosexually, what Sullivan (1953) terms the "lust dynamism" has finally awakened, demanding creative modes of coping with powerful sexual longings. The teenager, thus, is compelled by the changes from within to formulate new understandings of his or her bodily, sexual, and social selves. He or she has begun a new biological and psychosexual chapter. Puberty, thus, may mark a turning point in the adolescent's perceived developmental course, as childhood comes to represent, in the adolescent's mind, a bygone era.

Cognitive development, too, plays a critical role in the emergence of the identity issue. Piaget (Inhelder & Piaget, 1958) has argued that in adolescence many people enter the stage of *formal operations*. In this fourth and final stage in Piaget's model of cognitive development, the adolescent or adult begins to understand the world in highly abstract terms. In formal operations, one is able to reason about what is and *what might be* in terms of verbally stated propositions. Whereas the 10-year-old child adeptly categorizes and classifies a reality resplendent with variety and vicissitude, his or her thought remains embedded in that reality, bound to the concrete world of what is while oblivious to the abstract realm of what is not but what conceivably might be. We say, thus, that the typical 10-year-old knows the world via *concrete operations*. Ask one to recite the 50 state capitals, and he or she may score 100 percent. Ask what the capitals might be if the United States were divided into only 10 states, and he or she will probably have a lot of trouble. First, the child may argue that the proposition is inherently ridiculous because the United States *is* in fact made up of 50 states. Second, he or she may find it extremely difficult to devise a systematic plan for determining what the criteria of a capital should be in a hypothetical scenario. For the 10-year-old, *reality is all*, and the hypothetical is but an aberration. For the adolescent or adult in formal operations, on the other hand, reality is one possibility amidst an infinite array of hypothetical realities. In formal operations, what is comes to be seen as a subset of what might be. The real is merely an arbitrary manifestation of the hypothetical.

The adolescent or adult in formal operations, therefore, can systematically address hypothetical problems and possibilities and can proceed logically from a verbally stated proposition to derive hypotheses to be tested for their truth. In adopting a hypothetico-deductive strategy in solving problems, the formal-operational knower displays the analytic powers of logician and scientist. Propositional logic and scientific hypothesis testing emerge as potential *modi operandi* for solving problems. Furthermore, as one's ways of knowing become more and more abstract in formal operations, one comes to focus introspectively upon one's own thought processes. Thus, the adolescent or adult may take his or her thought as an object to reflect upon. According to Elkind (1981), the individual in formal operations is able to operate upon operations; to analyze the process of analyzing; to think about thinking.

With respect to identity, then, the adolescent or young adult who has entered Piaget's stage of formal operations comes to reflect upon his or her past and present and how they may or may not connect to a host of hypothetical futures. Further, he or she comes to reflect upon this process of reflecting. Approaching reflection from the perspective of the knower who is able to understand the nature of things both real and hypothetical, the individual may strive to bind together, in reflection, the reality of the past and present with an imagined hypothetical future. The construction of hypothetical "ideals" (Elkind, 1981)—ideal families, religions, societies, lives— may help launch the identity project. The individual discovers the striking contrasts between realities of the present and past and ideals for the future. The contrast may stimulate a campaign of concerted and sometimes painful questioning of the present and past. The targets of questioning may be previously unassailable beliefs and values as well as the significant persons who represent the sources of these beliefs and values. Breger (1974) summarizes the process:

> During the early years, the child has different selves and is not bothered by inconsistencies between them, by his lack of unity or wholeness. He may be one person with his parents, another with his friends, and still another in his dreams. The limitations of intuitive and concrete operational thought [Piaget's stages 2 and 3] permit such shifting about and contradictions. . . . [T]he idea of a unitary or whole self in which past memories of who one was, present experiences of who one is, and future expectations of who one will be, is the sort of abstraction that the child simply does not think about. . . . With the emergence of formal operations in adolescence, wholeness, unity, and integration become introspectively real problems. Central to the idealism of adolescence is concern with an ideal self. Holden Caulfield's preoccupation with phoniness is a striking example of this concern. He, and many young persons like him, become critical of those who only play at roles, who are one moment this and another moment that. This critical stance is taken toward themselves as well. Wholeness is, thus, an *ideal* conceived in late adolescence; a goal which may be pursued thereafter. (pp. 330–331)

But the biological, psychosexual, and cognitive changes which mark the adolescent years do not tell the whole story of identity's emergence as a central developmental issue. Paralleling the changes taking place within the individual are shifts in society's expectations about what the individual, who was a child but is now almost an adult, should be doing, thinking, and feeling. Erikson (1959) writes, "It is of great relevance to the young individual's identity formation that he be responded to, and be given function and status as a person whose gradual growth and transformation make sense to those who begin to make sense to him" (p. 111). In general, Western societies "expect" adolescents and young adults to bind their days together—the past, present, and anticipated future—by examining the occupational, interpersonal, and ideological offerings of society and eventually making a commitment to a personalized niche in the adult world. This is to say that both society and the young person are ready for the individual's identity experiments by the time he or she has in fact become a young person. As Erikson (1959) again describes it,

> The period can be viewed as a psychosocial moratorium during which the individual through free role experimentation may find a niche in some section of his society, a niche which is firmly defined and yet seems to be uniquely made for him. In finding it the young adult gains an assured sense of inner continuity and social sameness which will bridge what he was as a child and what he is about to become, and will reconcile his conception of himself and his community's recognition of him. (p. 111)

There is a tension in this. It is the tension between the "niche" carved out by society and the individual's desire to carve out his or her own niche. In constructing an identity that is integrated within a society's particular occupational, interpersonal, and ideological roles and expectations, the individual need not "sell out" and accommodate carte blanche to the dictates of his or her world. To achieve identity is *not* simply to conform, as the case studies of great revolutionaries such as Luther and Gandhi make clear. The individual and the society accommodate vis-à-vis each other, at least in the ideal Eriksonian scenario. The adolescent or young adult is neither victim nor master of his or her community. Neither is the adolescent or young adult victim or master of the past. Rather, the relationship between the "other" (one's past, the opportunities afforded by society) and the developing self is one of dynamic tension. Life histories blend together with historical moments, according to Erikson (1975), and even Gandhi, who transformed irrevocably our 20th-century world, could not break from that world, nor from the characteristic behavior and experience patterns laid down in the early chapters of his own life history.

Psychosocial Stages of Development

Though the issue of identity arises in the fifth of Erikson's eight stages of psychosocial development, Erikson maintains identity development cannot be fully understood without first understanding its relationship to all eight stages of the human life cycle. At each of Erikson's stages, changes within the individual and changes within the individual's social world combine to create a central conflict which defines the stage. The conflict must be addressed, though not necessarily "resolved," within the given stage, says Erikson, before the individual may move to the next stage. In a sense, the individual's experiences give rise to a unique *question* at each stage which is "asked" and eventually "answered" via his or her behavior. Though the question may not be consciously articulated as a verbal query, the overall pattern of the individual's behavior and experience within a given stage is structured *as if* the individual were asking a particular question.

Adopting a metaphor of the media, the central question in an Eriksonian stage constitutes developmental "front-page news" for that period, though the newspaper is certainly filled with other questions—other developmental issues—which merit consideration during the particular developmental stage. As the individual moves to the next stage, the central question of the previous period is eventually relegated to a latter page, replaced by a new lead story which has been developing all along in a less prominent column. Thus, developmental issues and questions wax and wane in significance across the life span, but rarely does a former front-page story completely vanish from the paper. Rather, early questions and issues linger on, and those that were especially troublesome during their first tenure as lead articles have a way of reemerging as hot news items later on. This is what it really means to be "fixated" (a very unfortunate and misleading word) at a given Eriksonian stage. In Erikson's scheme, although the late reorganizes the early, the early also continues to affect the late.

For the infant and its social world, the first psychosocial conflict is trust versus mistrust. Through behavior and experience, the infant is asking the most fundamental of all psychosocial questions: "How can I be secure?" Though other lines of development are beginning and a multitude of other developmental issues are simultaneously being raised, finding security is the number one question, and much of what happens developmentally can be understood as informing this question. Through the developing attachment bond with the care giver(s), the infant first sees its environment as a secure place that can be trusted (Ainsworth, 1969; Sroufe & Waters, 1977). During its first year, the infant develops from a relatively nonsocial and non-discriminating organism to emerge as a highly selective social creature who has formed clear preferences for certain salient people with whom it feels secure. These are the infant's attachment *objects*, usually one or both parents and/or other primary caregivers.

Furthermore, the infant learns its first lessons of mistrust or insecurity. In the second half of the first year, separation and stranger anxiety emerge as normal manifestations of mistrust (Bowlby, 1973; Spitz, 1965). Whereas the relaxed four-month-old may coo and smile at virtually any old face, the nine-month-old is not so promiscuous. The older infant's affections are reserved for a select few, and strange others may elicit anything from slight wariness to full-fledged terror. Thus, experiences of both trust and mistrust are front-page news for the infant, providing a thematic framework within which psychologists have come to understand a variety of cognitive, affective, and behavioral changes occurring in this initial chapter of human life.

With the establishment of a secure attachment bond, the individual and its world are now adequately prepared for a psychosocial period in which the person begins to define self and the world. This is the stage of autonomy versus shame and doubt, or what I am characterizing as the period in which the central developmental question becomes "How can I be independent?" In his psychosexual model of development, Freud called this period the anal stage because the libido, or psychosexual energy, of the human appears at this time to have migrated from its first home in the oral region to the anus. Thus, the holding on and the letting go of feces was seen as a sensual experience of increased tension followed by release or tension reduction.

It was the genius of Erikson to understand that the toddler's anal experiences are fledgling attempts at self-definition—expressions of the self struggling to become autonomous or independent vis-à-vis its world. In holding on and letting go of feces in situations both appropriate and inopportune, the toddler is asserting self over and against the surroundings. Through successful toilet training, the toddler learns the first lessons of self-control—how to be an effective and competent agent operating in a fashion partially independent (autonomous) of others and of his or her own bodily impulses. But anal expression and toilet training are small parts of a much larger second-stage story, as the toddler comes to experience autonomy through increasing abilities in the realms of locomotion, language, and exploratory play. The toddler is coming to understand what it means to be autonomous and effective in dealing with his or her world, but along the way he or she repeatedly encounters situations and scenarios in which the environment is simply too tough to deal with in any effective manner. Thus, experiences of shame and doubt—of being exposed, embarrassed, humiliated—are seemingly inevitable, though the most felicitous of environments are those which promote the toddler's independence and buoy his or her confidence when self-assertion and self-control occasionally give way to self-doubt.

The third psychosocial stage is defined by the conflict of initiative versus guilt. During this time in the life cycle, the preschooler is asking the central psychosocial question "How can I be powerful?" Freud viewed this stage—his favorite stage—as the setting for the universal power/sex tragedy of Oedipus, an unconscious drama of desire and eventual capitulation in which the young child-as-conqueror ultimately learns that he or she cannot have it all. Having merged with the world via the secure attachment bond of the first year and having subsequently separated itself from that merger via the autonomous assertion of self and the active exploration and manipulation of the environment in stage 2, the child is now about the business of dividing and conquering his or her world. As he or she desires the affections of the parent in the Oedipus complex, so does the preschooler seek to own and reign over a host of other things and people in his or her environment. As Erikson puts it, the young child in stage 3 is "on the make," gaining "pleasure in attack and conquest" (1963, p. 255). At stage 3, one begins to assert the self in a much more powerful way:

> The *intrusive mode* dominating much of the behavior of this stage characterizes a variety of configurationally "similar" activities and fantasies. These include the intrusion into other bodies by physical attack; the intrusion into other people's ears by aggressive talking; the intrusion into space by vigorous locomotion; the intrusion into the unknown by consuming curiosity. (pp. 87–88, italics in original)
>
> In the boy, the emphasis remains on the phallic-intrusive modes; in the girl, it turns to modes of "catching" in more aggressive forms of snatching or in the milder form of making oneself attractive and endearing. (p. 255)
>
> The danger of this stage is a sense of guilt over the goals contemplated and the acts initiated in one's exuberant enjoyment of new locomotor and mental power: acts of aggressive manipulation and coercion which soon go far beyond the executive capacity of the organism and mind and therefore call for an energetic halt on one's contemplated initiative. . . . The child indulges in fantasies of being a giant and a tiger, but in his dreams he runs in terror for his dear life. This, then, is the stage of the "castration complex," the intensified fear of finding the (now energetically erotized) genitals harmed as a punishment for the fantasies attached to their excitement. (pp. 255–256)

The resolution of the Oedipus complex serves as a prototype for the psychosocial adjustment that must be made on a very large scale if this stage is to be traversed expeditiously: The child must renounce the desire *to have* all in order *to be* like others. In Freud's terms, the object cathexis of the Oedipus complex gives way to identification and the establishment of the superego, and thus is resolved the Oedipus complex. In a more general sense, the child's power has been checked, and the resultant establishment of limits paves the way for the next stage in which the desire to be *good* pushes the desire to be *powerful* off center stage.

Freud's latency period of the elementary-school years has been reconceptualized by Erikson as the fourth stage of industry versus inferiority. Whereas Freud characterized the years following the resolution of the Oedipus complex up to puberty as a relatively quiescent time in which the libido simmers on a distant back burner, Erikson discerned a central psychosocial issue usually transacted for the first time during these years. The issue concerned the child's increasing competence in a growing social and instrumental world.

During these years, children in most cultures undergo some form of systematic instruction outside the family; some form of "schooling" designed to render the young boy or girl proficient in using the *tools* and assuming the *roles* of adulthood. The exemplar for this stage is the industrious schoolchild immersed in the "reading-'riting-'rithmetic" of his or her culture—learning the rudimentary skills required to be a productive member of society while being exposed to the proper modes and manners of conduct expected inside and outside the workplace. Erikson (1963) writes, "It is at this point that wider society becomes significant in its ways of admitting the child to an understanding of meaningful roles in its technology and economy" (p. 260). The elementary-school child is learning how to be a good worker, a good citizen, and a good member of a good society.

Because the learning applies to matters both material and moral, economic and ethical, I have chosen to characterize the central psychosocial question of this stage as "How can I be good?" It is during this highly formative developmental period that churches and schools deliver their most influential lessons on how to be a good boy or girl. And though we may be able to distinguish from a fairly early age the subtle differences between being good by getting an "A" on a spelling test and being good by telling the truth (Nucci, 1981), both involve *being good* and are heavily underscored in the experience of the schoolchild in Erikson's stage 4.

By the time the adolescent is ready to address the issue of identity versus role confusion (Erikson's stage 5), he or she has already negotiated tentative solutions to four more basic issues: security (trust), independence (autonomy), power (initiative), and goodness (industry). These negotiations have involved extensive two-way interactions with a variety of social worlds during the first decade and a half of the individual's life.

In Erikson's scheme of psychosocial development, the "psycho" and the "social," the internal and the external, develop in tandem, and with the resolution of each stage the two reach a new level of rapprochement. Thus, by the time the individual and his or her environment are ready for the questions "Who am I?" and "How do I fit into an adult world?" the two have traversed together an extensive developmental terrain. Identity versus role confusion becomes the focal point for a myriad of individual and societal changes (changes in societal expectations) which are given meaning and context in light of the young person's fledgling attempts to bind together the past, present, and future into an integration giving life unity and purpose.

Marcia (1966, 1980) has argued that the process of identity formation in adolescence and young adulthood follows a two-step sequence. The first step, *exploration*, involves the concerted questioning of beliefs, values, roles, relationships, and self-images grounded in the past and the active experimentation with new beliefs, values, roles, relationships, and images of self. During this time, the individual is in *psychosocial moratorium* (Erikson, 1959, 1963)—he or she has made a provisional break from the past but has yet to pledge any allegiance to a particular future. The second step, though, is *commitment*. Amidst the intimidating changes and insecurity occasioned by the break from the past, in light of all the questioning and doubt with respect to old means and old ends and in the face of mounting external pressures to "take a stand" and discover for oneself a self-defining niche, the individual comes to make long-term commitments to occupational, ideological, and interpersonal roles and, thus, to a new self and world—an adult world—of which he or she is now an integral part.

The outcome of identity exploration and subsequent commitment is a new configuration (Erikson, 1959), the components of which include "constitutional givens, idiosyncratic libidinal needs, favored capacities, significant identifications, effective defenses, successful sublimations, and consistent roles" (p. 116). The psychosocial legacy of successful identity resolution, or what Erikson (1964) terms the resultant *virtue* of the identity versus role confusion stage, is *fidelity*, or "the ability to sustain loyalties freely pledged in spite of the inevitable contradictions of value systems" (p. 125). Fidelity means taking a stand that is freely chosen in a world of pervasive relativism. In Erikson's ideal case, the individual who successfully resolves identity versus role confusion by passing through exploration and commitment phases moves on, psychosocially, to subsequent stages of adulthood: intimacy versus isolation, generativity versus stagnation, ego integrity versus despair.

Whether the identity issue can again rise to the psychosocial fore in the years following the young person's successful resolution is a matter of great theoretical controversy and confusion (Goethals, 1976; Levinson, 1978). Erikson himself appears somewhat ambivalent on the point. On the one hand, Erikson's eight-stage life cycle does not appear to afford a second identity crisis in which the individual launches a new and thoroughgoing reassessment of "Who am I?" and "How do I fit into an adult world?" Erikson's case studies of Gandhi

(1969), Luther (1958), George Bernard Shaw (1959), and others (1963) tend to frame personality changes in later adulthood in terms of an identity structure which, though flexible, appears laid down essentially in adolescence and young adulthood. Marcia (1966, 1980), too, writes that once the adolescent or young adult has passed successfully through identity exploration and commitment, he or she has "achieved identity." The latter term sounds quite irrevocable.

On the other hand, Erikson (1959) writes, "While the end of adolescence thus is the stage of overt identity *crisis*, identity *formation* neither begins nor ends with adolescence: It is a lifelong development largely unconscious to the individual and to his society" (p. 113). He also writes, "Ego identity could be said to be characterized by the actually attained but forever-to-be-revised sense of the reality of the Self within social reality" (1968, p. 210). Both statements are ambiguous. Identity involves fidelity, that is, commitments amidst relativism. Yet although commitments should be long term, identity is a "lifelong development" and "forever-to-be-revised." Identity means "continuity and sameness" (Erikson, 1963), and yet there appears considerable leeway for malleability and change.

The confusion over the relative stability of a person's identity configuration once consolidated in late adolescence or young adulthood is a function, in part, of the conceptual ambiguity surrounding the term *identity*. Psychologists have found it difficult to state exactly what identity is and, perhaps more importantly, what it is *not*. Because the concept cannot be delimited, it cannot be measured in any precise way. And because psychologists cannot measure it in individual lives, they will be unable to settle the controversy concerning its relative stability across the human life span.

Though psychologists have developed measures of the identity-formation *process*—phases of exploration and commitment—in adolescence and young adulthood (Grotevant & Cooper, 1980; Marcia, 1966, 1980; McAdams, Booth, & Selvik, 1981), they have generally avoided the question of what identity itself looks like once formed. That is, what is the *content* and *structure* of the identity *configuration* which binds together a particular person's past, present, and future and provides his or her life with unity and purpose? Can various identity configurations be grouped into categories based upon observable patterns of content and structure? Are there distinguishable types of identities? With respect to what criteria are different identities to be contrasted and compared? This book begins to address these questions.

Identity as Story

Power, Intimacy, and the Life Story explores the possibilities packed within a disarmingly simple metaphor—the *story* metaphor. It is an individual's story which has the power to tie together past, present, and future in his or her life. It is a story which is able to provide unity and purpose. It is a story which specifies a personalized "niche" in the adult world and a sense of continuity and sameness across situations and over time. This book examines the proposition that, beginning in late adolescence, we construct stories to integrate the disparate elements of our lives. With the advent of formal operations (Inhelder & Piaget, 1958), each of us becomes a self-biographer—a storyteller *par excellence*. The story is the answer to the questions, "Who am I?" and "How do I fit into an adult world?" *Identity is a life story.* The identity configuration to which Erikson alludes is a configuration of plot, character, setting, scene, and theme.

Individual identities may be classified in the manner of stories. Identity stability is longitudinal consistency in the life story. Identity transformation—identity crisis, identity change—is story revision. Story revision may range from minor editing in an obscure chapter to a complete rewriting of the text, embodying an altered plot, a different cast of characters, a transformed setting, new scenes, and new themes.

The problem of identity is the problem of arriving at a life story that makes sense—provides unity and purpose—within a socio-historical matrix that embodies a much larger story. A person's world establishes parameters for life stories. In this way identity is truly psychosocial: The life story is a joint product of person and environment. In a sense, the two write the story together. Jerome Bruner (1960) speaks of this story writing as the making of myths. He writes that the "mythologically instructed community provides its members with a library of scripts" against which the individual may judge his or her own "internal drama" (p. 281). He concludes, "Life, then, produces myth and finally imitates it" (p. 283).

Hankiss (1981) echoes Bruner in speaking of a "mythological rearranging" of life undertaken by each individual beginning in late adolescence. Hankiss writes, "Everyone builds his or her own theory about the history and the course of his or her life by attempting to classify his or her particular successes and fortunes, gifts and choices, and favourable and unfavourable elements of his or her fate according to a coherent, explanatory principle and to incorporate them within a *historical* unit" (p. 203). Similarly, Kohli (1981) asks the question, "How does the individual thematize his own life history in everyday life?" (p. 65). According to Kohli, the answer is not simply a matter of listing past accomplishments and predicting future ones. Instead, one's life is thematized within a "structured self-image." Kohli writes, "Life histories are thus not a collection of all events of the individual's life course, but rather 'structured self-images.' *This comes close to some notions of identity*" (p. 65, italics added).

This book encourages the reader to think about identity as a life story and to think about the person formulating identity as a story writer—a biographer of self. Leon Edel, renowned author of the five-volume biography of Henry James, asserts that the biographer's quest is not primarily to discover archives and materials pertaining to his or her subject of study. Rather, the biographer seeks to discover the personal myth which animates the subject's life. He writes, "When the biographer can discover a myth, he has found his story. He knows the meaning of his material and can choose, select, sift, without deceiving himself about the subject of his work" (Edel, 1978, p. 2).

Applying this insight to identity, one concludes that when the person finds (creates, constructs) a personalized life myth or story, he or she no longer "deceives" the self and world. The story provides a coherent narrative framework within which the disparate events and the various roles of a person's life can be embedded and given meaning. The story provides a pattern for the scattered identity pieces of the protean man. The story is an antidote for bad faith. Pachter (1979) writes that the "biographer probes in sympathy to define the myth that orders his subject's experience and that offers the key to his nature" (p. 14). Another student of biography, Olney (1972), states that "an autobiography is a monument of the self, a metaphor of the self at the summary moment of composition" (p. 35).

This book explores the kinds of life myths or stories that people construct to serve as their identities. In the following chapters, I examine life stories composed by men and women in the college years and at midlife and the ways in which these stories relate to other aspects of personality.

Drawing upon interviews, questionnaires, and psychological tests administered to these men and women, as well as a variety of theoretical and empirical sources inside and outside psychology, I have developed a working model of identity as a narrative construction or life story with predictable, interrelated features. The model specifies four major components of the life story and proposes how two personality variables influence and are influenced by the content and the structure of the story. In the following section, I will introduce my study by identifying it as an outgrowth of the personological tradition in the social sciences. This tradition is briefly described and its relationship to the present study outlined. Finally, I will preview the coming chapters in which the life-story model of identity is elaborated and illustrated.

A Personological Analysis

The approach I have chosen to take in this book is what I term a *personological* approach to inquiry. This is by no means the most dominant or popular methodological way of doing things in psychology. Historically grounded in the writings of Henry Murray (1938, 1955), personology has traditionally emphasized the study of the *whole person* in his or her sociohistorical context. In addition, personologists have traditionally adopted *biographical* approaches to the study of human lives and have often focused their inquiries upon fundamental human *motives*. Thus, the *whole person, biography,* and *motivation* are three major themes of the personological tradition in the social sciences, and each of these themes is apparent in my own inquiry into the life stories which make up human identities.

The Personological Tradition

In his landmark *Explorations in Personality* (1938), Henry Murray envisioned an exciting agenda for personology. Murray defined personology as the scientific study of the whole person. Whereas psychologists of other persuasions studied discrete processes and functions of the human organism, the personologist was to operate on a more molar and synthetic level, casting his or her empirical eye upon the overall pattern of an individual's unique adaptation to the world. The personologist was to search for recurrent thematic constellations which characterized the individual as a whole. This molar approach to inquiry sacrifices a certain degree of precision and predictive power at the molecular level to achieve theoretical coherence at the level of the person.

Thus, the emphasis on the whole person allied Murray's enterprise with the 19th-century tradition in the social sciences termed the *Geisteswissenschaften* ("moral sciences") and the early studies of the whole person found in the writings of Dilthey, Spranger, Stern, and (somewhat later) Allport. Dilthey (1900/1976), for example, argued for a holistic science of persons to serve as a counterpoint to the mechanistic and reductionistic natural sciences of his day. The major tool for inquiry in the *Geisteswissenschaften,* as Dilthey saw it, was *hermeneutics*, or the systematic interpretation of texts. In a hermeneutic investigation, the interpreter enters into a kind of dialogue with the object of study, be it a textual passage, some other human product, or another human (Radnitzky, 1973; Steele, 1982). The goal of the inquiry is to provide a careful description of the subject (interpreter) / object (interpreted) relationship, foreshadowing a traditional emphasis upon descriptive over and against predictive studies in personology.

Explorations in Personality reports the outcome of a series of studies at the Harvard Psychological Clinic in the 1930s. Fifty undergraduate men were studied longitudinally by a team of investigators representing a host of disciplines within the social and biological sciences and the humanities. Murray headed the team. Among the more notable collaborators were Jerome Frank, Robert White, Donald MacKinnon, Saul Rosenzweig, R. Nevitt Sanford, Samuel Beck, and Erik Homburger (who later changed his last name to Erikson). Over 200 pages of *Explorations* were devoted to describing innovative methods of assessing persons, including a number of tests of imagination. A new language and conceptual scheme for personology was delineated in great detail to provide a common theoretical framework within which to interpret the multidisciplinary, multidiagnostic investigation.

Personology flourished at the Harvard Psychological Clinic before and after World War II and in subsequent years was best embodied in the integrative and innovative research of Robert White (1952, 1996, 1975) and Jack Block (1971). The scientific study of the whole person, however, was never well integrated into the mainstream of American psychology in general, nor personality psychology in particular. In the 1950s and 1960s, the in-depth analysis of the individual life became almost the exclusive interest of the clinician who was concerned, for the most part, with abnormal personality. Personality psychologists studying normal persons tended to focus exclusively on single dimensions (such as a particular "trait" or "need") manifested in all persons. Thus, personality psychologists became experts in "extraversion" or the "need for achievement," but few deemed it worthwhile or profitable to become experts on "persons" (see the reviews provided by Adelson, 1969; Block, 1981; Carlson, 1971, 1975; Helson & Mitchell, 1978; Maddi, 1982; Singer & Singer, 1972).

In the late 1960s and early 70s, this approach to studying single personality traits or needs came under serious attack for its theoretical and methodological shortcomings (Argyle & Little, 1976; Fiske, 1974; Mischel, 1968, 1973). At about the same time, other critics began to ask, "Whatever happened to personology?" Carlson (1971) lamented the full-scale retreat of American psychology from the whole person during the 1950s and 60s, calling for a return to the person as a viable object of inquiry in personality psychology. Recent reviews suggest that Carlson's call is beginning to be heeded as a number of psychologists appear, in recent years, to have again taken up Murray's mission of studying persons as integrated wholes (Bertaux, 1981; Block, 1981; Carlson, 1975, 1981; Levinson, 1978; Maddi, 1982; Rabin, Aronoff, Barclay, & Zucker, 1981; Runyan, 1982; Schneidman, Barron, Sanford, Smith, Tomkins, & Tyler, 1982; Wrightsmann, 1981). Reflecting this significant shift in emphasis among a notable number of psychologists, Carlson has recently proclaimed that once again "Personology lives!" (1982, p. 7).

Murray placed prime importance upon biography in the study of whole persons. Personology, indeed, was to be a doubly biographical affair. First, the subjects whose lives formed the data for personological investigations were typically asked by Murray and his colleagues to reconstruct their own biographies which would then serve as starting points for subsequent interviews and other assessment procedures. Second, Murray envisioned a time when personologists themselves would be able to construct scientific biographies of their subjects, delineating and classifying common biographical forms across various human lives.

At the time of the publication of Murray's *Explorations*, the collection of biographies or life histories was a well-established methodology in European psychology and in the adjacent disciplines of sociology and anthropology. Working in Vienna, Bühler (1933) and Frenkel (1936) collected written life histories in order to chart general developmental principles manifest in adulthood. Going back to the 19th century, anthropologists had been collecting life histories orally delivered by the subjects themselves and supplementing these data with biographical information drawn from conversations. In sociology, the symbolic-interactionist school relied heavily on biographical investigations of such phenomena as "deviance" (Bertaux, 1981) to illuminate the interaction of social systems and persons. Sociologist John Dollard (1935) argued that a biographical account, when carefully interpreted by the investigator alert to the mirroring of society in the individual life, stands as a "deliberate attempt to define the growth of a person in a cultural milieu and to make theoretical sense of it" (p. 3).

Murray took this one step further with his statement that "The history of the organism *is* the organism," and therefore, "this proposition calls for biographical studies" (1938, p. 39). For Murray, biographical studies meant more than merely collecting life histories. The personologist was to construct biographies, too. Robert White (1981) describes Murray's view:

> Murray envisioned a time when scientific psychology would be able to write abstract biographies, expressed in a generalized notation derived from a common conceptual scheme. Such biographies would be the scientific contribution to understanding personality, in contrast to, though much indebted to, the literary contributions (p. 12).

Like the study of the whole person in general, biographical studies fell out of favor in the social sciences after World War II. They were seen as nonquantifiable, nongeneralizable, and lacking in rigor. And like the study of the whole person, biographical studies have recently enjoyed something of a renaissance in the social sciences. While sociologists have begun again to consider the life history a significant and unique form of data for their investigations of humans and societies (Bertaux, 1981), psychologist Daniel Levinson (1978, 1981) has undertaken explorations in biography in an attempt to delineate the "seasons of a man's life." Csikszentmihalyi and Beattie (1979) have collected life histories from blue-collar and professional men in their attempts to trace *life themes*, defined as "affective and cognitive representations of existential problems which a person wishes to resolve" (p. 45). Runyan (1978, 1982) has adopted a biographical orientation in his work on the *life course* as a sequence of person-situation interactions. Atwood and Tomkins (1976) have suggested a psychobiographical approach to personality theory, interpreting the ideas of personality theorists in light of the formative experiences of their lives. Howe (1982) has argued for the greater use of biographical evidence in exploring the development of outstanding individuals.

In a more interdisciplinary vein, a new journal focused exclusively on biography as a form of art and science has recently appeared under the name *Biography*. Numerous psychologists have contributed articles, among them R. Sears (Weiss-Bourd & Sears, 1982), Eysenck (1979), and Bigda-Peyton and Fine (1978). The latter write that "for every life a few central themes seem to predominate" (Bigda-Peyton & Fine, 1978, p. 37).

Strongly influenced by Freud and Jung, Murray contended that personologists should delve beneath the manifest surface of observable behavior to explore the latent motivational trends which serve as the springs to human action. Murray set forth a theory of personality which posited psychogenic *needs* or *motives* as underlying and goal-oriented forces within the individual which were assumed to energize, direct, and select human behavior and experience. Needs were to be inferred not from bodily action *per se* or what Murray termed *actones* but rather from *effects* or the consequences of action. Therefore, the individual may fulfill a particular need in many different ways, choosing a variety of behaviors which, on the manifest surface, appear very different but which are related on a latent level in that they serve the same end or goal. Murray delineated at least 20 psychogenic needs which appear to play energizing, directing, and selecting roles in human lives. Among these were included the need for achievement (*n* achievement), *n* affiliation, *n* dominance, *n* exhibition, and *n* play.

Of the many methods Murray developed for the assessment of human needs or motives, the most popular has traditionally been the Thematic Apperception Test or TAT (Morgan & Murray, 1935; Murray, 1938, 1943). In the TAT, the subject composes imaginative stories in response to picture cues. The stories are then analyzed for the prevalence of motivational themes or latent motifs which recur in the manifest narrative content. The method bears some resemblance to Freud's (1900/1953) interpretation of the manifest texts of dreams in terms of latent motivational motifs. The interpretive strategies for the

TAT, however, are typically much less involved and subjective than Freud's strategies for untangling the dream work.

The assessment of fundamental human motives via interpretation of the TAT has been refined and objectified by David McClelland and his associates (Atkinson, 1958; McAdams, 1980; McClelland, 1961, 1975; McClelland, Atkinson, Clark, & Lowell, 1953; Stewart, 1982; Winter, 1973) who have developed content coding strategies for human social motives (Murray's psychogenic needs) concerning achievement, power, and affiliation/intimacy. McClelland has conceived of a motive as an affectively toned cognitive cluster referring to a preference or readiness for a particular quality of experience. Thus, the person high in achievement motivation (*n* achievement) tends to prefer experiences of striving for success, accomplishing tasks of moderate challenge, and competing against an internalized standard of excellence over other classes of human experience—classes being defined by effects rather than actones. The recurrent preference for achievement experiences is hypothesized to be both pervasive and latent, and it comes to be known to both the psychologist and the subject via interpretation of narrative fantasy (e.g., TAT stories) rather than through conscious self-report such as questionnaires and adjective checklists (McClelland, 1980, 1981, 1984).

The Present Study

This book is a product of the recent revival of the personological tradition. Though a number of theories and empirical studies are highlighted in the following pages, the focal study around which the life-story model of identity is developed is first and foremost an exploration in personology. The study employs personological methods of inquiry from the perspectives of biography and motivation. Each chapter elaborates upon a particular aspect of the overall project. Methodological fine points are outlined in detail in the appendixes. A brief introduction examining the ways in which I have chosen to emphasize the whole person, biography, and motivation follows.

During the years 1981–83, my associates and I intensively studied two separate samples of subjects. The first sample (Sample A) consisted of 90 undergraduate students (57 women and 33 men) attending a moderately large private university in the midwestern United States. The majority of the students were sophomores in college. Sample B consisted of 50 adults (30 women and 20 men) between the ages of 35 and 50 years. Representing a cross-section of occupational groups, all participants in Sample B resided in or near Chicago, Illinois. Appendix A provides background information for both samples.

As part of class projects, the 90 undergraduates in Sample A were administered a number of personological measures including the TAT and a sentence-completion test (see Chapters 3 and 4 and Appendixes C and D). The undergraduates also completed a series of open-ended questionnaires comprising an "identity journal." The identity journals, reproduced in Appendix B, included questions about the students' earliest memories, significant life experiences, turning points in their lives, religious and ethical beliefs, significant personal relationships, and hopes and dreams for the future.

All participants in Sample B were administered the same personological measures, but rather than completing identity journals, these men and women were interviewed individually. Modelled after the identity journals, the identity interviews for Sample B are described in Appendix B. The interviews were tape recorded.

To the extent that a study explores a "greater part" of the *whole person*, it becomes more personological. Yet the amount of information collected on each individual is inversely related to the number of persons who can be studied. Therefore, a personological investigation that aims at even a modicum of representativeness must strike a balance between, say, the intensive case studies of White's (1975) *Lives in Progress* and the surveys of hundreds of persons so characteristic of trait psychology.

This book seeks such a balance. Though failing to tap as many different aspects of person's lives as do White's longitudinal case studies, the present project deals with a central issue in all lives which, by its very nature, concerns *how the whole person understands his or her "wholeness."* The issue is identity, and as I have already stated, identity is conceived as a life story which provides unity and purpose in human lives.

Like the work of Frenkel (1936) and Levinson (1978), this book adopts a *biographical* perspective on lives. Men and women are asked to relate their autobiographies by dividing their lives into significant chapters and detailing major turning points and trends. The theoretical model presented in the book states that individuals become biographers of self in late adolescence and early adulthood in order to integrate past, present, and future within a coherent narrative framework. Therefore, the inquiry into identity is doubly biographical in that it employs the method of biography while positing an image of human beings as organisms who, in their quest for identity, are impelled by the desire to construct their own biographies.

The central *motivational* themes in a person's life are major shapers of his or her identity. Chapter 3 highlights two fundamental human motives—the power and the intimacy motives—which appear to find their way into identity as significant influences upon the content of life stories. An individual's characteristic level of power and intimacy motivation is determined from content analysis of stories written in response to TAT pictures. The general proposition that the power and intimacy motives confer upon a person's identity a predictable thematic emphasis—an emphasis detectable in a variety of aspects and features of the life story—is explored throughout the book.

The Chapters Ahead

Chapter 2 considers in detail the proposition that one's identity is a life story by examining the structure and function of stories in both psychology and literature. Then the life-story model of identity is introduced. The four major components of the life story and the two classes of personality variables proposed as dominant influences upon the story—social motives and ego stage—are described and illustrated, in part via a reinterpretation of Erikson's (1958) classic study of the identity formation of Martin Luther. Eight general hypotheses are proposed, each specifying a connection between social motives or ego stage and one of the four components of the life story.

Chapter 3 entertains the thesis that the human social motives of power (Winter, 1973) and intimacy (McAdams, 1980) serve as organizing principles for life stories reflected in recurrent thematic lines in the story's text. This chapter deals with the meaning and measurement of intimacy and power motivation while providing some suggestions as to how these motives may influence and be influenced by life stories. For instance, individuals high in power motivation may emphasize themes of impact and strength (physical and mental) in their life stories, whereas those high in intimacy motivation may structure their identities by relationships with others characterized by warmth, closeness, and communion. This chapter argues that power and intimacy are two fundamental motives in human lives, capturing the motivational meaning in David Bakan's (1966) notion of *agency* and *communion* existing as the two basic modalities of living forms.

In Chapter 4, Jane Loevinger's (1976) stages of ego development are proposed as significant predictors of the degree of structural complexity in life stories. Thus, while the motives in Chapter 3 concern identity *content*, ego stages refers more to *structure*. The chapter deals with the meaning and measurement of ego development while providing some insight on how this variable may influence and be influenced by the life story. It is proposed that the life story of the person at higher stages of ego development will be much more differentiated and integrated (i.e., more complex) than the life story of individuals scoring at relatively low ego stages. Relationships between ego development and social motives are also explored.

Chapters 5–8 each consider one of the four major components of the life story. The chapters draw upon the personological data collected on college students and midlife men and women to evaluate and elaborate the proposed hypotheses concerning relationships between social motives and ego stage and each of the four story components. The first of the four components, *nuclear episodes* (Chapter 5), refers to critical scenes which stand out in bold print in the life story. Nuclear episodes include high points, low points, and turning points in life stories. As compressed and highly evocative scenes circumscribed within a particular time and place, nuclear episodes frequently illustrate how the person, in his or her own view, has remained the same over time as well as how he or she may have been radically transformed.

Chapter 6 introduces the concept of *imagoes*, personified and idealized images of the self playing *characters* in the story. Imagoes, thus, are akin to "subselves," personified parts of the "me" which act and interact over the course of the story to define the major plot line. Life stories can sometimes be characterized in terms of two conflicting imagoes arranged as narrative thesis and antithesis. Utilizing a taxonomy of imago forms derived from Greek mythology, imagoes can be classified according to their relative emphasis on power and/or intimacy.

Chapter 7 deals with the *ideological setting*, or the backdrop of personal beliefs and values which provides a context for the action. Like the temporal and spatial setting of a literature story, the ideological setting may be the most basic component of identity. Thus, ideological change may cause a major identity upheaval.

The *generativity script* (Chapter 8) is a future plan or outline concerning what one hopes to put into life and what one hopes to get out of it to fulfill the developmental mandate of *generating* a legacy (Becker, 1973; Erikson, 1963). Chapter 8 integrates Erikson's concept of generativity within the life-story model of identity while reconceptualizing some noteworthy aspects of adult development such as the midlife crisis.

The appendixes provide technical information concerning the collection and analysis of data described in the preceding chapters. This information is probably of most interest to professional researchers and clinicians, though the methods of analysis used and the statistics employed are not so sophisticated as to be beyond the reach of most educated laypersons.

Indeed, most of the ideas in this book, and most of the methods adopted to examine and evaluate them, are inherently rather simple.

My goal is to bring a straightforward and elegant theoretical frame to the complex and confusing stuff of human identities. Scientific inquiry aims at simplicity and elegance, and my inquiries into identity are no exception. The great risk, of course, is *oversimplification*. This book, therefore treads gingerly across the variegated landscape of human identities, drawing *tentative* distinctions and formulating *flexible* proposals. I offer what I believe to be a simple, illuminating and provocative way of looking at identity, for the clinician, researcher, and anybody else who has ever asked, "Who am I?" and "How do I fit into an adult world?"

Conclusions and Summary

This book is an *exploration* in personology. It ventures into the unmapped continent of human identity with a topographical hunch. The hunch is that the landscape takes the form of story. More accurately (and this is where the metaphor of geography breaks down), the hunch is that we—as scientists, therapists, and human beings—can come to comprehend the region of human identity *as if* it were laid out as a story. The "as if" reminds us that scientific models and theories are, by necessity, *fictions* we impose upon experience in order to render it more sensible; in order to transform the buzzing, blooming confusion of our confrontation with the cosmos into a relatively simple picture, a laconic statement, and an elegant framework. The picture, the statement, the framework—whatever you choose to term the product of scientific inquiry—is no *final* product at all: It is a tentative construction subject to considerable modification and eventual abandonment in the face of a better successor.

In this book, I offer the reader a tentative construction which, I sincerely hope, will be evaluated, criticized, modified, and eventually abandoned in light of something better. If this happens, we will have begun to think about human identity in a different way, generating new concepts and metaphors to make sense of how indeed we make sense of ourselves.

I began this chapter by considering some of our more haunting contemporary images of identity. Eliot's *walking dead,* Beckett's *zero identity,* Lasch's *narcissistic personality,* and Lifton's *protean man* are modern identity images inhabiting some of our best literary and social scientific works, reinforcing in the most disturbing fashion Langbaum's (1982) thesis that identity is "the spiritual problem of our time."

Identity is a sense of sameness and continuity which ties together our days anew. By integrating past, present, and an anticipated future, identity provides human lives with unity and purpose. Yet, these haunting contemporary images suggest that constructing a personalized identity—putting together the disparate elements of our lives into an integrated whole which journeys forward in a specified direction—is an extremely troublesome task for modern Westerners living in an age that has witnessed a host of destabilizing historical trends and events.

Though philosophers and psychologists have argued that finding unity and purpose in modern life involves extensive self-examination, they have differed radically on the issues of how that examination should proceed and how the ultimate product of that examination should connect, or not connect, to one's past and environment. Unlike those who would have us transform our identities with each "predictable crisis" and thus repeatedly emancipate ourselves from that which is old and constraining (e.g., Gould, Sheehy), Erik Erikson has argued that identity never loses touch with the past or the environment and is, rather, a phenomenon of the "late reorganizing the early," or the new reorganizing the old. A matter of both individuation and integration, of separation and connection, and of autonomy and interdependence, identity formation involves separating oneself from one's past and environment and, paradoxically, finding new connections to the separated.

The process of identity formation begins in adolescence and young adulthood, states Erikson. Psychosocial prerequisites include a certain level of biological and psychosexual maturation, the emergence of certain cognitive capacities, and society's expectation that the "time is right" for the young person's fledgling forays into the realm of identity exploration and eventual commitment. The beginning of the process ushers in Erikson's fifth stage of psychosocial development: identity versus role confusion. Where the process ends—and, therefore, when, if ever, identity is "achieved" or fully constructed—is a matter of considerable controversy among psychologists.

This book asserts that the process of identity formation proceeds throughout adulthood and that the outcome of the process—the created identity per se—is a dynamic, evolving *life story*. Beginning in late adolescence, we become biographers of self, mythologically rearranging the scattered elements of our lives—the different "selves," or what Erikson terms "identifications"—into a narrative whole providing unity and purpose. Thus, *identity is a life story*. The identity configuration to which Erikson alludes is a configuration of plot, character, setting, scene, and theme. It is, thus, a dynamic narrative configuration, taking initial shape in adolescence and continuing to evolve thereafter, that binds together past, present, and future, bestowing upon the individual that sense of inner sameness and continuity which Erikson sees as the great legacy of a well-formed identity.

My central mission in this book, then, is the examination of life stories. The approach I have taken to the inquiry is distinctively *personological*. At the end of this chapter, I put my inquiry into a historical context by discussing the *personological tradition* in the social sciences—the tradition to which this book owes its primary allegiance. Introduced to the scientific community in Henry Murray's (1938) *Explorations in Personality*, the personological approach to the study of human lives has historically emphasized three central themes: the whole person, biography, and motivation. Each of these themes is evident in the chapters ahead.

Though personology virtually ceased to exist as a viable approach to the study of human behavior and experience in the 1960s, the past 10 years have signalled a budding revival. A variety of trends suggests that the whole person, biography, and motivation are resurgent points of emphasis in contemporary psychology and adjoining disciplines as well.

My own personological inquiry into identity is a product of the revival. I ended this chapter by introducing my inquiry. In essence, I have adopted *biographical* methods of investigation to shed some light on the process of *whole persons* making sense of their whole lives. I am proposing that people make sense of their lives via narrative—by constructing life stories which serve as their identities. The life stories bear systematic relationships to other personality variables, especially to social *motives* concerning power and intimacy. The chapters ahead elaborate and illustrate a life-story model of identity by integrating a number of diverse theories and concepts in the social sciences and humanities and by describing and analyzing personological data collected from college students and men and women at midlife.

Chapter 2

Identity and the Life Story

We tell ourselves stories in order to live.

(Joan Didion, 1979, p. 11)

Erikson's Luther

When Martin Luther fell raving to the ground and roared like a bull *Ich bin nit! Ich bin nit!* (*I am not! I am not!*), he was a fledgling German monk in his mid-20s consumed by his own identity turmoil. The stage for young Martin's emotional outburst was the monastery choir at Erfurt around the year 1507. Witnesses to the event were three of Luther's contemporaries who reported that the monk screamed like one possessed after reading of Christ's cure of a man possessed by a *dumb spirit* (Mark 9:17).

Occurring during a period of profound religious doubt in the life of the monk, Martin's *Ich bin nit!* was a desperate cry of negation: I am not this, but I do not know what I am. The "fit in the choir" (Erikson, 1958) was the second of three dramatic and legendary episodes in Luther's life which mark a spiritual pilgrimage from a compulsive and silent orthodoxy to an explosive and garrulous reformulation of humankind's relationship to God. The pilgrimage was one of ideology and identity. At its conclusion in 1512 in the tower of Wittenberg, the 29-year-old Luther had found his way out of spiritual darkness into light. Replacing the negation in the choir was young man Luther's affirmation of who he was, who he had been, and who he was to become in the future.

An Ideological Journey

In his celebrated inquiry into identity entitled *Young Man Luther,* Erik Erikson (1958) begins with a critical event. The fit in the choir is the episode of departure for understanding how young Luther came to understand himself. From an analysis of this episode, Erikson moves backwards and forwards in Luther's life—backwards to Martin's earliest confrontations with the authority vested in his father Hans and forward to his epic battles with the religious orthodoxy in Rome—as he traces the tortuous route of Luther's extended moratorium and the eventual consolidation of his identity as the spokesman of a new religious order. Without reducing Luther's life to the predictable unfolding of stages, Erikson shows how psychosocial issues rooted in Luther's early years came to be negotiated against the backdrop of certain sociohistorical themes and trends in such a way that the man and the moment came together to effect an ultimate and irrevocable transformation of each other.

A cornerstone of Erikson's analysis is the assertion that this transformation should be seen in the context of the psychoanalytic concept of *anality.* As Luther exhibits many of the personality traits of the anal character type, argues Erikson, so does Luther's age—an age witnessing the demise of medieval feudalism and the birth of capitalism—manifest certain cultural motifs reminiscent of Freud's anal stage of development, which is Erikson's second stage of autonomy versus shame and doubt. This argument is complex and multileveled, encompassing Erikson's keen observations concerning Luther's preoccupation with the vicissitudes of the anus, his anal character traits such as obsessiveness and stubbornness, the symbols of anality in Luther's private life which included the dirty devil and the copper mines (the bowels of the earth) where Luther's father worked, and the "anal" character virtues extolled by the rise of capitalism and the Protestant Reformation in the West: thrift, cleanliness, punctuality, individualism. As the two-year-old attains anal mastery and strives for autonomy and independence vis-à-vis a secure familial world, suggests Erikson, so did parts of Europe cleanly break away from the economic orthodoxy of feudalism and the religious status quo of Rome during the years Martin Luther lived.

Martin Luther was born in the German town of Eisleben on November 10, 1483. Shortly thereafter the family moved to the mining center of Mansfeld, where Luther lived until 1497. Martin's father, Hans Luder, was a copper miner who had left the farm. Ambitious, thrifty, and especially severe, Hans Luder personified a tiny but growing social phenomenon in late 15th-century Europe—the former peasant turned first-generation capitalist, a newcomer to a rising middle class. Hans "was an early small industrialist and capitalist, first working to earn enough to invest, and then guarding his investment with a kind of dignified ferocity" (p. 53).

Hans was also a harsh disciplinarian who beat Martin with a frequency and vigor that appear to have exceeded even the customs of the day. When Martin was a teenager, his father's bullying took a more subtle form as Hans attempted to dictate his son's occupational future, pushing Martin towards the field of law and a subsequent position as a secular leader. Entering the University of Erfurt in 1501, Martin appeared destined to fulfill his father's mandate, studying grammar, logic, rhetoric, natural philosophy, philosophy, and physics.

Martin's journey to secular success was brought to a dramatic halt, however, on the road back to college one summer eve in the year 1505. As Martin later described it, he was only a few hours from Erfurt when he was seized by terror during a severe thunderstorm. A bolt of lightning struck the ground near him, perhaps hurled him to the ground, and threw him into what some biographers have claimed was a state of convulsion. Before he knew what was happening, Martin screamed out, "Help me, St. Anne . . . I want to be a monk." On his return to Erfurt, he entered the monastery, telling his friends that his experience in the thunderstorm affirmed a commitment to the church. This first critical event stands in marked contrast to the fit in the choir. In the thunderstorm, Martin affirms an orthodox Catholic identity: "I want *to be a monk.*" A few years later in the choir, he takes it all back.

Between the affirmation and the negation lie Luther's early years in the monastery at Erfurt. The would-be-lawyer-turned-monk was no ordinary religious novice. He prayed more than the other monks. He tortured his body and mind by denying himself even the simplest earthly comforts while ruminating day in and day out over the meaning of the scriptures. Erikson writes that the young monk's enthusiastic embracing of even the most mortifying practices of monkhood bordered on overkill and reflected a latent ambivalence about the Catholic Church:

> It makes psychiatric sense that under such conditions a young man with Martin's smoldering problems, but also with an honest wish to avoid rebellion against an environment which took care of so many of his needs, would subdue his rebellious nature by gradually developing compulsive-obsessive states characterized by high ambivalence. His self-doubt thus would take the form of intensified self-observation in exaggerated obedience to the demands of the order; his doubt of authority would take the form of an intellectualized

scrutiny of the authoritative books. This activity would, for a while
longer, keep the devil in his place (p. 137).

In the monastery at Erfurt, Luther struggled daily with the
Devil. No place was too mundane nor too sacred, no action was too
trivial nor too glorious to keep out the insidious interloper, "the old
evil foe" as Luther called him in verse. Faith was to be a mighty
fortress against the Devil, but in Luther's early years as a monk the
drawbridges were down and the castle walls filled with gaping holes
through which the Devil managed to find his way. Eventually, the
Devil was to find a home in Rome.

The seeds of Luther's discontent with the Roman Church were
sown in the monastery as he witnessed the enactment of church
policies that were decidedly contradictory and corrupt. The practice
of selling indulgences epitomized what Luther perceived as the moral
bankruptcy of the church. Through indulgences individuals were able
to buy time in heaven for themselves or for a deceased relative by
sending money to the church. The selling of indulgences was to
become a rallying point for the entire Protestant Reformation as it
came to represent both corruption in the church and the Catholic
view of salvation as a commodity to be bought through good works.
Luther did not believe that human beings were capable of good
works. Humans were like pitiful worms or filthy swine, in Luther's
view. Only Christ could perform a "good work" capable of redeeming
them.

The third critical event in Martin's life occurred in 1512 after
Luther had become a doctor of theology and delivered his first lectures on the Psalms at the University of Wittenberg. According to
Luther's own accounts (a dramatic reconstruction of his own life
story), his spiritual questioning and reformulation—which had filled
his daily thoughts since at least the fit in the choir and which had
exacerbated a chronic melancholia going back even to childhood—
culminated in a revelation of truth in the monks' toilet in the Wittenberg tower.

The truth was a new meaning, Luther's meaning, attributed to
the last sentence of Romans 1:17: "The just shall live by faith." In the
tower, Luther envisioned a new image of a God more directly accessible to the common person than the distant God of the Catholic
orthodoxy ensconced behind the retinue of Rome. Rather than the
God who met each man and woman on a future day of judgment at
which time He pronounced the final word concerning one's record on
earth, Luther's God administered justice in the here and now
through the Word which is Christ. Consequently, men and women
encounter God through his Son, who, as Luther understood it, proclaimed that one need only accept the Word in order to have faith. For

Luther in 1512 and for Lutherans today, faith precedes good works, not the reverse.

In keeping with the spirit of Freud's anal stage and Erikson's theme of autonomy versus shame and doubt, we can say that Luther's ideological reformation sought to *separate* the individual from the secure matrix of Roman orthodoxy and place him or her in direct relationship with Christ. Each individual is an *autonomous* agent with respect to Rome, claimed Luther, and with this autonomy comes the awesome responsibility of engaging Christ one-on-one. Though Luther saw the value of a collective and formal liturgy in Christian worship, he did not deem it appropriate that church elders and scholars should dictate Christian experience to the common people. Likewise, the common people should not rely solely on the church for the development of their faith. Rather, every single person should confront the Word directly, in some cases struggling with the Word, grappling and wrestling individually with God, as did Luther, Jacob, and many of the prophets before Luther. Thus, it was imperative, in Luther's view, that the Mass be recited in the language of the people and that the Bible, too, be translated into the vernacular.

Luther's successful resolution of ideological questions—questions centering on man's relationship to God—established a coherent backdrop of belief and value for the unfolding story of his life. The story, as Luther appeared to construct it himself, is his identity. It is a story punctuated by three dramatic episodes understood by Luther as turning points or epiphanies in an heroic quest for unity and purpose.

The biographical episodes in the thunderstorm, the choir, and the tower illustrate a dialectical development in ideology. From his affirmation of the church ("I want to become a monk") to his negation of what he had been ("I am not!"), Luther's ideological narrative runs from the Hegelian *thesis* to *antithesis*, from total identification with the orthodoxy to total rejection. *Synthesis* is the affirmation of an alternative ideology to take the place of the orthodoxy, an affirmation proclaimed in the humblest of environments—the monks' toilet. In Wittenberg's tower in 1512, young man Luther consolidated an ideological setting for his life story and thereby became an adult. As Erikson writes,

> To be adult means among other things to see one's own life in continuous perspective, both in retrospect and in prospect. By accepting some definition as to who he is, usually on the basis of a function in an economy, a place in the sequence of generations, and a status in the structure of society, the adult is able to selectively reconstruct his past in such a way that, step for step, it seems to have planned him, or better, he seems to have planned *it*. In this sense, psychologically we *do* choose our parents, our family history, and the his-

tory of our kings, heroes, and gods. By making them our own, we maneuver ourselves into the inner position of proprietors, of creators (pp. 111–112).

The Heroes of the Story

There is more to the story than Luther's spiritual pilgrimage between 1505 and 1512. Identity is more than ideology. The consolidation of the latter established a backdrop for the former, and consequently Luther's ideological movement from orthodoxy to reformulation establishes a setting of belief and value for a narrative of heroic action and conflict. The heroes of the drama are two superordinate personifications in Luther's life, *indeed two parts of Luther himself*, whose mighty deeds and monumental conflicts define much of the story's action. As I see Erikson's Luther, the two protagonists are the archetypal *Father* and the archetypal *Son*. The Son is split into two characters: the *Spokesman* and the *Mute*.

The initial manifestation of the Father is Martin's biological father, Hans Luder. We have already seen that Hans was a hardworking capitalist who proved to be a harsh disciplinarian at home. Hans, as the former peasant turned miner, appears to have represented to Martin the vulgarity and dirtiness of corporeal existence. But he was also the representative of a new breed of men who extolled thrift, order, and individualism as paramount human virtues. Hans and God were Martin's first wrathful judges, and his inability to satisfy either of them was a source of great sadness throughout Martin's childhood. Erikson writes, "Martin, even when mortally afraid, *could not really hate his father*, he could only be sad; and Hans, while he could not let the boy come close, and was murderously angry at times, *could not let him go for long*" (p. 65, italics in original).

In the monastery and after, a parade of authority figures was incorporated into the image of the Father. These included the Pope, God, and the Devil. Each was perceived as a ruthless tyrant who evoked fear and resentment in the Son. In childhood the name of God would turn Martin pale and terrified, "for I was taught to perceive him as a strict and wrathful judge" (p. 71). Repeatedly personified in Luther's life story, the Devil too evoked fear and trembling. Yet the Devil was typically cast in the role of tempter rather than judge. Associated with dirt, feces, evil, and unbridled passion, the Devil threatened to bring anarchy and total loss of control. Hans Luder's brother, Martin's uncle, was a drunkard and criminal who may have represented for young Luther an incarnation of the Devil within the Father, what Erikson terms a *negative identity*. The uncle, nicknamed "Little Hans," was cast by the family into the role of the "dirty peasant." Erikson writes, "We must add Little Hans to the concept of the 'dirty peasant' in the list of possible negative identities: as an evil uncle (who according to his name was a minor edition of the righteous father), he was a constant reminder of a possible inherited curse which potentially could lead to proletarization if there were any relaxation of watchfulness, any upsurge of self-indulgent impulse" (p. 59). The *Father* exists inside the life story of Luther and *is* thus *an integral part of Luther's identity.* As Luther grew older and became both the father of his own son (named Hans) and the father of a pervasive religious movement in central Europe, he often spoke, wrote, and behaved in ways *reminiscent of Hans, the wrathful God, and the Devil.* Erikson's analysis is full of examples, especially from the latter half of Luther's life. After the revelation in the tower, Luther as a doctor of theology at the University of Wittenberg lectured widely on the scriptures, delivering between 1513 and 1516 his great trilogy on the Psalms, Romans, and Galatians. In 1517 at the age of 32, Luther outlined his major critique of the Roman Church in the "95 theses," which he nailed to the church door in Wittenberg in order to stimulate a discussion among his colleagues. Marking the start of the Reformation as a whole, the 95 theses stimulated a good deal more than academic discussion. Following their publication and mass circulation in Germany, Luther

> grew elatedly into his role as reformer. How he thus changed identities—he who had defied his father's wish that he become a secular leader by choosing monastic silence instead—we can only sketch. It is clear, however, that the negative conscience which had been aggravated so grievously by Martin's paternalistic upbringing had only waited (as such consciences always do) for an opportunity to do to others in some measure what had been done to him. (Erikson, 1958, p. 222)

And in a pamphlet written in 1525 entitled *Against the Robbing and Murdering Hordes of Peasants,* Luther

> promised rewards in heaven to those who risked their lives in subduing insurrection. One sentence indicates the full cycle taken by this once beaten down and then disobedient son: "A rebel is not worth answering with arguments, for he does not accept them. The answer for such mouths is a fist that brings blood from the nose." Do we hear Hans, beating the residue of a stubborn peasant out of his son? (Erikson, 1958, p. 236)

Erikson implies that whereas Martin Luther rebelled against the wishes of his father Hans by turning his back on a secular career, Luther in later life appears to have internalized significant aspects of Hans' personality. Martin, thus, identified with his father to a certain extent, and that identification became part of Luther's identity. The identification with Hans is only a *part* of the whole, however, for as we saw in Chapter 1, identity serves to reorganize old identifications into a larger, integrative totality. In the narrative terms of this book, Martin's identification with his father serves as a component of a larger Father archetype or *imago* which exists as a personified and internalized hero who does battle with other heroes over the course of a larger life story which is Luther's identity.

The other heroes are two internalized and personified images of self as the Son. The Son's stance vis-à-vis the Father is perpetual and ambivalent rebellion. The mode of rebellion is either expulsive and noisy (the Spokesman) or retentive and silent (the Mute). Both modes of rebellion are derivatives of Freud's anal stage of psychosexual development, reframed by Erikson as the stage of autonomy versus shame and doubt.

Again, the theme of anality runs through much of Luther's story: revelation came to Luther on the monks' toilet in Wittenberg; "Ich bin nit!" recalls the "negativism" (Spitz, 1965) of the 18-month-old whose penchant for saying "no" through words and deeds is an active assertion of autonomy (versus shame and doubt) in the second stage of psychosexual development; Luther exhibited a number of character traits associated with the anal erotic personality including "suspiciousness, excessive scrupulosity, moral sadism, and a preoccupation with dirtying and infectious thoughts and substances" (Erikson, 1958, p. 61); Luther made liberal use of scatological imagery and metaphors in his writings and preachings ("Thou shalt not write a book unless you have listened to the fart of an old sow, to which you should open your mouth wide and say 'Thanks to you, pretty nightingale; do I hear a text which is for me?' " p. 33); Luther had a great capacity for "dirt-slinging wrath" (p. 206); Luther suffered life-long constipation.

The Mute is the first of the two Sons to emerge in Luther's life story. This is Martin the young boy who silently endured the beatings delivered by Hans. This is the obedient monk who piously and silently enacted the rituals of meditation, prayer, study, and self-denial in the austere confines of the monastery at Erfurt. This is the man possessed by a dumb spirit in Mark 9:17. Christ's casting out of the spirit frees the man to speak and stimulates in Luther the loud and anguished cry, "I am not": I am not the obedient son of Hans; I am not the obsequious servant of the church; I am not the Mute.

Throughout Luther's life, silence was one of two recurrent reactions to threat from the Father. Typically accompanied by chronic sadness, which Erikson terms the "overall symptom of his youth" (p. 40), silence often covered a seething resentment toward others in authority. Replacing words were obsessive-compulsive rituals and bouts of passive aggression. The Mute—who appears in the story again when Luther visited Rome in 1510 and ended up uninspired and with nothing to say—is "mentally and spiritually constipated" (p. 170).

The Son as Spokesman, on the other hand, is Luther nailing the 95 theses on the church door. He is the Luther who appealed the Pope's bull threatening excommunication in 1518, publicly burned the bull, wrote his great pamphlet "On the Freedom of a Christian Man" in 1520, and appeared before the Diet of Worms in 1521 to deliver his famous speech with the climactic ending: "Here I stand; I can do no other. God help me."

Whereas the rebellion of the Mute against the Father is a seething silence accompanied by obsessive-compulsive rituals and passive aggression, the rebellion of the Spokesman is defiant noise—revolutionary *words*. After the revelation in the tower, Luther

> became God's "spokesman," preacher, teacher, orator, and pamphleteer. This had become the working part of his identity. The eventual liberation of Luther's voice made him creative. The one matter on which professor and priest, psychiatrist and sociologist, agree is Luther's immense gift for language: his receptivity for the written word; his memory for the significant phrase; and his range of verbal expression (lyrical, biblical, satirical, and vulgar) which in English is paralleled only by Shakespeare (Erikson, 1958, p. 47).

Luther's vision of man's relationship with God was an affirmation of voice and word as instruments of faith. In translating the Bible from Latin into German, Luther brought the Word to the masses. Positioned as the intermediary for God and man in Luther's reformulated ideology was Christ and his Word. Christ, in fact, may have represented for Luther an idealized image of the Spokesman who was the Son. Indeed Christ rebelled against the established authority by uttering *words* that mystified, enraged, and inspired. According to Luther's reformulated ideology, faith was a matter of internalizing, in a sense, the Son of God via the encounter with his Word. Erikson writes, "Christ now becomes the core of Christian identity: *quotidianus Christi adventus*, Christ is today here, in me" (p. 212).

Though Erikson does not explicitly say it, I would submit that most of the major events in Luther's life which inform, for us and for Luther, his identity are manifestations of the great deeds of and conflicts between the superordinate and internalized characters of the Father and the Son. Each is a protagonist in the life story, but neither is completely identified with Luther *per se*. Rather, Luther is identified with the story within which the protagonists duel. In other words, Luther's identity is not the Father, nor is it the Son. Luther's identity is the story.

The story is in part a narrative integration of the personifications of Father and Son. In young adulthood, according to Erikson, men

FIGURE 2.1 Protagonists in the Life Story of Erikson's Luther

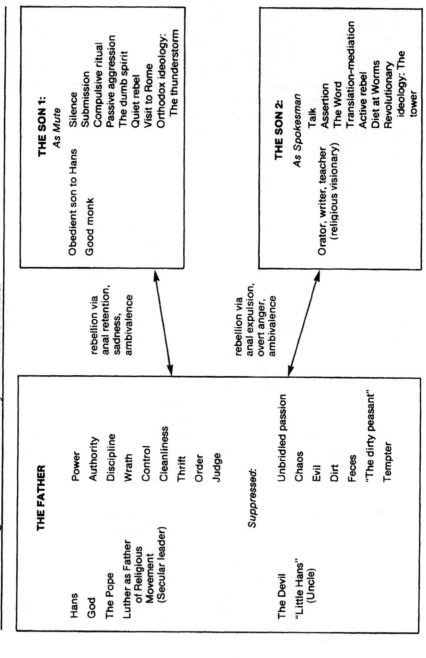

and women come to see "life in continuous perspective, both in retrospect and in prospect," "selectively reconstructing" the past such that "we *do* choose our parents, our family history, and the history of our kings, heroes, and gods" (p. 112). In Luther's life story, the Father and the Son are alternatively kings, heroes, and gods (and devils). Their personified components, personality attributes, and interrelationships are diagramed in Figure 2.1.

The Empirical Study of Identity

In *Young Man Luther,* Erikson focuses a psychoanalytic eye upon the life and times of one great man in order to view and to understand the formation of an identity which shaped and was shaped by a decisive historical epoch. In examining closely the complex totality of Luther in an effort to discover general patterns and themes underlying the manifest biographical data, Erikson is investigating the construct of identity in a personological way. Though many readers may believe that, upon reading *Young Man Luther,* they have come to see with Erikson the order and pattern behind the chaos of Luther's tormented and magnificent life, most would acknowledge that Erikson's manifesto does not speak *directly* to the general business of identity formation as transacted by relatively normal young men and women today.

Erikson integrates biographical data into elegant idiographic propositions, generating concepts and hypotheses that may generalize beyond the life of Luther but, then again, may not. More empirically minded psychologists have attempted to operationalize some of these concepts and test some of the implied hypotheses in order to assess their generalizability and relevance vis-à-vis contemporary young adults in the process of constructing their own identities. Some of their best efforts are now reviewed.

Identity Statuses

Since the publication of Erikson's major theoretical works on identity (Erikson, 1958, 1959, 1968), empirical research on the topic has been dominated by James Marcia's approach to "identity statuses" (Bourne, 1978a, 1978b). Employing a semistructured interview which can be administered to an individual in a half hour, the investigator using Marcia's (1966) methodology inquires into the processes of *exploration* (questioning, experimentation) and *commitment* (resolving questions, deciding on a role or niche) in the salient identity areas of occupational choice and ideology. By dividing identity formation into two discrete steps of exploration and commitment, Marcia has formulated a neat Eriksonian scheme with four possible outcomes or statuses: *identity achievement,* or the person who has gone through significant occupational and ideological questioning or exploration and has subsequently made occupational and ideological commitments (exploration, yes; commitment, yes); *moratorium,* or the person in the midst of exploration who has not yet made commitments (exploration, yes; commitment, no); *foreclosure,* or the person who has foregone exploration and made premature commitments to occupation and ideology (exploration, no; commitment, yes); and *diffusion,* or the person who has neither entered exploration nor made occupational and ideological commitments (exploration, no; commitment, no).

Because of Marcia's explicit scoring rules for determining identity statuses, the methodology has proven fairly reliable (Bourne, 1978a; Marcia, 1980). Recent elaborations on Marcia's original method have included interview questions concerning friendship, dating, and sex roles, on the assumption that these, like occupation and ideology, are legitimate identity arenas within which young adults explore and make commitments (Grotevant, Thorbecke, & Meyer, 1982; Tesch & Whitbourne, 1982).

The word *status* implies something mutable—something that can be changed. Identity statuses have been understood as frozen snapshots of a person's ceaseless identity activity. They are static pictures of the transient here and now. If the photograph is taken a year later, it is indeed possible that the picture will look much different: the person may have attained a new status.

Waterman (1982) argues that the statuses should follow a progressive sequence over an individual's lifetime. From the diffusion status, one may move directly to either moratorium (beginning exploration of possible occupations and ideologies) or foreclosure (bypassing exploration and making premature commitments). From foreclosure one may move into moratorium by renouncing early commitments and initiating exploration. From moratorium one is expected to move, once occupational and ideological questions have been given provisional answers, into identity achievement. Little mention is made of regression in identity formation, or what happens to the person who decides to rework his or her identity at a later date.

Most of the research employing Marcia's methodology and classification scheme for identity statuses has sought to test relatively discrete hypotheses derived from Erikson and common sense. Typically the Marcia interview, or some variant, is administered along with some other kind of measure—be it a measure of interpersonal functioning, task effectiveness, cognitive style, personality traits, etc.—in order to examine mean differences in the second variable as a function of the four statuses. College students usually serve as subjects. A representative example is a study of identity status and conformity (Toder & Marcia, 1973) in which identity-achievement and foreclosure women were shown to conform less than their counterparts in moratorium and diffusion in a standard laboratory task. As such, this kind of research is not particularly personological. Exceptions to this generalization are the probing explorations of identity formation in women undertaken by Josselson (1973, 1982) and the idiographic studies of Donovan (1975).

Identity Achievement

Identity achievers wear the white hats throughout most of the literature on identity statuses. Josselson's (1973) psychodynamic portrait of women classified as identity achievers highlights the striving for internalized goals and reliance upon one's own skills and capacities, which appear as identity hallmarks of the young man or woman who has explored various occupational and ideological options and now knows who he or she is and is not. Less concerned with winning their parents' love than are subjects in some of the other statuses, identity achievers may perceive their parents in balanced though somewhat ambivalent terms (Jordan, 1971; Josselson, 1973). Having lived through and partially rejected traditional social forms, women in identity achievement see themselves as competent, assertive, and yet capable of demonstrating care for others in a noncompulsive way (Donovan, 1975; Josselson, 1973).

Several studies indicate that identity achievers are more academically inclined than persons in other statuses. Cross and Allen (1970) showed that identity achievers received higher grades in college courses. Marcia and Friedman (1970) found that, among women, identity achievers chose more difficult college majors. Orlofsky (1978) found that identity achievers and moratoriums scored higher on the TAT measure of achievement motivation than did foreclosures and diffusions. Another result linking together identity achievers and moratoriums is the general finding that these two statuses are accompanied by higher stages of moral reasoning, in which the individual premises moral decisions on abstract principles of justice and social contract which transcend conventional laws of societies and egocentric concerns of individuals. Foreclosures and diffusions tend to score at lower moral stages (Podd, 1972; Poppen, 1974; Rowe, 1978). Similarly, Hayes (1977) employed Hogan's (1973) measure of moral attitudes in a study which demonstrated that identity achievers and moratoriums were more highly ethical, empathic, and socialized than were individuals classified as foreclosure or diffusion.

In the realm of interpersonal relations, identity achievement has been associated with highly satisfactory and intimate friendships and love relationships for both men (Orlofsky, Marcia, & Lesser, 1973) and women (Tesch & Whitbourne, 1982). Ideally, according to Erikson, identity formation (stage 5 in his scheme) should precede intimacy (stage 6), for one should not give oneself to another until one understands who one is (Erikson, 1963).

It is probably instructive to consider the positive psychological variables with which identity achievement has not been associated. Despite their perceived competence and demonstrated academic achievement, identity achievers do *not* consistently score higher on measures of self-esteem (Marcia, 1966, 1967; Marcia & Friedman, 1970; Schenkel & Marcia, 1972). Evidence for a positive relationship between internal locus of control—a set of beliefs and expectations that the control over one's life and behavior is located within oneself rather than in the external environment—and identity achievement has been mixed (Bourne, 1978a; Matteson, 1975). Finally, within college populations, intelligence (IQ) appears unrelated to identity status.

Moratorium

Involved in the active exploration of alternative occupational and ideological possibilities, young men and women in moratorium, according to Marcia, do not yet know who they are and know that they do not know. The latter realization can be accompanied by pervasive uneasiness and uncertainty about the future, fomenting for some, like Luther in the monastery, a full-blown identity "crisis." But the moratoriums of the present should become the identity achievers of the near future as they pass from exploration to commitment and thereby form a coherent image of self. Consequently, identity achievers and moratoriums are often paired off against foreclosures and diffusions in studies of moral reasoning, self-esteem, and interpersonal relations (especially when the subjects are male). Marcia (1980) terms identity achievement and moratorium the "higher" identity statuses.

Marked ambivalence is probably the best term to describe the characteristic relationship between the young man or woman in moratorium and his or her parents. In moratorium, the person may seek greater psychological distance from the family of origin, rejecting old identifications, ingrained values and beliefs, and setting up the parents or other authority figures as temporary negative identities (Erikson, 1959). These negative identities, like Luther's "dirty peasant," serve as much maligned antagonists in the battle to discover what one believes and how one is to live. Consequently, it is not surprising that parental relations in moratorium can be highly ambivalent.

Jordan (1971) observed that moratorium sons perceived their parents' attitudes toward them as both highly accepting and highly rejecting. Furthermore, the greatest discrepancies between parents' and sons' views of parental attitudes occurred between moratorium sons and their mothers. In her investigations of female identity formation, Josselson (1973) found that moratorium women suffered considerable guilt over rejecting their mothers and renouncing dependency. Many appeared to have identified more strongly with their fathers, evidenced in their strivings to fulfill instrumental ambitions. Further, Josselson observed that other interpersonal relationships in the lives of moratorium women were relatively intense and ambivalent. Josselson remarked that there was a quality of "wanting everything" about the moratorium status, and yet for all the ambivalence and the longing, the moratoriums emerged as the most sensitive, insightful, and likable of all four statuses in this study.

In keeping with the general uncertainty pervading this identity status, moratoriums tend to score high on measures of anxiety. Marcia (1967) showed that moratoriums scored highest of all four statuses on the Welsh Anxiety Scales (Welsh, 1956). Oshman and Manosevitz (1974) documented a comparable relationship employing the Pt scale on the Minnesota Multiphasic Personality Inventory (MMPI). And Podd, Marcia, and Rubin (1970) interpreted the moratoriums' unusually long reponse latencies in a laboratory game as indicative of high anxiety.

Foreclosure

The individual in foreclosure has failed to meet the identity challenge. Rather than risk the uncertainty that might accompany a thoroughgoing reevaluation of past identifications, the young person in foreclosure has opted for the security afforded by the orthodoxy that was childhood. Roles, values, beliefs, expectations, inculcated in the years of trust versus mistrust through industry versus inferiority, are transported intact and unsullied into late adolescence and adulthood. One's occupational aspirations and ideological formulations—pat answers derived from childhood identifications—are rarely questioned and never "worked through." Not surprisingly, foreclosure subjects report that they are very close to their parents, especially sons to fathers. Parents are typically seen as accepting and encouraging (Jordan, 1971). Donovan (1975) and Josselson (1973) found that foreclosures described their homes as loving and affectionate, while reporting that they sought to recreate this harmonious state of affairs in current interpersonal relationships.

Foreclosures appear the "best behaved" of the statuses (Donovan, 1975; Marcia, 1980). College students in this status tend to study diligently, keep regular hours, and appear happy—even in the face of upsetting circumstances (Donovan, 1975). The good behavior may be grounded in traditional and sometimes authoritarian value systems adopted carte blanche from parents and other authority figures.

A number of studies have documented a strong relationship, among men and women, between the foreclosure status and authoritarianism (Marcia, 1966, 1967; Marcia & Friedman, 1970; Schenkel & Marcia, 1972). Typically assessed via the California F Scale (Adorno, Frenkel-Brunswik, Levinson, & Sanford, 1950), authoritarianism refers to a constellation of traits and attitudes centered around a submission to and reverence for powerful authority, conventional societal values, and rigid standards of right and wrong, good and bad. One of the possible consequences of authoritarianism is blind conformity behavior in the face of authority. Podd (1972) had subjects administer electrical shocks to a "victim" in the Milgram obedience task. (Unknown to the subjects, the shocks were not real and the victims were confederates working for the experimenter.) Among subjects in all statuses who had delivered what they thought to be the maximum electrical shock to the victim, only foreclosures showed a significant willingness to do so again. In fact, all foreclosures who delivered the maximum shock agreed to do it again!

With respect to other personality variables, foreclosures score the lowest among the statuses on the Edwards Autonomy Scale (Orlofsky, Marcia, & Lesser, 1973). They also indicate a high need for social approval, scoring highest of the statuses on a measure of social desirability (Orlofsky and others, 1973). They score the lowest on anxiety (Marcia, 1967; Marcia & Friedman, 1970). Finally, Marcia (1966) observed that undergraduates in the foreclosure status tended to manifest unrealistically high levels of aspiration, showing the highest discrepancy between their predicted and actual level of performance on a concept attainment task.

Diffusion

Marcia's fourth identity status remains the most enigmatic. Like foreclosures, individuals in the diffusion status have yet to enter exploration, but unlike foreclosures they have yet to make commitments. Thus, with few strong allegiances to the past and fewer explicit commitments to a particular future, these young men and women appear afloat in a sea of ambiguity, without anchor to a bygone yesterday nor anticipated tomorrow. Empirical findings which distinguish these subjects from the other three statuses are scant because the samples in most studies contain only small numbers of diffusions (Bourne, 1978b).

Bourne (1978b) concludes that the best word to summarize the few findings on diffusion is *withdrawal*. Bob (1968) observed that diffusions' most common response to a stressful situation was withdrawal. Donovan (1975) found that diffusions tended to feel out of place and socially isolated from the world. They conceived of their parents as distant and misunderstanding, and they approached friends and acquaintances with excessive wariness. Aggressive feelings were projected onto others or translated into fantasy. Josselson (1973), too, points to fantasy and withdrawal as favorite coping strategies of women classified diffusion. Summarizing the little available data, Marcia (1980) concludes that the diffusions "seemed to sense little past to integrate, little future for which to plan; they were only what they felt in the present" (p. 176).

Luther Revisited

The research program launched by James Marcia is particularly significant for the facility with which the complex concept of identity has been operationalized for nomothetic research. The coding of semistructured interviews for identity statuses appears to produce the kind of data capable of speaking to the rather holistic construct of ego identity. In this sense, Marcia's empirical transformation of Eriksonian identity is a worthy successor to *Young Man Luther*. Nonetheless, a good deal is still lost in the translation. With the exception of studies by Josselson (1973, 1982) and Donovan (1975), identity research has eschewed personology. The intricate identity tapestry of Erikson's Luther is difficult to apprehend through the empirical lenses of identity achievement, moratorium, foreclosure, and diffusion.

The present inquiry into identity differs from Marcia on at least three fundamental points. First and foremost, the central study in this book is an exercise in personology. In the language of Chapter 1, it incorporates biographical and motivational methods and constructs in a detailed investigation of whole persons. The aim is to do with a moderate number of normal Americans on a limited scale what Erikson did with Luther in a very big way. Though it is absurd to expect that a number of men and women could be studied in the kind of detail employed by Erikson, I would submit that it is quite possible to apprehend more fully the unique and multifaceted nature of the individual identity than has been accomplished in studies of identity statuses. Bringing together the personological tradition of Murray and the study of identity inspired by Erikson, the present inquiry attempts to apprehend and comprehend identity from an integrated and holistic perspective.

Second, this book proceeds from the premise that identity is not "achieved" in any final sense in late adolescence, but that it remains a lifelong and dynamic process which, beginning in late adolescence, may undergo alternating periods of relative stability and marked change. Periods of stability in adulthood may share similarities with Marcia's identity achievement, times when the individual is no longer questioning but is instead living out commitments previously made. Periods of marked change may correspond to Marcia's moratorium, as the individual comes to reevaluate past commitments and experiment with possibilities for new ones.

Third, the focus of this inquiry is more upon the dynamic configuration of identity—what identity looks like—than the process of forming the configuration. Marcia's work speaks exclusively to the process assumed (by Marcia) to come to an end once identity is "achieved." The question of the identity configuration, however, is rarely addressed outside the single case study. A good deal of scientific light may be cast upon the identity configuration if it is seen as adopting a narrative form.

Thus, the configuration of identity which provided unity and purpose to the life of young man Luther was a narrative—a life story—that Luther both composed and lived by. The story contained critical scenes or turning points (the revelation in the tower, the fit in the choir), an ideological setting (established early as a backdrop for subsequent action or plot), and heroic characters (the Father, the Son as Mute, the Son as Spokesman) whose exploits and conflicts determined the narrative line. To examine further the concept of identity, therefore, we must explore the phenomenon of *story* as a general form in art and in life. Remembering the identity of Erikson's Luther as a life story, we will address the following questions: What is a story? What is the function of story? What forms can stories take?

The Meaning of Stories in Literature and Lives

What Is a Story?

Virtually everyone over the age of five knows intuitively what a story is. Children and adults show remarkable agreement when judging whether or not a given passage of prose qualifies as a story (Stein & Policastro, 1984). It is consequently somewhat surprising that social scientists, who of late have become enamoured with stories and story comprehension, have found it difficult to agree on a definition for the story. Stein and Policastro (1984) claim that their survey of the psychological, anthropological, and linguistic literatures yielded at least 20 different definitions. A major controversy concerns the goal-directed nature of story action. One group of definitions states that a story need include a *state-event-state change* sequence but that the sequence need not specify goal-directed action. A second set of definitions emphasizes the goal-directed behavior of an animate protagonist who acts to attain an end and then reacts to its consequences.

The most explicit example of the state-event-state change defini-tion is that offered by Prince (1973). For Prince, a text containing all the necessary features of a story could be as brief as three statements. In the first statement, a given state of being is described: "Bill is happy," or "All was quiet on the Western front." In the second, an event occurs which transforms the state: "Bill fell off his bicycle," or "Two armies arrived on the scene." The third statement depicts the change in the state occasioned by the preceding event: "Bill cries," or "There followed a senseless, bloody battle." Though most minimal stories include an animate protagonist (Bill, the two armies), Prince maintains that any kind of state-event-state change sequence qual-ifies as a story, even one devoid of protagonists: "The weather was warm; a cold front arrived; the weather turned cooler." Empirical research conducted by Stein and Policastro (1984), however, indicates that most children and adults insist that a passage contain reference to a specific animate protagonist if it is to be considered a story.

Definitions focusing on goal-directed action in stories are typi-cally couched in story grammars (Buss, Yussen, Matthews, Miller, & Rembold, 1983; Johnson & Mandler, 1980; Mandler & Johnson, 1977; Stein, 1979; Stein & Glenn, 1979; Trabasso, Secco, & Van Den Broek, 1984). According to this view, the story's essence is a protagonist motivated to carry out some type of goal-directed behavior. The pro-totypical structure of a story, then, is a grammar of goal-directed action which includes six major constituents: (*a*) the setting, (*b*) the initiating event, (*c*) the internal response, (*d*) the attempt, (*e*) the consequence, and (*f*) the reaction. The six constituents represent an idealized schema existing in the reader's head. If a given story does not include one or two of the constituents, the reader may fill in the information himself or herself. Therefore, a passage need not explic-itly set forth each of the six grammatical constituents but may, for some of them, merely hint at the information.

The grammatical constituents which make up the goal-directed story are connected in a causal chain (Stein & Policastro, 1984; Tra-basso and others, 1984). Therefore, each constituent is understood, by the listener, to give rise to the following constituent. That is, the preceding element (e.g., initiating event) causes the following ele-ment (e.g., the internal response). According to Trabasso and others (1984), the listener automatically encodes (organizes) the narrative into a causal chain in which story elements give rise to new elements which give rise to new elements and so on. "Good stories" are readily assimilated to a causal chain or network of casual chains: Most of the events are causally related, and therefore, there is minimal super-fluity. These stories present the listener with a coherent pattern or Gestalt which is easily remembered. "Bad stories," on the other hand, contain a number of events which do not connect to each other in a causal chain. There are numerous narrative cul-de-sacs and loose ends. The endings of bad stories typically fail to bring together the various story elements. These stories are often difficult to remember, appearing haphazard and incomplete. Bad stories lack an integral wholeness. Compare the following two stories.

Story A:

Once there was a little boy who lived in a hot country. One day his mother told him to take some cake to his grandmother. She warned him to hold it carefully so it wouldn't break into crumbs. The little boy put the cake in a leaf under his arm and carried it to his grand-mother's. When he got there the cake had crumbled into tiny pieces. His grandmother told him he was a silly boy and that he should have carried the cake on top of his head so it wouldn't break. Then she gave him a pat of butter to take back to his mother's house. The little boy wanted to be very careful with the butter so he put it on top of his head and carried it home. The sun was shining hard, and when he got home the butter had all melted. His mother told him that he was a silly boy and that he should have put the butter in a leaf so that it would have gotten home safe and sound.

Story B:

There was a fox and a bear who were friends. One day they decided to catch a chicken for supper. They decided to go together because neither one wanted to be left alone and they both liked fried chicken. They waited until nighttime. Then they ran very quickly to a nearby farm where they knew chickens lived. The bear, who felt very lazy, climbed upon the roof to watch. The fox then opened the door of the hen house very carefully. He grabbed a chicken and killed it. As he was carrying it out of the hen house, the weight of the bear on the roof caused the roof to crack. The fox heard the noise and was frightened, but it was too late to run out. The roof and the bear fell in, killing five of the chickens. The fox and the bear were trapped in the broken hen house. Soon the farmer came out to see what was the matter.[1]

Story A is a "good story" in which most of the events are connected in a coherent causal network. Story B might be termed a "bad story." Events do not connect well to each other and there is a good deal of superfluous information. Whereas the first story leaves the reader with a satisfying sense of wholeness and completion, the second story appears scattered, partial, and without good form.

Story Functions

For more than 2,000 years, philosophers and poets have puzzled over the underlying function of stories. In the last 100 years, psychologists have joined them. Though most would agree that stories are in some very fundamental way important for human beings, there has historically been a number of competing theories as to why. The question to be considered then is, "What do stories do?" The answers can be grouped into five classes: stories provide (*a*) mundane pleasure, (*b*) sublime pleasure, (*c*) moral instruction, (*d*) psychological instruction, and (*e*) integration.

Plato did not hold stories in very high regard. Like other forms of art, stories for Plato were merely imitations of the material world. And the material world was an imitation of a higher reality. Thus, stories were imitations of imitations. The individual who listens to stories is analogous to the prisoner in Plato's cave who, shackled and forced to look straight ahead, can only see the shadows of people walking behind him and the statues of animals they carry—shadows cast onto the wall directly in front by the light from the fire directly behind (*The Republic*, Book VII). Therefore, stories and other art forms are a number of steps removed from truth, representing distorted semblances of the material world which itself is a distorted semblance of the ideal and abstract world of truth. To make matters worse, stories tend to arouse base appetites in the listener. The pleasure experienced by the listener is a mundane and primitive pleasure which pales in comparison to the higher delights of reason and the abstract mind.

Among the many questions raised by the Romantic poets of the 19th century is one that could have been addressed to Plato 2,000 years before: "What is so bad about pleasure, anyway?" For Keats, Wordsworth, and Shelley, the pleasure experienced by the man or woman who encounters a good story is akin to a divine ecstasy. Wordsworth asserted that poetry and prose give pleasure through an affirmation of human vitality and volition and the union of humans with their natural world. Shelley understood stories as the record of the best and happiest moments of the happiest and best minds (Daiches, 1981). Contemporary men and women of letters, such as Vladimir Nabokov, likewise celebrate the sublime pleasure of the story. In his *Lectures on Literature* (1980), Nabokov writes

> a wise reader reads the book of a genius not with his heart, not so much with his brain, but with his spine. It is there that occurs the telltale tingle even though we must keep a little aloof, a little detached, when reading. Then with a pleasure which is both sensual and intellectual, we shall watch the artist build his castle of cards and watch the castle of cards become a castle of beautiful steel and glass (p. 6).

Stories delight, and they also instruct. Sir Phillip Sidney, writing in the 16th century, was the first to underscore the pedagogical value of story (Daiches, 1981). Sidney defended stories on the grounds that they often teach the listener a moral lesson—a lesson about what the world ought to be and what ought to be the relations among its inhabitants. From Aesop's fables to *The Book of Exodus*, stories tell us how to live, what values to hold, what is right, and what is wrong. According to this view of story function, the listener may improve his own moral stature by imitating the deeds of the heroes and heroines in narrative. A similar justification of story was provided first by John Dryden, in the 17th century, who argued that stories provide instruction about psychological truth and reality as well as moral worth (Daiches, 1981). Stories provide the listener with insights into human nature, revealing invaluable clues concerning the workings of the human mind, the normal course of development, interpersonal relationships, and the fine lines between genius and lunacy.

A fifth answer to the question of story function goes back at least to Aristotle and incorporates a number of ideas from such influential 20th-century thinkers as Bruno Bettelheim and Claude Levi-Strauss. According to this view, the story's primary function is integration. The integration may occur on the level of the individual or society. Aristotle implies such an interpretation in the *Poetics* when he introduces the idea of catharsis. The audience observing the enactment of dramatic narrative on stage comes to identify with the protagonist(s) and thereby comes to experience vicariously the vicissitudes of the emotion experienced. The resultant release of emotion, termed catharsis, is akin to an affective purgation which leaves the audience, in the case of very good drama, emotionally transformed and enlightened. Observing a dramatic narrative, therefore, introduces new experiences into the everyday experience of the observer. In this sense, the mundane and the sublime, the pedestrian and the exalted, life and drama are synthesized through an active kind of participant observation in which the observer "lives through" the story as it unfolds on stage.

A similar view is adopted by the psychoanalyst Bruno Bettelheim (1976) in his analysis of fairy tales. Children listening to the classic fairy tales, according to Bettelheim, unconsciously identify with the protagonists, who are typically little boys or girls who lived once upon a time in a far away place. The heroic actions of Little Red Riding Hood or Jack (and the Beanstalk) portray conflicts and fears that are very salient in the unconscious lives of the four- and five-year-old children so fascinated by the tales. These conflicts and fears, according to Bettelheim, typically concern power and love, the two fundamental dynamics of the Oedipus complex. By identifying with the protagonist in the fairy tale, the child vicariously experiences the dramatic struggles between the wicked witch and the little girl, the ferocious ogre and the little boy and, like the protagonist, emerges victorious (lives happily ever after) in the end. In exceedingly subtle ways, fairy tales speak encouragement to the child whose confidence has been shaken by the dramatic Oedipal tragedy he or she is experiencing on the unconscious level. Fairy tales thereby promote psychosocial growth and integration for the young child who lives an analogous story of power and love unconsciously.

Coming from perspectives less Freudian, students of narrative, such as Stein and Policastro (1984), Labov and Waletsky (1967), and Sutton-Smith (1976), agree with Bettelheim in arguing that stories function to solve personal problems by integrating unconnected segments of information into more cohesive representations. Similarly, Hunt and Hunt (1977), in describing the experience of divorce, suggest that the construction of a story, involving the reconstruction of past experience, is often an essential task for emotional survival of the divorced individuals. Rainer (1978) and Progoff (1977) offer similar arguments for the writing of diaries or personal stories. Explicitly composing one's story in a diary is a therapeutic exercise which helps the individual solve personal problems while facilitating growth and personality integration. In all of these examples, stories function to put together previously disconnected elements enabling the listener (or the story writer) to put together his or her life.

Moving from the individual to the society, Levi-Strauss (1969) has suggested that certain kinds of stories—what he terms a society's myths—function to integrate ideas and facts pertaining to the society's collective understanding of itself and the universe around it. Myths are "constitutive units" or "classificatory schemes" for the ongoing business of making sense of the perceived universe. They encode in narrative form the traditional beliefs, values, and outlooks of the people who tell them. Like Bettelheim's fairy tales, a society's myths mirror the salient issues with which the society is preoccupied, functioning to tie together a motley host of elements which collectively help to preserve a society's integrity and assure its continuity. Like fairy tales, myths suggest answers to mysteries. As fairy tales and other stories promote personal integration, so do traditional myths promote the integration of societies.

Story Forms

To paraphrase two personologists (Kluckholn & Murray, 1953), every *story* is (*a*) like all other stories, (*b*) like some other stories, and (*c*) like no other story. Though all stories share a general Gestalt which identifies them as members of the genre "story" (like all other stories), each story offers something unique which cannot be found, in its exact form, in any other story (like no other story). But there are recurrent patterns, striking similarities among stories which enable the reader to arrange them into groups. Brontë's *Jane Eyre* and Austen's *Mansfield Park* have a lot more in common than either one has with Dostoyevsky's *The Idiot*. Stories which are like some other stories can be classified, albeit somewhat roughly, into groups. A number of scholars have observed recurrent narrative patterns in stories which have led to the delineation of taxonomies of story forms. Two intriguing classification schemes have been developed by literary scholars Northrop Frye (1957, 1963) and Lawrence Elsbree (1982).

Mythic Archetypes. In his landmark volume entitled *Anatomy of Criticism*, Northrop Frye (1957) attempts to classify the great stories of antiquity and the modern day. Taking his lead from Aristotle's *Poetics*, Frye proceeds inductively by noting commonalities of plot in a variety of the most renowned narratives. The result is the delineation of four fundamental story forms, or what he terms four "mythic archetypes." The archetypes comprise a primitive periodic table for stories: Each story is seen as either a compound of two or more of the archetypes or as nearly a pure manifestation of a single archetype. Frye's four mythic archetypes are *comedy*, *romance*, *tragedy*, and *irony*.

Comedy is the archetype of dawn, spring, and the birth phase. Stories of the hero's birth, of revival and resurrection, of creation, and of the defeat of the powers of darkness, winter, and death come under this heading. In the classic comedy (which may or may not be funny or "comic"), a young man wants a young woman, or occasionally vice versa, but his (her) desire is thwarted by some opposition, often a parent or some figure of authority. At the end of the story, some twist in the plot enables the hero to have his (her) will.

Thus, the movement in comedy is toward eventual union between people as the hero proceeds from one kind of society (say, his family of origin) to another (union with a lover). The obstacles standing between the hero and his (her) desire form the action of the comedy, and the overcoming of these obstacles, a comic resolution. The resolution and subsequent entry of the hero into a new society are marked, in many comedies, by a ritual, such as the wedding in Shakespeare's *As You Like It*. Consequently, comedy usually has a happy ending. At the story's conclusion, the reader or audience feels that things have turned out the way they should and that all shall now live happily.

Romance is the archetype of the sun's zenith, summer, and the triumph phase. Stories of the hero's great exploits, of apotheosis, and of entering into paradise are manifestations of this mythic archetype. The essential ingredient in romance is adventure. The action consists of a series of heroic exploits as the protagonist oftentimes proceeds on a perilous journey, encounters fierce rivals, and emerges triumphant and exalted in the end. Subordinate characters in the story are divided between those for and those against the hero's quest. A proto-typical romance is Homer's *Odyssey*.

The mythic archetype of sunset, autumn, and the death phase is *tragedy*. Included in tragedy are stories of "the fall," dying gods and heroes, violent death, sacrifice, and isolation. In the classic tragedy, the hero finds himself separated in some fundamental way from the natural order of things. This separation makes for an imbalance of nature, and the righting of the balance is the tragic hero's nemesis. Like Oedipus, the tragic hero may be supremely proud, passionate, and of soaring mind; yet, these extraordinary attributes are exactly what separate him from common people and bring about his eventual downfall. Frye remarks that tragedy evokes in the listener "a para-doxical combination of a fearful sense of rightness (the hero must fall) and a pitying sense of wrongness (it is too bad that he falls)" (1957, p. 214). Though it is inevitable that the tragic hero encounter defeat, he is nonetheless perceived as a victim of his nemesis, more wronged than wrong, and in many cases his fall may be followed by the at-tainment of some kind of wisdom, as happens with the blinded Oedipus who eventually becomes a sage and is finally able to "see" the truth (Ross, 1982).

The archetype of darkness, winter, and the dissolution phase is *irony*. Included in this category are stories of floods and the return of chaos: of the triumph of forces which bring mystery and confusion. Frye writes that irony attempts "to give form to the shifting ambigui-ties and complexities of existence" (1957, p. 223). The hero of irony can assume numerous forms. One favorite is the successful rogue of the picaresque novel who employs satire (what Frye calls "militant irony") to expose the absurdities underlying convention. Another is the antihero of some modern novels whose world appears devoid of opportunities for comedy, romance, or tragic heroism but instead manifests itself as a swirl of double meanings, ambiguities, and am-bivalence, a puzzle or mystery which will never be understood.

Romance and, to a lesser extent, tragedy are probably the two mythic forms most readily observed in the life story which is Martin Luther's identity. The epic battles between the Father and the Son define a series of heroic adventures—comprising a spiritual and psy-chosocial journey—in which the Son triumphs and is then defeated again and again. The major battles in the story include the following: Martin (Son as Mute) versus Hans (Father); Martin (Son as Mute) versus God (Father); Luther (Son as Mute and Spokesman) versus the Pope and the Roman orthodoxy (Father); Luther (Son as Mute and Spokesman) versus the Devil (Father); Luther (Father) versus his fol-lowers (Son as Mute); and Luther (Father) versus the peasants and others threatening to push the Reformation too far (Son as Spokesman). One might expect to observe traces of romance, tragedy, comedy, and irony in the life stories of contemporary American adults. We shall consider further this possibility in Chapter 3.

Generic Plots. Lawrence Elsbree (1982) provides a different taxonomy of story forms. He begins with a fundamental question: Why are stories—originating in different times, places, and cultures, and adopting various media, genres, and styles—even intelligible? Elsbree's answer: "I now believe it is in part because all narratives participate in one or more of a few archetypal actions" (1982, p. vii). These archetypal actions are understood as generic plots—universal action sequences intelligible to all people in all cultures which "are felt by the audience to have something like the authority of those rituals which articulate basic phases of human growth and express primary human needs" (p. vii). Furthermore, each of Elsbree's generic plots can be treated in a comic, romantic, tragic, or ironic mode. According to Elsbree, there exist in narrative at least five generic plots.

The first of these is *establishing* or *consecrating a home*. The basic action is (literally or figuratively) the making of the garden, the building of the house, the sustaining of the human community. The actor creates order out of chaos—separating light from darkness, land from water, male from female, task from task, leaders from followers, phases of work from phases of play. The justification for the action is the fostering of growth, individuation, and the continuity of human societies. The dominant rhythm is work; a dominant image is the garden. Examples are readily observed in *Genesis, Robinson Crusoe,* Golding's *Lord of the Flies,* and Carl Sandburg's paeans to Chicago.

The second generic plot is *engaging in a contest* or *fighting a battle.* Here the actor is asserting and protecting the integrity of the self through combat and contest, often vis-à-vis members of the opposite sex. The dominant rhythm is building excitement and subsequent release. As Elsbree puts it, hostility is "provoked, encountered, intensified, then discharged, conquered, pacified, or transformed by love" (1982, pp. 25–26). Examples are observed in stories such as *Taming of the Shrew* and *Pride and Prejudice.*

Taking a journey is the third universal action sequence. In the *Odyssey, Exodus, Pilgrim's Progress,* and *Alice in Wonderland,* the protagonists set out to find a new home, a new identity, or a new commitment. Whether the actors are seeking a better future or fleeing an intolerable past, the journey upon which they embark is sure to be full of discovery and surprise, making for temporary involvements (moments of relative stability) followed by quite sudden movements onward. The rhythm is often a kind of restless propulsion—inexorable forward momentum which propels the actors through a linear series of episodes, settings, and entanglements.

A very common generic plot is Elsbree's fourth, *enduring suffering*. Examples are legion: *Job, King Lear, The Scarlet Letter,* most of Dostoyevsky, Beckett's *Waiting for Godot.* The essential movement is the testing of one's fidelity to the choices one has made. The rhythm of the action is essentially centripetal as the world comes to exert mounting pressure on the sufferer to give in or to change.

Elsbree's final generic plot is the most inclusive. It is the action of *pursuing consummation,* and it is often combined with one of the other four plots, serving as an ultimate aim of the action. Most stories, however, fall short of full consummation. Exceptions, according to Elsbree, include *Revelation, The Divine Comedy, War and Peace,* and Eliot's *The Waste Land.* The basic action is seeking transcendence. As Elsbree describes it, the pursuit of consummation can take many forms—from shedding all earthly desires and thereby purifying the soul to exacting the ultimate vengeance of a Captain Ahab who cannot rest until he destroys the white whale. In the pursuit of consummation, the hero transcends the self and merges with something larger and all encompassing. The rhythm of the action is that of the hunt, the chase, and the relentless striving for something perceived by the protagonist as transcendently good, true, or beautiful.

Elsbree suggests that the five generic plots apply not only to great stories found in literature, but also those stories that make up our lives. He writes:

> We not only borrow other people's and culture's basic plots and stories and adapt them to our purposes; we resort to stories as ultimate kinds of personal evidence. When we really want to explain why we married or divorced, left a job or chose a school, became pacifists or hawks, accepted a faith or became skeptical, we tell a story or series of stories. After our abstractions and generalities have failed to convince or to be clear, we recite the parable of our personal experience (p. 12).

We will search for evidence of Elsbree's generic plots in the life stories of American adults in Chapter 4.

A Life-Story Model of Identity

My central proposition is that identity is a life story which individuals begin constructing, consciously and unconsciously, in late adolescence. As such, identities may be understood in terms directly relevant to stories. Like stories, identities may assume a "good" form—a narrative coherence and consistency—or they may be ill-formed, like the story of the fox and the bear with its cul-de-sacs and loose ends. Examples of the latter might include life stories produced by Lasch's narcissists and Lifton's protean men (Chapter 1) as well as some of the foreclosed identities studied by Marcia. Like stories, furthermore, identities may serve many functions, but their primary function is likely to be that identified by Bettelheim and Levi-Strauss: integration, or the putting together of disparate parts. Like stories, identities may be grouped into classes according to form. This book experiments with the classification systems of Frye and Elsbree and presents a life-story model of identity which attempts to classify according to four story components and two higher-order variables. The life-story model of identity suggests how the personologist, or anyone else seeking to understand the whole person, may apprehend identity in narrative terms. Furthermore, the model suggests hypotheses about identity which can be tested in research and, less rigorously, in personal experience.

Related Concepts

A number of psychologists have proposed theoretical concepts bearing some resemblance to the idea of life story. Alfred Adler proposed the concept *fictional finalism* to denote the final goal or destination that each person imagines for his or her life (Adler, 1927, 1930; Ansbacher & Ansbacher, 1956). Adler was strongly influenced by philosopher Hans Vaihinger who published in 1911 *The Psychology of "As If."* Vaihinger contended that human beings structure their lives around purely fictional ideas which bear little resemblance to reality. These fictions, such as "honesty is the best policy" and "all persons are created equal," are untestable assumptions that guide human behavior "as if" they were true. Breaking from the Freudian doctrine that the major determinants of behavior lie in the person's buried past, Adler followed Vaihinger's lead in suggesting that men and women are more motivated by their expectations for their own futures—expectations purely subjective and not amenable to empirical test. Future goals comprise a fiction, that is, an ideal which is impossible to realize but which nonetheless serves as a catalyst for life striving. Adler wrote, "Experiences, traumata, sexual development mechanisms cannot yield an explanation, but the perspective in which these are regarded, the individual way of seeing them which subordinates all life to the final goal, can do so" (Adler, 1930, p. 400). Though most all persons live by fictions, psychologically healthy individuals are able, according to Adler, to emancipate themselves from these hypothetical story endings when reality demands, though the neurotic cannot.

A similar idea is found in the writings of Eric Berne and other proponents of the brand of psychotherapy termed *transactional analysis* (Berne, 1964, 1972; Steiner, 1974). These clinical psychologists and psychiatrists argue that much of human behavior can be conceptualized in terms of games that people play and the life scripts within which these games are embedded. Games are ritual patterns of behavior that individuals repeatedly enact in normal social intercourse. In arguing with his wife, the frustrated middle-level executive may play the game "if it weren't for you," a recurring scenario in which the wife gets the blame for the husband's failings. Games appear to be segments of larger patterns of interaction termed *life scripts*. Steiner writes:

> A script is essentially the blueprint for a life course. Like theatrical tragedy, the life script follows Aristotle's principles of drama. According to Aristotle, the plot of good tragedy contains three parts: prologue, climax, and catastrophe (1974, p. 60).

Though life scripts vary from the highly dramatic to the banal and from the relatively harmless to the destructive, scripts in general are understood as detriments to authentic living. Berne argues that scripts are the result of the repetition compulsion, Freud's concept which postulates that people have a tendency to repeat unpleasant events from their past. The aim of script therapy, then, is the freeing of people from their compulsions to relive old stories. As Steiner (1971) puts it, the therapist seeks to "close the show and put a better one on the road" (p. 16). Therefore, Adler and the transactional analysts agree that life narratives get in the way of healthy and spontaneous living. The life-story model of identity proposed in this book suggests a less jaundiced view of narrative.

David Elkind (1981) observes that the adolescent may construct a heroic scenario about his or her life course which proclaims the greatness and uniqueness of the protagonist. Elkind terms the phenomenon *personal fable*, a story which the adolescent tells and which is not true. Elkind finds evidence for personal fable in adolescent diaries which often appear to be "written for posterity in the conviction that the young person's experiences, crushes, frustrations are of universal significance" (p. 93). Personal fable is understood as a passing event in the teenager's life, and subsequent identity work in late adolescence and early adulthood forces one to cast aside these fantastical stories of self.

Hungarian psychologist Agnes Hankiss (1981) focuses, too, on adolescence. Implying that Elkind's personal fable gives way to more realistic stories about one's life as one grows older, Hankiss suggests that throughout late adolescence and into adulthood individuals engage in a "mythological rearranging" of their pasts in light of changing future expectations. In so doing, persons construct *ontologies of the self*, which are narratives that tell who a person is and why. In her surveys of life stories, Hankiss finds that people typically adopt one of four different strategies for understanding who they are (and why they are who they are) through narrative. In the first, termed the *dynastic* strategy, the person's view of his or her present situation is generally positive, and the view of the past is also positive: a story in which the good begets the good. In the *antithetical* strategy, the person's present situation is positive but the past is seen as negative—variations of the "rags-to-riches" theme. The *compensatory* strategy employs a negative view of the present but a positive view of the past. Finally, the *self-absolutory* strategy presents a negative present situation born out of a negative past. In delineating different ontologies of the self, Hankiss follows the literary lead of Frye and Elsbree who have attempted to classify stories according to form.

An Overview of the Model

The life-story model refers solely to identity and not to more encompassing terms, such as *personality* and *character*. The model implies no particular theory of personality functioning. If personality refers to the overall organization of a person's behavior and experience as well as the individual differences in general functioning among various persons (Hall & Lindzey, 1970; Liebert & Spiegler, 1978), identity refers to something smaller, a part of personality but not its totality. Though healthy identity may be associated with the well-adjusted personality, the two are hardly synonymous. It is quite conceivable that an individual suffering from a serious disturbance in overall adjustment might find very little with which to be concerned in the province of identity. This is to say, pathology in persons' lives cannot routinely be reduced to problems of identity, though the latter may, in some cases, make a significant contribution.

The central metaphor of the model is the life story. It is proposed that beginning in adolescence, with the advent of formal operational thinking (Inhelder & Piaget, 1958), the person becomes a biographer of self. Early biographical accounts constructed by adolescents may take the form of Elkind's (1981) personal fable—a dramatic and highly unrealistic saga of personal heroism and uniqueness. With time, the stories individuals construct may become more realistic, more tempered, as past experiences and future goals are better integrated so as to confer upon the person's life Erikson's (1963) sense of "sameness and continuity" (p. 261). At this point the individual may have "achieved" identity in Marcia's (1980) sense. Yet the story telling continues, and stories may change markedly in adulthood, corresponding to transformations in identity which occur many years after a late-adolescent stabilization.

Figure 2.2 represents the model. A person's identity (life story) is divided into four major components: *nuclear episodes, imagoes, ideological setting,* and *generativity script.* Two second-order variables are

FIGURE 2.2 A Life-Story Model of Identity

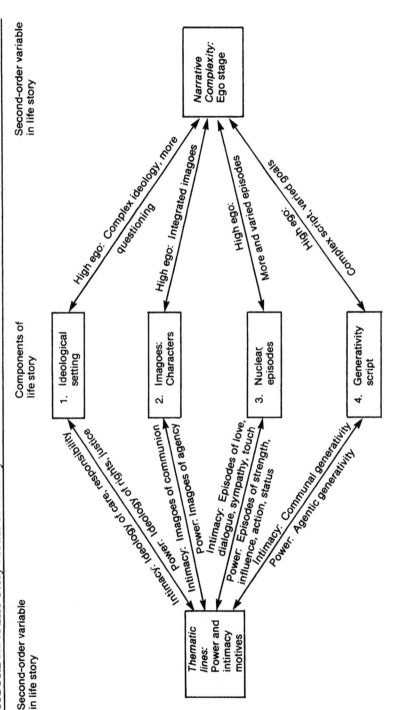

thematic lines and *narrative complexity.* Associated with thematic lines of life stories are power and intimacy motivation—two personality dimensions measured via the TAT. Associated with narrative complexity is ego development—measured via a sentence-completion test. Figure 2.2 provides eight kinds of relationships between motives (thematic lines) and ego development (narrative complexity), and the four story components. These eight correspond to eight general hypotheses which will be considered in subsequent chapters of this book.

Thematic Lines. Thematic lines are recurrent content clusters in stories, analogous to recurrent melodies in a complex piece of music. Though the kinds of thematic lines we might hear in listening to people's life stories are probably infinite, the life-story model asserts that two dominant content clusters center around the themes of *intimacy* (feeling close, warm, and in communication with another) and *power* (feeling strong, having impact on one's environment). These two general themes share conceptual space with Bakan's (1966) constructs of *communion* and *agency*, which in his personality scheme exist as the two fundamental modalities of living forms.

The salience of intimacy and power themes in people's thoughts can be measured via thematic coding of stories people write in response to pictures (Murray's Thematic Apperception Test, or TAT). TAT scores on intimacy motivation (McAdams, 1980) and power motivation (Winter, 1973) are utilized in the present inquiry as predictors of the degree of intimacy and power content in persons' life stories. It is expected, therefore, that a person's score on intimacy and power motivation assessed via the TAT will relate in meaningful ways to the recurrent content themes in the life story which exists as his or her identity.

Narrative Complexity. Though stories differ in content, they also differ in complexity. Some are relatively simple, containing few characters, a straightforward action line, and minimal subplots. Others are more complex. In speaking of a story's complexity, one refers to the overall organization of the story's content, or what might be termed the story's *structure.* It is assumed that the structures of people's life stories vary greatly, from the simple to the complex. Complex life stories are highly differentiated (the storyteller incorporates many elements, makes many distinctions) and highly integrated (the story teller makes many connections among the various elements, synthesizing them within hierarchical patterns of organization). Developmental studies (Applebee, 1978; Botvin & Sutton-Smith, 1977) have shown that children, as they grow older, tell more highly differentiated and integrated stories.

Employed as an index of narrative complexity is Jane Loevinger's (1976) construct of *ego stage*. Measured via a structural analysis of a person's responses on a sentence-completion test, ego stage refers to the integrative framework of meaning an individual imposes upon his or her experience. At lower stages of ego development, the individual's framework of meaning is relatively simple, incorporating global, black-and-white understandings of self and society. At higher stages, one's understandings become much more differentiated and hierarchically integrated so that, eventually, paradox and ambiguity are tolerated and the individuality of others is accepted, even "cherished" (Loevinger, 1976). It is expected, therefore, that a person's stage of ego development, assessed via Loevinger's sentence-completion test, will predict the level of complexity in his or her particular life story or identity.

Nuclear Episodes. The revelation in the thunderstorm, the fit in the choir, the vision of faith encountered in the monks' toilet—these are three critical scenes in the life story which is Martin Luther's identity. The scenes exist as specific autobiographical events which have been reinterpreted over time to assume a privileged status in the story. In Luther's identity, these events are turning points or chapter markers. Such experiences, as they are reconstructed in our own life stories, tend to be understood and felt as uniquely "ours." There is a sense of ownership we experience in reviewing the great moments in our past. Such moments will be called nuclear episodes, which serve as highlighted scenes in life stories.

Hypothesis 1 in the present inquiry is that intimacy and power motivation (thematic lines) will relate in meaningful ways to nuclear episodes. More specifically, persons high in intimacy motivation will report more nuclear episodes characterized by love, dialogue, sympathy, and touch; persons high in power motivation will report nuclear episodes characterized by themes of strength (physical or mental), impact on others, vigorous action, and heightened status. Hypothesis 2 links ego stage (narrative complexity) and nuclear episodes. It is predicted that individuals at higher ego stages will report a greater number of nuclear episodes (greater differentiation). These hypotheses are evaluated in Chapter 5.

Imagoes. In Luther's life story, the Father, the Son as Mute, and the Son as Spokesman exist as diverse personifications of Luther and his world—dominant characters in a story of conflict and high adventure. These three prominent characters, the derivatives of which reside within Luther and his world, are imagoes. Chapter 6 entertains the notion that imagoes tend to arrange themselves in a dialectical fashion in life stories. This is to say, they exist as perceived opposites (the Father, the Son), contradictory images of self (thesis and antithesis) which, in some stories, strive for full expression through some kind of reconciliation or superordinate integration (synthesis).

Hypothesis 3 specifies relationships between thematic lines and imagoes. It is predicted that individuals high in intimacy motivation will present imagoes of *communion* whereas those high in power motivation will present imagoes of *agency*. Communal imagoes are those centered around noncontractual, reciprocal, and harmonious interaction with others in which, as Bakan (1966) puts it, there is "the participation of the individual in some larger organism of which the individual is a part" (p. 15). These include images of self as helper, lover, counselor, caregiver, and friend. Agentic imagoes, on the other hand, bespeak "self-protection, self-assertion, and self-expansion" in which the individual separates self out from context in "the urge to master" (Bakan, 1966, p. 15). These include imagoes of movement, action, and force, such as the traveler, master, father, and sage.

Hypothesis 4 connects narrative complexity and imagoes. A high ego stage should be associated with greater integration among imagoes such that, for example, imagoes from childhood and adolescence are synthesized in more articulated imagoes of adulthood, making for hierarchic integration of imagoes.

Ideological Setting. Erikson has written that identity and ideology are two sides of the same coin. The adolescent in the throes of moratorium searches for answers to ultimate questions concerning truth (epistemology), rightness (ethics), and being (ontology) (Erikson, 1963). The emergence of ideology in adolescence is probably dependent upon the acquisition of Piagetian formal operations with its attendant capacity for unlimited abstraction through thinking about thought.

Underscoring this developmental precedent in adolescence, Hankiss (1981) writes that the life stories of adolescents and adults embody an ontological quality which makes them qualitatively different from the concrete stories of self that might be offered by children. For Hankiss, and for some other investigators of ideology in lives (Fowler, 1981), ideology is something like a backdrop for the identity story. Generally, it is established fairly early in the story (adolescence) and remains in the background, fairly resistant to change. If, however, one encounters major ideological questioning in the adult years, the life story may be in for profound transformations necessitating a reworking of most of its other major components (e.g., imagoes, nuclear episodes). This would suggest that the most tumultuous identity crises are ideological in that the entire background or setting of the story, previously assumed to be given, is transformed. This is the kind of identity crisis we witness in Luther's spiritual pilgrimage from Catholic orthodoxy to the Protestant reformulation of faith. Fowler (1981) speaks of ideology as "faith" and one's "view of the ultimate environment." He writes, "You might say that our image of the ultimate environment determines the ways we arrange the scenery and grasp the plot in our lives' plays" (p. 29).

Examining sex differences in ideological development, Carol Gilligan (1982) speaks of two contrasting ideological approaches: that based on rights and abstract principles of justice and that based on interpersonal responsibilities and concrete exigencies of care. Gilligan's research suggests that the first is a particularly masculine orientation, whereas the second is feminine.

The present inquiry explores the possibility that this difference may in part be mediated by the motives of intimacy and power (thematic lines). For Hypothesis 5, it is predicted that individuals high in intimacy motivation will tend to couch their life stories within an ideological setting based on responsibility and care, whereas individuals high in power motivation will manifest ideological orientations centered around rights and abstract principles of justice. For Hypothesis 6, high ego stage should be associated with (a) greater degree of ideological questioning or rearranging of the ideological setting in life stories and (b) greater complexity in belief and value.

Generativity Script. Although Erikson (1963) depicts generativity as an adult issue confronted *after* one has consolidated identity and intimacy, the life-story model suggests that generativity may be incorporated within identity, which is to say in order to know *who I am* (my life story) I should also have a sense of what I am going to do as an adult in order to fulfill the developmental mandate of generating a legacy. Generativity is a profound concept which bears striking resemblances to (a) the passing on of a genetic legacy understood by biologists as the sine qua non of species survival throughout the animal kingdom and (b) the offering to the next generation of a self-justifying life product which confers meaning or authenticity upon human existence (Becker, 1973). The generativity script is a vision of exactly what one hopes to put into life and what one hopes to get out of life before one is too old to be generative. The so-called midlife crisis (Levinson, 1978), I would submit, is usually a crisis in generativity rather than a thoroughgoing identity crisis which would entail a complete rewriting of the life story along different thematic lines and incorporating new imagoes, nuclear episodes, and ideological settings.

In Erikson's portrayal of Luther, it is difficult to perceive the outlines of Luther's generativity script. A major reason for this obscurity is that Erikson is focusing on *young man* Luther. Though the religious and political movement championed by Luther in midlife was surely an example of generating a life-justifying legacy, Luther appears to have been reluctant to free his legacy of dictatorial control. In generativity, one generates a product and then one, ideally, offers it to the world. The step of offering implies a relinquishing of control which frees the generated product to assume its own somewhat autonomous identity. The prototype is the raising of children. The limited evidence we have in Erikson's account suggests that Martin Luther's approach to the generated products in his life story was not unlike the perceived approach of Hans. As paradoxical as it may seem, one might suspect that the Father imago in Luther's life story was the major obstacle to the construction of a script of true generativity.

Two hypotheses concerning relationships between thematic lines and narrative complexity on the one hand and generativity script on the other will be considered in Chapter 8. In Hypothesis 7, it is predicted that individuals high in intimacy motivation will present generativity scripts centered around significant interpersonal relationships in their present lives or foreseen for the future (generativity as communion), whereas individuals high in power motivation will present generativity scripts centered around personal accomplishments and expansion of the self (generativity as agency). In Hypothesis 8, higher stages of ego development are predicted to be associated with greater complexity in generativity scripts manifested by a greater number and variety of future generative goals.

Summary

In this chapter, I considered in detail the proposition that identity is a life story. Reinterpreting Erikson's classic *Young Man Luther*, I argued that Luther's identity could be understood as a life story containing dramatic *scenes* perceived as turning points (the thunderstorm, the fit in the choir, the revelation in the tower), an ideological backdrop or *setting* of beliefs and values which is transformed or rearranged at various points in the story, and a plot line dominated by the actions and interactions of competing images of self residing partly within and partly outside Luther—the main *characters* of the Father, the Son as Mute, and the Son as Spokesman. I contrasted Erikson's personological portrait of identity in *Young Man Luther* to the nomothetic research tradition on *identity status* inaugurated by James Marcia. Though Marcia's empirical work on identity exemplifies a systematic and highly successful attempt to operationalize a very complex topic, few studies in this tradition are particularly personological—few emphasize the whole person, biography, or motivation.

Next, I considered the various meanings of story in literature and philosophy. Modern scholars have attempted to delineate the minimum requirements of a story. One school of thought holds that the most basic story is composed of a state followed by an event which gives birth to a change in this state. Another school conceptualizes stories in terms of grammars of goal-directed action. Stories are structured such that events come to be seen as "causing" subsequent events, the action being arranged in causal chains. A "good story" may be one in which most events are well assimilated to a coherent causal chain. A "bad story," on the other hand, may leave the reader with the sense that the narrative has "too many loose ends" or that it "fails to hang together."

Going back at least to Plato, scholars have argued about the primary functions of story. Five classes of opinions have been offered: Stories may provide mundane pleasure, sublime pleasure, moral instruction, psychological instruction, or integration. In the latter, stories serve to put together previously disconnected elements enabling the listener (and the story teller) to put together his or her life.

Literary scholars have also attempted to catalogue basic story forms. Northrop Frye offers a fourfold taxonomy of *mythic archetypes* which is akin to a narrative periodic table. For Frye, the four basic kinds of stories are comedy, romance, tragedy, and irony. Lawrence Elsbree takes a slightly different approach in arguing that all stories, regardless of genre or medium, present variations on one or more of five *generic plots:* establishing, consecrating a home; engaging in a contest, fighting a battle; taking a journey; suffering; and pursuing consummation.

Like stories in literature, identities or life stories can serve a variety of story functions—the prime function being integration—and can be classified according to fundamental story forms. It may even be possible to conceptualize life stories in terms of causal chains and thereby make inferences concerning "good" and "bad" life stories. A number of psychologists have proposed theoretical concepts bearing some resemblance to the general notion that life is like a story, amenable to a quasi-literary analysis. Adler put forth the concept of *fictional finalism* to denote a hypothetical story ending serving as a telos of human striving. Berne has spoken of *life scripts,* which resemble Aristotelian tragedy. Elkind has observed the *personal fable* as it manifests itself in adolescent diaries and personal correspondence. Hankiss has proposed *ontologies of the self,* personal narratives "mythologically rearranging" the past in light of future expectations. These narratives are constructed by the individual in an attempt to know who he or she is and why.

I concluded this chapter with a brief overview of the life-story model of identity. A person's identity (life story) is divided into four major components: *nuclear episodes, imagoes, ideological setting,* and *generativity script.* Reflected as recurrent *content* clusterings in life stories, two central thematic lines in human identity concern power and intimacy, and each is reflected in content analysis systems applied to the Thematic Apperception Test (TAT) in the assessment of power and intimacy motivation, respectively. Narrative complexity, on the other hand, refers to *structure*. Stories range from the structurally simple to the complex. The relative complexity of one's life story should be a function of one's level of ego development, which refers to one's overall framework of meaning for making sense of one's experience and world. At the end of the chapter, I offered eight general hypotheses concerning relationships between motives (power and intimacy) and ego development, and each of the four life-story components. One of the functions of the following chapters is to empirically evaluate each of these hypotheses.

NOTES

[1] Trabasso, T., Secco, T., & Van Den Brock, P. Causal cohesion and story coherence. In H. Mandl, N. L. Stein, and T. Trabasso (Eds.), *Learning and comprehension of text*. Hillsdale, N.J.: Lawrence Erlbaum Associates, 1984.

Chapter 3

*T*hematic Lines[1]

*Starting from speculations on the beginning of life and from biological paral-
lels, I drew the conclusion that, besides the instinct to preserve living substance and to join into even larger units, there must exist another, contrary
instinct seeking to dissolve those units and to bring them back to their
primeval, inorganic state. That is to say, as well as Eros there was an instinct of death. The phenomena of life could be explained from the concur-
rent or mutually opposing action of these two instincts.*

(Sigmund Freud, 1930/1961, pp. 65–66)

Flourishing around 440 B.C. on the south coast of Sicily was one
Empedocles, a pre-Socratic philosopher who asserted that *love* and
strife existed as the two organizing principles of the cosmos. The first
to establish earth, air, fire, and water as the four fundamental elements of the universe (Russell, 1945), Empedocles contended that
these were mixed in different proportions to produce all matter in the
world according to the dynamic laws of love and strife. Specifically,
elements were combined by love and separated by strife. Love and
strife, therefore, corresponded to the forces of union and division
in realms as diverse as the movement of clouds and human
relationships.

For Empedocles, history, too, obeyed this dynamic duality.
There were periods in which love was ascendant and others when
strife reigned supreme. In the golden age, love was triumphant, and
humans paid sole homage to the Cyprian Aphrodite; but in subsequent epochs, strife asserted its power to divide element from element, thing from thing, person from person. History proceeds, therefore, in cycles. After love brings things together, strife gradually sorts
them out again until all is divided. Then love again begins to reunite.

In Empedocles' vision of a universe in constant flux, the forces
of love and strife account for all motion and change. Love and strife,

to anthropomorphize for a moment, constitute the *motivation* for the action of the universe in that they exist as underlying forces which set things into motion. More than 2,000 years after Empedocles, Sigmund Freud proposed a similar dichotomy of motivation in Eros and Thanatos.[2] As two distinct groups of underlying forces (what Freud termed *instincts*) impelling the human organism to act (move) and thereby change, Eros and Thanatos, like love and strife, work at cross purposes. Whereas Eros unites so as to harken back to a primordial union of opposites, Thanatos divides in seeking the primordial inorganic state, or the death that preceded life. In Freud's 20th-century view, men and women encounter psychic conflict at virtually every behavioral junction, for not only do their instinctual desires conflict with society and the superego, but they also conflict with each other. Even at the instinctual core, we are torn by a dichotomy of motivating forces which unconsciously exert their powerful influence upon our behavior and our experience.

The life stories which make up our identities are surely shaped by underlying motivational forces acting in concert with a host of other personological and situational factors. In the stories' texts, these forces can manifest themselves as recurrent content clusters, or what shall be termed *thematic lines*. Thematic lines are general content motifs which appear again and again in a life story. Though depicting the countless themes running through the countless life stories men and women have composed sounds like an impossible task, this chapter follows the lead of Empedocles and Freud in pursuing a dualism in lives. The dualism is couched in the terms of intimacy and power, two broad thematic clusterings in the texts of our identities. No claim is made that this is *the* dualism in life, nor that intimacy and power motivation are the fundamental motives in living. There are many different ways to understand lives. I believe the dichotomy proposed in this chapter is *useful*. Further, it makes some intuitive sense. Finally, it bears some resemblance to schemes proposed by other theorists who have expressly endeavored to frame *the* dichotomy.

Thematic Lines as Human Motives

A motive speaks to the question of *why* in human behavior and experience. When one asks the question, "Why did Johnny put a thumbtack on the third-grade teacher's chair?" or "Why did Luther nail the 95 theses to the church door in Wittenberg in 1517?" one inquires into the underlying reasons for behavior. Though the reasons are typically many in number and kind (Johnny seeks attention from his classmates; the teacher has recently given Johnny a low grade; Luther felt impelled by God to speak the "truth"), motivational psychologists have focused their attention primarily upon the *internal* factors—variables *within* the individual which have traditionally been conceptualized in terms of force: instincts, needs, drives, incentives, motives. William James (1890) referred to these internal factors which serve as reasons for behavior as the "springs of action."

Motivational psychologist David McClelland (1951, 1984) has argued that the internal springs of human action exist within the person as affectively toned cognitive clusters centered around general preferences. This is to say, constellations of ideas (cognitive clusters) which refer to desired goals and goal states in living (experiential preferences) come to be infused with emotion (they become affectively toned) so as to form a particular motive. The motive is a personality disposition for the individual. Thus, a given motive is a relatively stable constellation operating in various and sundry ways in a person's daily behavior and experience. A motive serves to *energize, direct,* and *select* behavior and experience within the context of constraints and opportunities afforded by the environment.

The achievement motive serves as a case in point. McClelland and associates (1953) defined the achievement motive as a recurrent preference for experiences of doing well on instrumental tasks of moderate challenge. The general experience of achieving is the goal state of the motive, the desired aim of behavior. The person who is high in achievement motivation, therefore, will reveal a richer and more articulated network of associations (e.g., specific personal memories of success and failure, general attitudes and beliefs about "doing well") to an achievement cue (e.g., a challenging task) than will the person low in achievement motivation. The network of associations is laden with positive affect (joy, excitement, interest) such that opportunities for "doing well," as they present themselves in daily living, come to be emotionally arousing and, thereby, consistently preferred. Consequently, the person high in achievement motivation may engage in challenging tasks with marked enthusiasm (the motive as energizer). He or she may choose to spend more time establishing and working toward the achievement of instrumental goals than, say, talking with friends, caring for children, or enjoying the arts (the motive as director); and the person may attend more closely to achievement-related events and process more efficiently achievement-oriented information than events and information concerned with other goal states, such as intimacy and power (the motive as selector).

Of all the terms used by psychologists to refer to the underlying springs of action, the term *motive* is probably the most generic. Most of the others connote meanings peripheral to the core idea of serving as the spring of action, or the force behind behavior. For instance, the term *instinct* commonly suggests a biological underpinning, some kind of inborn genetic blueprint for action rooted in the species' evolution. The term *drive* has often suggested the same as well as implying that the underlying springs of action exist in some amount which is used up through consummatory behavior, that is, behavior which serves the drive. The motivational theories of Freud and such behaviorists as Miller and Dollard (1941) have been called "drive-reduction theories" because they propose that a given drive within the individual builds up to produce greater and greater tension, which is subsequently reduced through goal-directed behavior. Tension reduction is experienced as pleasurable. Drives have traditionally been understood as relatively generalized sorts of things which serve to arouse the person to action (energize behavior) but which have little to say about the particular direction a person's behavior will take (direct and select behavior) (Atkinson, 1964). The term *need*, on the other hand, has typically referred to more specific phenomena. One's behavior may, for instance, be energized and directed by a need for achievement, a need for affiliation, a need for succorance, and so on. Nonetheless, need, like drive, also suggests tension reduction. Murray (1938) posited that needs tend "to transform in a certain direction an existing unsatisfying situation" (p. 124). This is to say that need deprivation (going without fulfillment of the need for a long time) produces an unsatisfying situation (tension) which calls for a remedy. Behavior servicing the need, therefore, moves the organism from an unsatisfying state to a satisfying one. As tension is reduced, the need is temporarily sated, and behavior in service of the need, one would predict, should stop.

Instinct, drive, and need are variations of the generic idea of motive as an underlying spring of action. To avoid excess connotations, the term *motive* will be most often used in the rest of the book. Like its three analogues, motive refers to *preference*. This is to say, the kinds of behaviors and experiences which are set into motion—energized, directed, and selected—by a given motive are recurrently preferred by the individual who is dispositionally high on the motive. Thus, motives concern what people like to do—what they enjoy experiencing. They do *not* speak directly to the issue of what people do well. Though a person may score high in achievement motivation, he or she may or may not be very effective in achieving. In talking about what people do well, psychologists often employ such terms as *skills* and *competencies*. Motives are not skills; motivation does not imply competence. Though there are numerous examples in the empirical literature of motives being associated with skills, the two domains of recurrent preference and competence should remain conceptually independent.

Personality theorists who have posited a circumscribed set of motivational constructs which energize, direct, and select human behavior and experience fall into three camps: (*a*) those suggesting a large number of basic human tendencies (e.g., McDougall's (1908) 12 instincts, Murray's (1938) 20 psychogenic needs); (*b*) those arguing for the primacy of a single motive (e.g., Adler's (1927) striving for superiority, Rogers' (1951) self-actualization); and (*c*) those proposing motivational dichotomies. Psychologists of the latter ilk have typically asserted that two primary forces in the personality exist in a dialectical tension. Dualistic theories commonly imply that humans are, by their motivational nature, beset with conflict, and that the telos of development and therapy is reconciliation of opposites.

Over the course of about 20 years, Freud (1900/1953, 1920/1955) moved from a twofold vision of motivation embodying the life-maintenance instincts (such as hunger) and the pleasure-inducing instincts (libido) to a more polarized view of life instincts (Eros) in conflict with death instincts (Thanatos). Eros seeks union through pleasure. In childhood, Eros instincts are expressed through oral, anal, and phallic behavior which produces sensual pleasure. After puberty, the genital organs assume dominance, and Eros is directed towards the preservation of the species through the coming together of man and woman in the act of making progeny. Assumed to underly the compulsive repetition of unpleasant experiences as well as aggression directed toward self and others, Thanatos seeks separation and ultimate peace through the dissolution of the organism and a return to the inanimate from the animate. Thus, the death instincts aim at the destruction of the organism, though they are often directed outward in behavior aimed at destroying or injuring others, that is, aggression against others. Both Eros and Thanatos are conservative in that they seek to conserve or reinstate an earlier epoch in the history of the human species. Thanatos seeks to reinstate the organic state of death: "We shall be compelled to say that 'the aim of all life is death' and, looking backwards, that 'inanimate things existed before living ones'" (Freud, 1920/1955, p. 38). Eros seeks to reinstate the original bisexuality of humans, a unity in sexuality that Freud hypothesized was a hallmark of the earliest organisms on earth.

Otto Rank (1936) and Andras Angyal (1941) have proposed motivational dichotomies similar to Freud's. Rank maintained that fear of life and fear of death were the two primary forces in human lives. Angyal suggested the need for autonomy and the need for surrender. In a compelling synthesis, David Bakan (1966) has argued that two fundamental "modalities" exist in all living forms. The first, *agency*, refers to the separation of the individual from others and from context; the second, *communion*, refers to the coming together of individuals and a merger with context. Bakan writes:

> I have adopted the terms "agency" and "communion" to characterize two fundamental modalities in the existence of living forms: agency

for the existence of an organism as an individual, and communion for the participation of the individual in some larger organism of which the individual is a part. Agency manifests itself in self-protection, self-assertion, and self-expansion; communion manifests itself in the sense of being at one with other organisms. Agency manifests itself in the formation of separations; communion in the lack of separations. Agency manifests itself in isolation, alienation, and aloneness; communion in contact, openness, and union. Agency manifests itself in the urge to master; communion in noncontractual cooperation. (1966, pp. 14–15)

To be an *agent* is to assert oneself without regard to the integrity of the surroundings and in so doing to master one's environment and make it his or her own. In the animal kingdom, Bakan points to the cancer cell as the paradigmatic case of "unmitigated agency." The cancer cell continues to grow, divide, and multiply without regard to limits or boundaries. Eventually it completely dominates the embedding context but in so doing destroys the context, kills the host, and itself dies. In healthy living, however, communion mitigates agency. The individual organism is embedded in a larger context, conceived by Bakan as a structured "organism" in itself, and a definition and function (an identity) is conferred on the individual by the context in terms of *relatedness*. Whereas agency recalls Empedocles' strife and Freud's Thanatos in promoting separation and mastery, communion recalls love and Eros in its emphasis upon contact, openness, union, cooperation, and a sense of being at one with other organisms. Though healthy human adaptation presupposes a dynamic tension between the agentic and the communal, Bakan maintains, individual differences in motivational dispositions can be understood in part according to which of the two tendencies is given priority in behavior and experience (Maddi, 1980).

In what follows I will introduce the power and intimacy motives as two personality dispositions upon which individuals differ. Power and intimacy motivation capture the essential meaning of Bakan's agency and communion respectively, and as such their conceptual lineage can be traced to Empedocles' strife and love. Individual differences in power and intimacy motivation can be readily measured through Murray's Thematic Apperception Test (TAT), whereby the psychologist applies basic principles of content analysis to the interpretation of imaginative stories written by individuals in response to ambiguous picture cues.[3]

Intimacy Motivation

Theory and Scoring

I submit that the TAT method of assessing intimacy motivation is a sensitive measure of the relative strength and salience of Bakan's communion in human lives.[4] Intimacy motivation, like Bakan's communion, refers to a particular quality of experience in which the self merges with others. Among other 20th-century scholars who have described this quality of experience and its significance for the development and adaptation of the whole person are Abraham Maslow, Martin Buber, and Harry Stack Sullivan.

The humanistic psychologist Abraham Maslow (1954, 1968) documents the unconditional and noninstrumental merger with another in reported experiences of *Being-Love* (B-Love). Devoid of desperate seeking, B-Love is characterized by a welcoming of the other into a mutually enjoyed, reciprocal union. The tone of the interaction is "gentle, unintruding, undemanding, able to fit itself passively to the nature of things as water gently soaks into crevices" (1968, p. 41). The emphasis upon "being" differentiates B-Love from D-Love *(Deficiency-Love)* in which "doing" (striving) is predominant. D-Love is characterized by striving to fill a void, to satisfy a lack in the individual's interpersonal world. B-Love, on the other hand, "may be enjoyed without end" and usually "grows greater rather than disappearing." B-Love is "intrinsically enjoyable"; it is "ends rather than means" (1968, p. 42). Moreover, Maslow insists that B-Love can enhance psychological growth for all individuals involved, providing experiences profoundly therapeutic in times of distress.

Although he explicitly denies writing about love or intimacy *per se*, Martin Buber (1965, 1970) has been a lyrical spokesman for a dialogical philosophy which undergirds the present approach to intimacy motivation. Buber is concerned with dialogue or communication between people. The *I-Thou* relation is characterized by a special and rare form of dialogue in which each partner is completely absorbed in what the other has to offer, and yet each remains a completely unique and separate communicator. The dialogue is what Sullivan (1953) has termed *syntactic* experience at its best, an exchange of information in which all symbols and signals are fully comprehended by both partners. Of course, such a happening is an ideal only approached in the most reciprocal and egalitarian exchanges. Buber maintains that these exchanges or encounters present themselves in a myriad of situations in everyday life, and as a theologian, Buber points to them as opportunities for making the mundane sacred:

> When I confront a human being as my Thou and speak the basic word I-Thou to him, then he is no thing among things nor does he consist of things. He is no longer He or She, limited by other Hes and Shes, a dot in the world grid of space and time, nor a condition that can be experienced and described, a loose bundle of named qualities. Neighborless and seamless, he is Thou and fills the firmament. Not as if there were nothing but he; but everything else lives in *his* light. (1970, p. 59)

The I-Thou is a momentary dialogical vignette in people's lives in which each focuses unswervingly on the other. It is not a type of long-term relationship in the sense that a marriage, siblingship, or love affair is. The dialogic message, rather, is that episodes of intimate exchange are possible between all kinds of people, and at virtually any time.

The psychiatrist Harry Stack Sullivan (1953) offers a developmental perspective on the capacity to engage in episodes of intimate exchange. According to Sullivan, the *need for interpersonal intimacy* first arises in the human life cycle during the brief but crucial stage of preadolescence. At this time, the appearance in the child's life of the same-sex "chum" may mark a critical transition in the development of the individual's orientation towards interpersonal relations. The hallmark of chumship is the preadolescent's preoccupation with the well-being of the chum. The emergence of chumships precedes the onset of puberty and what Sullivan calls the awakening of the "lust dynamism." Hence, the need for interpersonal intimacy is somewhat independent of genital sexuality, although the two must be successfully integrated in the mature heterosexual union between adults.

Concomitant with the emergence of the intimacy need are the first experiences of loneliness or the vexing condition of living outside an intimate relation. Sullivan remarks that "loneliness, as an experience which has been so terrible that it practically baffles clear recall, is a phenomenon ordinarily encountered only in preadolescence and afterward" (p. 261). The opposite pole of loneliness is intimacy—the "collaborative" relation with another first encountered, for many, in the chumship. The capacities to experience these two phenomena—loneliness and intimacy—develop in tandem.

In sum, the writings of Sullivan, Bakan, Buber, and Maslow converge upon a particular quality of interpersonal experience. The experience can be described as an egalitarian exchange between (among) persons characterized by:

1. Joy and mutual delight (Maslow).
2. Reciprocal dialogue (Buber, Sullivan).
3. Openness, contact, union, receptivity (Bakan, Maslow).
4. Perceived harmony (Buber, Sullivan).
5. Concern for the well-being of the other (Sullivan).
6. Surrender of manipulative control and the desire to master in relating to the other (Bakan, Buber, Maslow).
7. *Being* in an encounter which is perceived as an end in itself rather than *doing* or striving to attain either a relationship or some extrinsic reward (Bakan, Buber, Maslow, Sullivan).

The seven themes define the ideal intimate exchange which serves as the preferred experience or goal state of the individual high in intimacy motivation. In sum, the intimacy motive is defined as *a recurrent preference or readiness for experiences of warm, close, and communicative exchange*—interactions with others deemed ends rather than means to other ends. Intimacy motivation energizes, directs, and selects behavior in certain situations. Individual differences in the strength of intimacy motivation can be measured via content analysis of narrative responses on the TAT.[5] To score a TAT story for intimacy motivation, the psychologist determines the presence or absence of each of 10 explicitly defined intimacy themes. Each of the themes refers to a particular quality of the relationships among the characters in the story. The total number of these themes observed in an individual's TAT stories constitutes his or her total score on intimacy motivation. The 10 themes comprising the intimacy motivation scoring system are described in detail in Appendix C and in the complete scoring manual (McAdams, 1984c), which also includes 210 practice stories and specific scoring rules.

Spontaneous Thought and Behavior

During the course of a normal waking day, men and women high in intimacy motivation spend more time thinking about interpersonal relationships than do their counterparts low on the motive. Support for this proposition comes from a study conducted by McAdams and Constantian (1983) in which 50 college students carried electronic pagers ("beepers" of the sort worn by physicians) for a week during which time they were paged seven times a day. Each participant in the study agreed to wear a pager between 9:00 A.M. and 11:00 P.M. each day for one week. The individual was subsequently paged (beeped) seven times a day according to a computer-generated random number sequence, one paging taking place sometime within each of the seven two-hour intervals between the time the subject put the pager on in the morning and took it off at night. When individuals were paged, they stopped doing what they were doing, if at all possible, and filled out a very brief questionnaire asking for a record of thoughts, feelings, and behaviors which were being experienced or emitted at the exact moment of paging. Over the course of the week, then, the participants reported on as many as 49 random samples of daily experience and behavior. This method of collecting data about a person's daily life via the pagers—the "experience sampling method"—has proven a valuable research tool in previous studies conducted by Csikszentmihalyi and Larson (Csikszentmihalyi, Larson, & Prescott, 1977; Larson & Csikszentmihalyi, 1978, 1980).

We scored each account of what the person was thinking about when paged for interpersonal content, giving a score of 1 when the person said he or she was thinking about specific people or interpersonal relationships in his or her life. Accounts of thoughts which made no reference to specific people or relationships received scores of 0. Examples of responses that might score 1 include "my boy-friend," "the obnoxious guy sitting next to me in class," "my father's retirement," "a friendship," "whether to have lunch with my room-mate or alone," "people around me at a party." Intimacy motivation scores determined by a prior administration of the TAT were strongly correlated ($r = +.52$) with frequency of interpersonal thoughts, over the course of the 49 pagings. In other words, the higher a person's TAT score on intimacy motivation—indicating a strong recurrent pre-ference or readiness for experiences of warm, close, and commun-icative interaction—the higher the number of interpersonal thoughts collected over the course of the week via the random pagings.

The same study speaks to the issue of spontaneous behavior. Men and women high in intimacy motivation were more likely to report, when paged, that they were engaged in behavior indicative of warm and close interpersonal relations: conversations and letter writ-ing ($r = +.40$). Furthermore, subjects high in intimacy motivation reported more positive affect (feeling "happy," "carefree," "alert," etc.) when engaged in some form of interpersonal interaction than did subjects scoring low in intimacy motivation. In sum, college stu-dents in McAdams and Constantian's (1983) study who scored high in intimacy motivation spent more time over the course of the week (*a*) thinking about people and relationships, (*b*) talking with people or writing to them, and (*c*) feeling good about their interactions with people, than did their counterparts scoring low in intimacy motivation.

McAdams and Powers (1981) examined further the relationship between intimacy motivation and spontaneous behavior in an un-usual investigation in which college students met in small groups to enact dramatic scripts. The method was derived from the work by Moreno (1946) on psychodrama. Traditionally, psychodrama has been employed in group therapy as a method of acting out psychosocial problems and effecting in action emotional resolutions. In the classic psychodrama scenario, one group member (the *protagonist*) is desig-nated the main character in his or her own *action drama*. The drama is enacted in the space available (the *stage*), and other members of the group may serve as either *actors/actresses* or *audience*, as the psycho-drama *director* (therapist) monitors and interprets the proceedings. In McAdams and Powers' study, volunteers meeting in small groups were instructed by a trained psychodrama therapist in the basics of the method and then led through a one-hour sequence of action games and discussions designed to lower anxiety and promote an atmosphere of openness and sharing. Following this warmup period, each subject in turn came forward to enact a minipsychodrama, using the group members and room to illustrate in spontaneous action any issue or theme he or she deemed appropriate. The psychodrama scenarios did not generally touch on profoundly personal issues, as they might in traditional clinical settings, and were not elaborated into therapeutic explorations.

Over the course of six weeks, five psychodrama groups were run, yielding data on 43 subjects. All of the proceedings were video-taped. Coding the tapes in a variety of ways designed to measure the quantity and quality of warm and close interpersonal interaction in the groups, McAdams and Powers found that psychodrama protagonists scoring high in intimacy motivation structured dramatic scenarios which contained more (*a*) positive affect (joy, happiness, etc.), (*b*) reciprocal dialogue, (*c*) spontaneous participation among equals (group members were allowed to adopt individualized roles in the protagonist's scenario, and their actions were not controlled or dictated by the protagonist), and (*d*) nonthreatening, tender touching. Furthermore, these high-intimacy protagonists, compared to their peers low in intimacy motivation, made more references to "we" or "us" when referring to themselves and the group, issued fewer commands to their peers, stimulated in the group more outbursts of laughter, and positioned themselves in closer physical proximity to other group members when enacting their dramatic scenarios.

Personal Relationships

Though the two studies reviewed above document significant relationships between intimacy motivation and spontaneous thought and behavior centered around warm, close, and communicative interaction, they do not address directly the kind of ongoing relationships exhibited and experienced by persons high in intimacy. A second set of studies (McAdams, 1984a); McAdams, Healy & Krause, in press; McAdams and Losoff, 1984; McAdams & Vaillant, 1982) pursues this topic by investigating intimacy motivation in marriage and friendship.

This research supports the general proposition that men and women high in intimacy motivation tend to be engaged in meaningful personal relationships which exhibit many of the hallmarks of Bakan's (1966) communal mode of human existence. Bakan's communion implies a gentle and delicate approach to significant personal relationships. In communion, the self merges with another as boundaries between egos are blurred and each interactant surrenders manipulative control in the spontaneous process of relating. In surrendering control, the communal individual focuses upon *being* over *doing* in a relationship. He or she is especially sensitive to the possibilities of reciprocal sharing with others—of the spontaneous kind of dialectic in relationships described by Martin Buber as the I-Thou encounter. Numerous theories of love and friendship state that a blurring of ego boundaries through a surrender of control in the process of relating is a sign of the harmonious and mature inter-personal relationship (Balint, 1979; Erikson, 1963; Guntrip, 1973; Maslow, 1968).

Sampling students' friendship episodes over the course of two weeks, McAdams and others (in press) discovered that intimacy motivation was associated with (*a*) dyadic as opposed to large-group friendship encounters (episodes between two friends rather than among a large number of friends) and (*b*) self-disclosure and listening in interactions with friends. The latter finding was particularly strong. Men and women high in intimacy motivation consistently reported that, when they got together with friends, they spent a good deal of time talking about relatively personal issues, such as individual feelings, emotions, needs, wants, fantasies, strivings, dreams, hopes, plans for the future, fears, and self-awareness. Further, these high-intimacy subjects, compared to those low in intimacy motivation, were more likely to report conversations with friends which dealt explicitly with the topic of the friendship itself. In interacting with their friends, the high-intimacy men and women were not reluctant to adopt the passive role of listener. On the contrary, they appeared to invite the role, readily assuming a receptive orientation in which they said or did little, but listened much.

The findings on self-disclosure and listening suggest that the individual high in intimacy motivation is more apt to surrender control in the process of relating to close friends, adopting the receptive communal mode of interaction. In the communal mode, relationships are understood as egalitarian. Two equals open up to each other, neither stifled by any fear of exposing vulnerabilities. Bakan states that the communal mode is characterized by "participation of the organism in some larger organism of which the individual is a part" (1966, p. 15). The "larger organism" in this case is the friendship itself—the relationship which partially subsumes individuality as it spontaneously unfolds.

Evidence for a significant link between intimacy motivation and self-disclosure in friendship was garnered in another investigation in which college students were asked to review the history of the closest friendship they had ever experienced (McAdams, 1984a). A series of open-ended questions guided their review. In one question, the students were asked to describe in some detail a concrete incident from that history in which the student and his or her friend found that their friendship bond was strengthened. This could be seen as a high point or peak experience in the friendship history. Students high in intimacy motivation overwhelmingly described these high points as including some kind of personal revelation—an incident of significant self-disclosure—on the part of one friend and the acceptance of that disclosure on the part of the other. Here are two verbatim examples:

> In junior year in high school, I went on a class trip to California and I roomed with Sandy and two other girls. Sandy and I paired up together for most of the activities during the trip, and during that time we became rather close, each of us telling each other boyfriend troubles. I was glad that I found someone that was interested in what I had to say and was sincere and honest in her replies. At the same time I was very interested in listening to her and trying to understand her.

> This is not really very dramatic. I think what got us together so that we understood each other and laughed and yelled about the world and our feelings was not one particular thing but something that happened on several different occasions. These occasions were when we started writing crazy sayings—poems—of our day's events. We kept a diary-type journal in this class and we each felt confident enough to share the journals with each other. During the course of the year, we would exchange these notes—even up until our graduation we made it a weekly kind of thing to read each other's poems. I guess this is a silly and strange thing to do, but I never grew so close to anyone else.

In describing a "low point" in the friendship history or a concrete incident which weakened or tested the friendship bond, the high-intimacy students tended to focus on *betrayals of trust*—episodes in which one of the friends broke an implicit pact of the friendship. Examples included breaking a promise, disclosing a secret to some third person, and failing to show warmth or understanding to the other. In a number of cases the violation involved a failure in candor, indicating that honest self-disclosure and confidentiality were extremely important issues in these friendships. Individuals high in intimacy motivation were more likely, furthermore, to accept at least partial blame for the friendship low point and to indicate that the two friends subsequently worked towards a resolution. Finally, in describing fears they frequently experienced in the presence of the best friend, students high in intimacy motivation tended to focus on *separation* from the friend as a possible result of such uncontrollable happenings as geographic moves, divergent courses of development, injury, or death.

Another study has investigated children's friendships. McAdams and Losoff (1984) modified the intimacy motivation scoring system to make it appropriate for the coding of stories told in response to pictures by fourth and sixth graders at a private elementary school. The modified intimacy motivation scores were positively associated with (a) reporting more factual information about one's best friend in an interview, (b) emphasizing sharing and cooperation with friends in explaining why one likes particular others, (c) having the same best friend over a long period of time, and (d) teacher ratings of "friendly," "affectionate," "cooperative," "sincere," and "popular."

Only one study has examined intimacy motivation in marital relations, and it dealt only with middle-aged men. McAdams and Vaillant (1982) rescored TAT stories written by 57 male graduates of Harvard University at age 30 (in 1950–1952) for intimacy motivation. The men were contacted regularly between the ages of 30 and 47, providing a wide variety of data on overall functioning. A psychiatrist reviewing the longitudinal information on each subject then gave a numerical score to the variable "marital enjoyment" for each. Further analysis revealed that these scores were significantly correlated with intimacy motivation, $r = +.38$, for 57 subjects. Men high in intimacy motivation at age 30, therefore, were more likely to report happiness and stability in their marriages at midlife. Other motives assessed via coding the TATs, such as power and achievement motivation, were unrelated to marital enjoyment.

Adaptation to Life

McAdams and Vaillant's (1982) longitudinal study of midlife men provides further information concerning the relationship between intimacy motivation and overall psychosocial adjustment. The researchers calculated an overall adult adjustment index based on the interview and questionnaire data collected between ages 30 and 47. Focusing, for the most part, on behavioral indexes that were relatively concrete and thereby reliably measured, the adjustment index was a sum of ratings on nine dimensions: income level, occupational advancement, recreational activities, vacations, job enjoyment, number of psychiatric visits, drug or alcohol misuse, days of sick leave, and the aforementioned marital enjoyment. The nine ratings were assumed to be well representative of implicit standards of psychological adaptation in this group of middle-class, well-educated, white men growing up in the 1930s and entering midlife in the 1960s. Characteristics of the men in the sample are described fully in Vaillant (1977) and Vaillant and McArthur (1972).

Intimacy motivation assessed at age 30 predicted overall psychosocial adjustment 17 years later at statistically significant levels ($r = +.39$). Other TAT motives were not associated with overall adjustment, though achievement motivation revealed a nonsignificant trend in the positive direction. The results are in keeping with the many theoretical and clinical statements suggesting that a desire and a capacity to engage in intimate relationships with others is a virtual sine qua non of psychosocial adaptation in the adult years (see Erikson, 1963; Fairbairn, 1952; Levinson, 1978; Sullivan, 1953). Given the small size of the sample and its limitations with respect to sex, age, socioeconomic status, and ethnic background, however, broad generalizations concerning intimacy motivation and psychosocial adaptation are not warranted. Yet the findings suggest a possible connection that should be fleshed out in future research.

Other Findings; Sex Differences

In two separate studies, college students scoring high in intimacy motivation, compared with those scoring low, were rated by their friends and acquaintances as significantly more "sincere," "loving," "natural," and significantly *less* "dominant" (McAdams, 1980; McAdams & Powers, 1981). Another study (McAdams, 1979) provides tentative support for the hypothesis that individuals high in intimacy motivation are more sensitive to changes in facial behavior than are those scoring lower. McAdams, Jackson, and Kirshnit (in press) explored the relationship between intimacy motivation and nonverbal behavior in videotaped dyadic interviews. In convivial and nonthreatening interviews, students high in intimacy motivation showed increased smiling, laughter, and eye contact compared to those scoring low.

No consistent results concerning sex differences have as yet been obtained in intimacy motivation research. Though one might expect women to score higher on the motive than men, TAT data collected thus far do not support this expectation. Because most research has been conducted with college students and because the intimacy motive is a relatively new personality construct, the jury is still out on the possibility of a sex difference in motive strength. Though not statistically significant, females have tended to score slightly higher than males on intimacy motivation in more traditional settings, such as the two colleges in the midwestern United States where much of the research has been undertaken. Results from Harvard University, however, have generally produced slightly higher scores for males, reflecting perhaps a greater repudiation of traditional sex-role stereotypes concerning the communal nature of women and the agentic nature of men in this setting. Still, these differences were not statistically significant.

Power Motivation

Theory and Scoring

I submit that the TAT method of assessing power motivation is a sensitive measure of the relative strength and salience of Bakan's agency in human lives. Power motivation, like agency, refers to a particular quality of experience in which the self masters the surrounding environment, emerging separate and autonomous vis-à-vis its world. Agency unmitigated by communion means unlimited expansion and conquest. This is the ideal goal state—the preferred experience—for the person high in power motivation. Therefore the power motive can be understood as a *recurrent preference or readiness for experiences of having impact and feeling strong (potent, agentic) vis-à-vis the environment.* Like intimacy motivation, the power motive manifests itself as an affectively toned cognitive cluster which energizes, directs, and selects behavior in certain situations.

Precursors to the modern understanding of power motivation appear in the psychologies of Nietzsche and Adler. Deploring all religious and psychological views of humans extolling universal love and meekness, Nietzsche (1844–1900) celebrated the *will to power* as an ethical, religious, and psychological imperative in lives. Forged through Spartan discipline and not self-indulgence, the will to power inspires *men* (Nietzsche was a blatant sexist) to passion and pride, revenge and anger, adventure, war, destruction, and (strangely enough) *knowledge.* All things, all people, all ideas are the objects of conquest. Nietzsche's hero, the *noble man,* is essentially the incarnate will to power. The prototype is the governing aristocrat who is both a ruthless tyrant and a man of high culture espousing a passion for the arts and for the pursuit of knowledge. Most men, however, are made of meaner stuff. Flacid, obsequious, and proletarian, they walk through the world as the *collective men,* occasionally rubbing against each other to produce just a little warmth and paltry pleasure.

Adopting what became a Freudian doctrine 12 years before Freud, Adler (1908) argued for an inherent aggressive drive in human lives that was on equal footing with Freud's libido or sexual drive. Manifestations of the aggressive drive were first identified in attempts to compensate for perceived physical inferiority. Somewhat later, Adler came to consider a whole host of psychological inferiorities for which men and women compensated by cultivating such personality traits as impudence, stubbornness, rebelliousness, impertinence, courage, and defiance. The aggressive drive came to be understood as a general striving for superiority—an inherent biological urge toward self-expansion, growth, and competence. This is Adler's most agentic formulation of the fundamental human motive, and it shares many similarities with the modern view of power motivation. In later theorizing, Adler (1927, 1930) settled on a less agentic motivational construct—a striving for perfection through the fulfillment of a fictional life goal—which blended themes of identity, intimacy, and power.

In more recent years, McClelland (1975) has enriched our understanding of power motivation by presenting a provocative argument for four distinct classes of power experience and expression. Each of the four is linked to a Freudian psychosexual stage: oral, anal, phallic, genital. In the first class (stage 1, oral: "It strengthens me"), the individual experiences power vicariously by associating himself or herself with outside agents of strength (father, God, leaders, friends). This is power through dependence upon powerful others, a passive orientation anathema to the likes of Nietzsche. In the second class (stage 2, anal: "I strengthen myself"), the source of power is experienced as within, and the individual comes to feel strong through self-assertion and self-control. McClelland associates this power orientation with disciplining the self and collecting (anal hoarding) prestige possessions to enhance the power of self. Closest to Nietzsche's will to power, the third class (stage 3, phallic: "I have impact on others") is similar to the second in that the source of power is experienced as within, but it is different in that the object (the target) of power strivings is no longer the self but others. One seeks to control, persuade, change others, and in so doing expand one's domain of influence. The fourth class (stage 4, genital: "It moves me to do my duty") is considered by McClelland the most mature form of power experience. In this manifestation of power, the source of power is again perceived, as it was in stage 1, as outside the self (God, society, laws, my group), but the individual seeks to use that power to serve or influence his or her world in a beneficial way. This is the power of the manager, the scientist, and the healer.

To score a TAT story for power motivation, the psychologist determines the presence or absence of each of 11 explicitly defined content themes. Each refers to ways characters in the stories have impact upon each other and their environments. The total number of times these themes occur in an individual's TAT stories constitutes his or her total score on power motivation.[6]

Instrumental Behavior

Winter and Stewart (1978) write:

> The essence of power is the ability to make the material world and the social world conform to one's own image or plan for it. This is a complicated process, involving steps such as forming a plan, articulating it, rallying support and amassing resources, convincing others, checking the implementation, using positive and negative sanctions, and so forth. In social units that have grown beyond the simplest stages, seeking and getting power takes place within the framework of rules and procedures for each step of the process: Power is said to be institutionalized in leadership roles or *offices*. Therefore, we would expect that the power motive should predict office seeking and office holding. (p. 400)

Research suggests that it does, to a certain extent. Winter (1973) found that officers in university student organizations did score higher on TAT power motivation than nonofficers. Students high in power motivation also tended to become dormitory counsellors, members of important faculty-student committees, and staff workers on the university newspaper and radio station (Winter, 1973). Among working-class adults, high power motivation has been associated with office holding in organizations (McClelland, Wanner, & Vanneman, 1972). Among middle-class and upper-class adults, however, this relationship does not hold (Winter & Stewart, 1978). Power motivation has been associated with careers in which the individual has the opportunity or duty to direct the behavior of others in accordance with established plans and to use positive and negative sanctions in doing so: business executive, teacher or professor, psychologist, clergyman, and journalist (Winter & Stewart, 1978).

Fodor and Smith (1982) investigated how people high in power motivation direct the behaviors of others in group decision making. Forty groups of undergraduates containing five students each met to discuss a business case study which concerned whether a company should market a new microwave oven. In each group a leader was appointed. Half the leaders scored extremely high in power motivation and half extremely low. All group members were given fact sheets to guide the discussions. Those groups whose leaders scored high in power motivation tended to bring less factual information from the sheets into group discussion and considered fewer alternative action proposals than did those groups whose leaders were low in power motivation. The authors interpreted the findings as supporting the notion that leaders high in power motivation promote *groupthink* (Janis, 1972), a form of hasty decision making characterized by diffusion of responsibility, failure to consider long-term ramifications, and domination by one or two strong leaders whose opinions are not challenged.

Support for this interpretation comes from another simulation experiment in which business administration students acted as supervisors directing the labors of a work crew (Fodor & Farrow, 1979). Supervisors high in power motivation were more likely than those scoring low in power to react favorably to workers who ingratiated themselves. High-power supervisors also perceived themselves as exerting greater influence over the work group than did those low in power motivation.

Personal Relationships

Research into power motivation and significant interpersonal relationships converges on two tentative conclusions: (*a*) men high in power motivation appear to have problems in love relationships, and (*b*) men and women high in power motivation appear to adopt relatively agentic (Bakan, 1966) orientations toward friendships.

Stewart and Rubin (1976) conducted a longitudinal study of 63 dating couples living in the Boston area. At the time of the initial testing, high power motivation in the males was significantly associated with greater expressed dissatisfaction with the relationship on the part of both members of the couple and greater anticipation of future serious problems in the relationship among the men. Two years later, 50 percent of the couples in which the man was high in power motivation had broken up and only 9 percent had married. In those couples in which the male was low in power motivation, 15 percent had broken up and 52 percent had married over the two-year span. Additionally, males high in power motivation were more likely to report that during the two years immediately preceding the start of this dating relationship, they had been seriously involved in a romantic relationship that eventually terminated. The authors concluded that men high in power motivation manifest marked instability in romantic relationships, moving from one serious involvement to the next in relatively rapid succession. Bolstering their claims are the findings of Winter (1973) in which power motivation among men was positively associated with number of sexual partners and frequency of sexual activity. According to Winter, the archetypal representation of the high-power-motive man in Western folklore is Don Juan, the expansive and profligate womanizer.

Winter, Stewart, and McClelland (1977) related power motive scores determined from TAT protocols collected in 1960 among undergraduate men to the career levels attained by these men's wives in 1974. Among the 51 husbands studied, power motivation assessed in 1960 was significantly and negatively associated with wife's career level 14 years later. In other words, well-educated men high in power motivation were likely to marry women who chose *not* to pursue professional careers (over whom, presumably, they could exercise considerable influence and control).

A contrasting study undertaken with women (Winter, McClelland, & Stewart, 1981) found that well-educated women high in power motivation tended to marry successful men. Similarly, Veroff (1982) reports that power motivation in *women* is associated with marital *satisfaction*, whereas other studies have associated power motivation in *men* with a higher divorce rate (McClelland, Davis, Kalin, & Wanner, 1972) and a greater degree of marital dissatisfaction (Veroff & Feld, 1970). At the root of the high-power man's apparent dissatisfaction and instability in romantic heterosexual relations may be a latent fear of women and the control they may exert. Slavin (1972) has shown that men high in power motivation express more themes of feminine evil in fantasies than do men lower on the motive. These themes include females harming men through physical contact, females exploiting men, females rejecting men, females proving unfaithful in relationships, and females triumphing over men. In keeping with this image of Medea, Winter and Stewart (1978) report that men high in power motivation, when asked to draw pictures of women, produce sometimes frightening and bizarre sketches of females with exaggerated sexual characteristics.

In the arena of friendship, McAdams and others (in press) discovered that power motivation was associated with (*a*) interactions with friends in large groups as opposed to dyads and (*b*) agentic striving in friendship episodes. Agentic striving was defined as an active, assertive, or controlling role assumed by the individual when interacting with friends. Examples included taking charge of a situation, assuming responsibility, making a point in a debate or argument, helping another, giving advice, making plans, organizing activities, and attempting to persuade others. In these agentic friendship episodes, the subjects perceived their roles as dominant, guiding ones. They were actively *doing* something, behaving as an agent.

In McAdams' (1984a) investigation of the history of a person's relationship with a best friend, students high in power motivation often described the friendship's high point as an incident in which one or the other friend offered *help* to the other. Helping—whether a heroic act or quiet counsel—is an active assertion of the self: It intervenes in the environment and effects a significant change. Helping temporarily transforms a relationship into one between relative unequals. For the moment, the helper is dominant; the helped is submissive. The relationship is hierarchical rather than egalitarian. Helping is highlighted in these two verbatim accounts of friendship high points, written by a young woman and man, respectively, both high in power motivation:

> One incident where my friend and I grew closer was when I became ill and began to lose a great deal of weight. I had no appetite and went a long time without eating. It did not happen in a specific event, but rather I began to feel sick and she noticed how much I was changing and tried to console me. Others noticed that I began to look thinner and act a bit different than I normally did, but they really did not say much to me and acted just the way they did before (these were other classmates). This incident occured when I was a sophomore in high school. I really was not aware of the changes at the time.

> I was working at the _____ as a waiter. A lunch rush hit and the cook (my friend) was in trouble. He and I figured out the situation and took on the problem. Within 45 minutes we were able to serve lunch to 75 people. The best part was that we handled it so smoothly that there were no complaints.

In describing low points in the history of their relationships with best friends, individuals high in power motivation tended to focus on incidents in which the other friend acted in a socially inappropriate or obnoxious way, usually in a public arena. High-power persons appeared to be highly concerned about how they and their friends appeared in public. Any boorish action on the part of a friend might be seen as a humiliation lowering the prestige of all involved. Consequently, a public display of self would become an embarrassment for the agentic individual who desires an approving audience to affirm self-display.

The interpretation is supported by the additional finding that high-power men and women tend to report that they fear *conflict* in their relationships with best friends. In fearing conflict, the high-power individual may be expressing concern over a possible clash between active agents. For agentic relationships to work well, the friends must tolerate, even condone, each other's agentic striving, each other's ventures of self-expansion, self-assertion, and self-display. Conflict threatens the breakdown of equilibrium which has nurtured the agentic strivings of the friends. The findings are consistent with Winter's (1973) report that high-power men tend to avoid carefully the possibility of conflict in their relationships with peers.

Adaptation to Life

Research findings concerning the relationship between power motivation and overall psychosocial adjustment are highly equivocal. Winter (1973) provides data on working-class men suggesting a positive association between high power motivation and the expression of anger via "aggressive" behaviors, such as throwing things around a room and stealing towels from hotels. The finding has not been replicated, however, among middle-class men nor among women. Employing power motivation and another TAT measure designed to assess "activity inhibition," McClelland (1979) has argued that a high power motive score combined with high activity inhibition indicates a high level of suppressed anger. Clinicians have long observed that individuals who are chronically angry but unable to express their anger may be high-risk candidates for hypertension (high blood pressure). In three separate samples, McClelland found a significant relationship between the suppressed anger profile on the TAT (high power motivation and high activity inhibition) and high blood pressure levels in men. In one sample followed longitudinally, the suppressed anger profile as measured in TAT stories written when the men were in their early 30s significantly predicted elevated blood pressure and signs of hypertensive pathology appearing 20 years later. Other studies have documented rather complex relationships among high power motivation, stress, and susceptibility to illness

(McClelland, Alexander, & Marks, 1982; McClelland, Floor, Davidson, & Saron, 1980; McClelland & Jemmott, 1980). These investigations hint at a possible relationship between high power
motivation and high levels of stress on the one hand and a breakdown
of the body's immune functions because of increased activation of the
sympathetic nervous system on the other.

Power motivation has also been linked to alcohol consumption.
McClelland and others (1972) found that moderate drinking increases
dramatically the power motive scores of men. TAT stories written
after consumption of even a few ounces of alcohol contained significantly more power images and themes than those written by men
who had not recently had a drink. Correlations between general levels of alcohol consumption over long periods of time and dispositional
power motivation, however, have been low. On the other hand, a
content analysis of folk tales from 44 independent cultures from all
the world continents indicated that those societies whose folk tales
emphasized themes of power (such as those making up the power
motivation scoring system) and deemphasized inhibition or control
exhibited high levels of per capita consumption of alcohol (McClelland and others, 1972).

Other Findings; Sex Differences

A number of empirical investigations of power motivation fall
into a miscellaneous category. High power motivation has been associated, in at least one study, with all of the following: participation in
and viewing of competitive sports among young men (Winter, 1973);
collecting prestige possessions, such as credit cards (McClelland and
others, 1972; Winter, 1973); reading magazines concerned with sex
and aggression among men (Winter, 1973); taking extreme risks in
order to gain visibility (McClelland & Teague, 1975; McClelland &
Watson, 1973); getting into more arguments (McClelland, 1975); and
writing letters to the university newspaper (Winter, 1973).

Reviewing the entire literature on power motivation with an eye
towards sex differences, Stewart and Chester (1982) conclude that
there is little evidence available to suggest that one sex typically
scores higher in power than another. They add that relationships
between the power motive and behavioral correlates concerning organizational leadership, career preferences and pursuits, and emotional
experiences tend to be similar for both sexes. In the areas of (a)
aggressiveness and impulsiveness and (b) personal relationships,
however, results differ markedly as a function of gender. Though
various studies have documented connections between impulsive
and aggressive behavior in men and high power motivation, in-

vestigations with women have not produced these connections. And as observed in the present chapter, power motivation has been associated with instability and dissatisfaction in love relationships among men, but not among women.

An Exploration: Mythic Archetypes

Motives and Myths

Let us return to the concept of identity as a life story. Intimacy and power have been set forth as two superordinate content clusterings (thematic lines) in the texts of identities. Assessed via thematic coding of stories written in response to pictures (the TAT), intimacy and power motivation have been proposed as empirical predictors of the relative salience and significance, in life stories, of these two thematic lines. Men and women scoring high in intimacy motivation, therefore, are predicted to frame their identities in terms which emphasize close, warm, and communicative interaction with others. In Bakan's words, their identities should be more communal. Men and women high in power motivation, on the other hand, are predicted to couch identity in terms more agentic. Their life stories should emphasize having impact and feeling strong.

Four of the eight hypotheses introduced at the end of Chapter 2 specify ways in which the intimacy and power motives are predicted to relate to the content of life stories. For instance, I hypothesized that high power motivation should be associated with nuclear episodes framed in terms of strength, influence, action, and status, whereas high intimacy motivation should correlate with nuclear episodes highlighting love, dialogue, sympathy, and touch (Hypothesis 1). Likewise, the imagoes inhabiting the life stories of men and women high in power motivation should include the agentic figures of the sage, warrior, and traveler, whereas the imagoes for life stories of individuals high in intimacy motivation are expected to include communal protagonists like the caregiver, friend, and lover (Hypothesis 3). These hypotheses relate the four components of the life-story model of identity—nuclear episodes, imagoes, ideological setting, and generativity script—to the social motives of power and intimacy described in the present chapter. These hypotheses are examined and evaluated in Chapters 5–8.

In what remains of the present chapter, I will engage in a brief exploration of the relationship between power and intimacy motivation on the one hand and particular story forms on the other. Introduced in Chapter 2, Northrop Frye's story forms are tragedy, comedy, romance, and irony (1957). Though these story forms do not find an explicit place in the life-story model of identity I have proposed, they represent an alternative and highly interesting system for conceptualizing life stories and one which can be meaningfully related to the fundamental motives of power and intimacy.

Frye calls the four forms mythic archetypes. Each corresponding to one of the four seasons of the year, the mythic archetypes suggest general thematic lines or content clusterings which arise again and again in the great stories of antiquity and the present day. The following is my thematic delineation of Frye's four story forms in terms of the story's central problem, general sentiment, recurrent emotions, status of the protagonists, and moral or lesson. This scheme will be applied to the life stories which make up human identities.

Comedy

Central problem: How to find happiness and stability in life and with others by minimizing interference from environmental obstacles and constraints.

General sentiment: Optimistic.

Recurrent emotions: Generally positive, joy, contentment.

Status of protagonists: Common; the ordinary person coming together with other ordinary persons, seeking the simple and pure pleasures while avoiding pain.

Moral: The person is given the opportunity to achieve happiness that is free from guilt and anxiety and to provide a happy ending to his or her own story on earth.

Romance

Central problem: How to move onward and continue growing through life's journey so as to emerge victorious.

General sentiment: Optimistic.

Recurrent emotions: Generally positive, excitement, interest, joy.

Status of protagonists: Elevated; the extraordinary adventurer, ever-moving, ever-growing in the quest.

Moral: The person embarks on a long and difficult journey in life in which circumstances constantly change and new challenges continually arise.

Tragedy

Central problem: How to avoid or minimize the dangers and absurdities of life which threaten to overwhelm even the greatest human beings.

General sentiment: Pessimistic, ambivalent.

Recurrent emotions: Mixed negative and positive, sadness, fear.

Status of protagonists: Elevated; the extraordinary victim pursued by life's nemesis.

Moral: The person confronts inescapable dangers and absurdities in which he or she finds that pain and pleasure, happiness and sadness are always mixed.

Irony

Central problem:	How to solve some of the mysteries of life, to gain some perspective on the chaos, ambiguities, and contradictions of human living.
General sentiment:	Ambivalent, pessimistic.
Recurrent emotions:	Mixed positive and negative, sadness, fear, interest.
Status of protagonists:	Common; the ordinary person confused by life's mysteries, seeking a modicum of perspective and understanding.
Moral:	The person encounters ambiguities and contradictions in life which are larger than him or her and which are, for the most part, beyond comprehension.

In bringing together people and thereby consolidating happiness and stability, comedy seems to speak a language of intimacy and communion. Frye notes that comedies are often punctuated by social rituals marking the coming together of characters previously apart. The prototype is marriage, a favorite happy ending in comedy.

Romance and tragedy, on the other hand, appear to highlight power and agency. In both, extraordinary protagonists duel with the world around them, emerging triumphant in the case of romance and defeated in tragedy. Unlike comedies, romances and tragedies are typically stories of great deeds achieved by great heroes, agents attempting to separate themselves from their environments and, in so doing, to gain mastery over them.

Irony, finally, is more difficult to characterize. Like comedy, the protagonists are relatively common, ordinary folk who do not seek to separate themselves from their worlds. Yet the characters do not typically come together in alliances. Thus while comedy manifests thematic connections to intimacy, and romance and tragedy likewise to power, irony remains true to its nature, that is, ambiguous.

I offer, somewhat cautiously, the following hypothesis: Persons high in intimacy motivation will tend to manifest identities of comedy, and those high in power motivation, romance and tragedy. The hypothesis is explored by examining data provided by the 50 midlife adults (30 women and 20 men) designated in Chapter 1 as Sample B. The characteristics of Sample B are described in Appendix A.

Intimacy and power motivation scores for Sample B were obtained in the standard fashion (McAdams, 1980; Winter, 1973).[7] Following the administration of the TAT, each person was individually interviewed by a female graduate student. In these one- to two-hour interviews, the person essentially recounted his or her own life story, described his or her hopes and plans for the future, and related his or her "philosophy of life" and "underlying theme" of the life story. The interview questions are reproduced in Appendix B. Two research assistants then listened to the tapes of all of the interviews and coded each for the relative strength and salience of Frye's four mythic archetypes. The scoring system was modelled after the thematic delineation of comedy, romance, tragedy, and irony presented above. For each of the four mythic archetypes, a score of 1, 2, or 3 was given per interview. A score of 1 denoted little or no evidence of the particular story form; 2 denoted a moderate degree of evidence; and 3 denoted strong evidence for the dominance of the particular story form. The scorers were trained using practice tapes in order to establish reasonable interscorer reliability.[8]

The results of the analysis are presented in Table 3.1. Men and women scoring high on intimacy motivation had significantly higher comedy scores in their life-story interviews than did men and women low on intimacy motivation, F (1, 46) = 4.68, p < .05. Romance, tragedy, and irony, on the other hand, were not systematically related to level of intimacy motivation. A comparable analysis employing power motivation supported the hypothesis concerning power and romance but not that concerning power and tragedy. As predicted, midlife adults high in power motivation had significantly higher romance scores than those scoring low, F (1, 46) = 4.35, p < .05. Tragedy, comedy, and irony scores, however, did not differ as a function of power motivation. Furthermore, gender appeared to have little influence on the results. Men and women did not differ significantly on any of the four mythic archetypes, and they did not differ significantly on power or intimacy motivation.

The following case summaries illustrate life stories of comedy and romance drawn from Sample B. The first case of comedy is from a woman scoring moderately high in intimacy motivation as measured via the TAT, and the second case of romance is presented by a woman scoring very high in power motivation (and moderately high in intimacy).

Sandy M.

The archetype of comedy is especially prominent in the life story of Sandy M.,[9] one of the midlife adults in Sample B. A 39-year-old nurse, unmarried and well traveled, Sandy grew up on a farm in Iowa but now lives in a middle-class Chicago suburb. She is white, Protestant, and earned between $40,000 and $50,000 in 1982. Sandy's intimacy motivation score on the TAT was moderately high (50.3), and her power motivation was very low (39.7). She was one of only three subjects to receive a rating of 3 for comedy.

From the earliest chapters of an idyllic youth, through 10 years of travel around the world, and up to the last five years as a "staff nurse anesthetist" in Chicago, Sandy's story exudes optimism and

TABLE 3.1. Mean Mythic Archetype Scores of Midlife Adults According to Sex and
Motivation Classification

Motive Classification[a]	N	Mythic Archetype[b]			
		Comedy	Romance	Tragedy	Irony
High power					
Male	12	1.58	1.75	1.50	1.42
Female	14	1.57	1.64	1.57	1.57
Total	26	1.58	1.69	1.54	1.50
Low power					
Male	8	1.50	1.25	1.25	1.63
Female	16	1.81	1.31	1.75	1.25
Total	24	1.71	1.29	1.58	1.38
High intimacy					
Male	11	1.73	1.45	1.36	1.27
Female	15	1.87	1.60	1.80	1.40
Total	26	1.81	1.54	1.62	1.35
Low intimacy					
Male	9	1.33	1.67	1.44	1.78
Female	15	1.53	1.33	1.53	1.40
Total	24	1.46	1.46	1.50	1.54
All subjects					
Male	20	1.55	1.55	1.40	1.50
Female	30	1.70	1.47	1.67	1.40
Total	50	1.64	1.50	1.56	1.44

[a] High power motive scores are greater than or equal to 49.0. Low power motive scores are
less than 49.0. High intimacy motive scores are greater than or equal to 50.0. Low intimacy motive
scores are less than 50.0.
[b] For each archetype, a score of 1 denotes little or no evidence for its presence; 2 denotes a
moderate degree of evidence; and 3 denotes strong evidence for the dominance of the archetype in
the life story.

affirmation of life. In her childhood years, she was a tomboy who was
extremely popular with the girls in her class. In high school, she
delighted in the pure and simple experiences so often associated with
life in the country: nature hikes, hayrides, ice-cream socials. Active in
numerous extracurricular organizations and pursuits in high school,
Sandy found that she was very adept at playing the role of the clown.
She was the improvisational comic with her friends, frequently eas-
ing tensions by inducing people to laugh. The role of clown remained
dominant even through her very difficult college years in which she
found disciplined studying to be supremely onerous but unfortunately the only available avenue to a nursing degree. Though
college marked the first negative chapter in her life story, Sandy
underscores the fact that she rarely felt depressed or anxious during
this time and that throughout it all she never lost her sense of humor.
    Shortly after completing college, Sandy fell in love with a grad-
uate student and planned to marry. Due to a major change in his

career plans which necessitated spending many more years in school than originally expected, Sandy's fiancé broke off the engagement and suggested that she "go travel around the world" because "you will never be completely happy if you don't." Though Sandy reports that she was "crushed" after the breakup, the next chapter in her story—a 10 year stint of virtually continuous travel—is filled with happiness and joy. During this period, Sandy financed her travels by taking on a series of nursing jobs in the United States, Europe, and the Orient. She reports having more fun during this period of her life than even during her golden years in Iowa. Indeed, the "peak experience" of her entire life occurred on a 4300-mile boat trip across the Atlantic in which she became very close friends with four men—a German, South African, Englishman, and an "American surfer."

Sandy expresses a strong desire to help others—"to do my bit for mankind," as she puts it. Her many attempts to put this desire into action include volunteer nursing in Viet Nam and a one-year tenure with the "Hope Ship." In both, she reports, she ended up having more fun than she ever dreamed possible and even came to feel somewhat guilty about not experiencing more hardship herself in these situations in which so many others were in pain. Now that Sandy has settled down in the Midwest, she is finding that her job and relationships with friends (she corresponds regularly with every roommate she has ever had—at least 25 in all!) are rich sources of joy and satisfaction. Though a number of her peers in the nursing profession report that they eventually experience "burn out," Sandy maintains that she still "loves" her job and "would not trade it for the world."

In Shakespeare's comedies, a favorite happy ending involves the coming together of protagonists through marriage. A foreshadowing of this kind of happy "ending" is evident in Sandy's life story. Through an unlikely set of circumstances, Sandy and her former fiancé have resumed their relationship and are now living together. As she tells it, he is the brooding intellectual; she, the carefree clown. While he is the thinker, she is the doer. Sandy asserts that this disparity in personality style is viewed by both as highly complementary rather than conflictual. Sandy's dreams for the future include getting married, traveling, buying a larger condominium, and "doing something for others." Throughout it all she fully expects to have fun.

Jessica C.

Jessica C. tells a contrasting life story. Her narrative is a romance, one of only five life stories in our sample to receive a rating of 3 for romance. A partner with her husband in a graphic design corporation, Jessica is a 35-year-old, white, Protestant female who is also working toward a master's degree in Business Administration. Her power motive score (70.9) was the second highest in our sample. Intimacy motivation was also relatively high (55.8).

Jessica's life story reads like an adventure. She is the ever-moving, ever-changing heroine in quest of the new, the beautiful, and the true. Jessica reports that at an early age she was preoccupied with "where she stands in the world." She adds that she is still preoccupied. In her mind, the preoccupation stems from her ethnic lineage, half German (her mother) and half Sicilian (her father). Even in childhood she was very concerned with where she stood in relation to this essential duality in her life. Was she more the rational and orderly German or the passionate and impetuous Sicilian? Was she some kind of unique combination of the two? In Jessica's life story, the two sides of her nature, as she sees it, are played off against one another, and major turning points or chapter markers typically involve a temporary reconciliation between the two. It is essential to note that these reconciliations are only temporary. In Jessica's mythology, she continues to grow and change with each new experience. As she describes it, she is much the artist and her life is an unfinished work of art, constantly transforming itself into new and unpredictable configurations of color and form.

Like Sandy's, Jessica's life story is framed in relatively optimistic terms. But whereas Sandy's optimism is grounded in simple pleasures, good friends, and happy experiences, Jessica reveals a taste for the exotic and the extraordinary. Like Sandy, Jessica enjoys traveling. But whereas Sandy's story is marked by a coming together of quite "ordinary" mortals (the renewed relationship with her former fiancé is the perfect example), Jessica appears to see herself as a heroine larger than her peers—a characterization she attributes to her being a "spoiled, only child"—and as the consummate traveler whose most significant sojourns have been more psychological than physical. In her description of a trip to Egypt, she focuses not on the good times, the fun, or the friends, but rather upon a kind of spiritual awakening, a powerful and expansive adventure of the mind:

> One of my peak experiences was the actualization of a dream. For reasons quite unknown to myself, I have always been drawn to the culture of the Egyptians. At seven when I heard there was a King Tut exhibit at the Field Museum, I begged and wheedled my parents into taking me, and it was like I knew everything there. I have since read extensively on the subject and seen exhibitions in London, New York, and I hope to see Boston. My husband and I are soul mates when it comes to traveling. It makes us happy to challenge the unknown places. In an attempt to find an inexpensive vacation, we went to a Greek travel agent who curiously asked if we'd like to see Egypt, too. We both lit up like she had said Xanadu and thought of

nothing else for days. Of course we scraped the money together and held our breaths until the day—fearing it would not be as we dreamed. But it was more than imagined—in Cairo I saw the ancient and the modern world as if they existed on the same plane—a definite déjà vu. A sense of time coming together. Of the world as it was and will be. I felt small and great at the same time. Part of the whole.

In the classic romance such as the *Odyssey*, the hero or heroine learns lessons about life, love, and power through his or her adventures. At the end of the story, the protagonist is glorified as stronger, wiser, or more beautiful than before. In modern psychological terms, the protagonist attains "self-actualization." Jessica is quick to point to what she has learned from each of her life adventures, the negative and the positive. With each new lesson, she moves closer to self-fulfillment or what she describes as finding a "balance" and "knowing where I stand." "Life goes from achievement to achievement," Jessica asserts. "You don't just sit there with what you've been given." She adds, "You can always do better tomorrow." For Jessica's identity quest, this realization gives her "hope" and keeps her moving.

Summary

Though our lives are doubtlessly shaped by a host of inner forces, two fundamental springs of human action are the general desires to feel *close* and to feel *strong* vis-à-vis other human beings and our environments. This motivational dichotomy goes back as far as Empedocles' delineation of love and strife as the two basic forces of the cosmos, and it is brought forward to the 20th century in the theories of human motivation espoused by such psychologists as Freud (Eros versus Thanatos), Rank (fear of life versus fear of death), Angyal (need for surrender versus need for autonomy), and Bakan (communion versus agency). In this chapter, I adopted this basic dualism in lives by introducing the intimacy and power motives as two measurable personality dispositions approximating most closely Bakan's conceptualization of communion and agency, respectively. Intimacy and power motivation are internal preferences for certain classes of experience, and these preferences energize, direct, and select behavior in certain situations. Both motives are measured via content analysis of responses to the TAT.

Intimacy motivation is a *recurrent preference* or *readiness* for experiences of *warm, close,* and *communicative interaction* with others. Intimacy motivation is theoretically rooted in the writings of Maslow on Being-Love, Sullivan on the need for interpersonal intimacy, Buber on the I-Thou encounter, and, of course, Bakan on communion. In scoring TAT stories for intimacy motivation, the psychologist assesses the quality of the interpersonal interaction manifested by the characters in the subject's story in terms of 10 explicitly defined content themes. A number of recent studies suggest substantial construct validity for the TAT measure of intimacy motivation. For instance, individuals high in intimacy motivation have been shown to spend more time thinking about relationships with others, to engage in more conversations with others, and to experience more positive affect when interacting with others than individuals scoring low in intimacy motivation. In a laboratory psychodrama, students high in intimacy motivation behaved in ways which promoted warm and egalitarian exchange among group members. Students high in intimacy motivation were rated by their peers as especially "loving" and "sincere." Intimacy motivation has been positively associated with (*a*) self-disclosure among friends; (*b*) higher levels of smiling, laughter, and eye contact in interviews; and (*c*) better psychosocial adjustment among middle-aged men. Possible sex differences in intimacy motivation are at present unclear.

Power motivation is a *recurrent preference* or *readiness* for experiences of feeling *strong* and *having impact* upon one's environment. Among the theoretical antecedents to the modern understanding of power motivation are the writings of Nietzsche and Adler. In scoring TAT stories for power motivation, the psychologist assesses the presence or absence of 11 explicitly defined content themes having to do with forceful action and its consequences. Power motivation has been empirically associated with a host of other variables and measures. For instance, individuals high in power motivation have been shown to adopt authoritarian leadership strategies when supervising decision-making groups. Among working-class adults, high power motivation has been associated with holding offices in organizations. Power motivation has also been positively associated with (*a*) pursuing careers affording opportunities for exerting influence over others, (*b*) collecting prestige possessions, such as credit cards, and (*c*) taking extreme risks in order to gain notoriety. Men do not score consistently higher or lower than women in power motivation. However, sex differences have been observed in correlates to the motive. Among men, power motivation has been positively associated with (*a*) aggressiveness and impulsiveness and (*b*) problems in intimate personal relationships. These empirical connections have not generally manifested themselves in studies of women.

In the context of the life-story model of identity, intimacy and power motivation are conceptualized as predictors of particular thematic lines or content motifs in identity. At the end of this chapter, I described an initial exploration into the relationships between intimacy and power motivation on the one hand and content motifs in life stories on the other. Coding the 50 life-story interviews collected from the midlife men and women comprising Sample B for the relative prevalence of each of Frye's four mythic archetypes, I predicted that intimacy motivation would be positively associated with life stories emphasizing comedy, whereas power motivation would correlate positively with romance and tragedy. In bringing together people and thereby consolidating happiness and stability, comedy seems to speak the language of intimacy and communion. Frye notes that comedies are often punctuated by social rituals marking the coming together of characters who were previously apart, as in the ritual of marriage, a favorite happy ending in comedy. Romance and tragedy, on the other hand, appear to highlight power (agency). In both, extraordinary protagonists duel with the world around them, emerging triumphant in the case of romance and defeated in tragedy.

The results of the analysis indicated that life stories can be usefully conceptualized in terms of Frye's story forms and that significant relationships between intimacy motivation and comedy and between power motivation and romance in life stories do appear to exist as predicted, at least in this small sample of midlife adults. No empirical relationships was observed, however, between TAT power motivation and scores on tragedy obtained from the life-story interviews. The chapter concluded with two brief case studies: Sandy M., whose life story exemplifies comedy; and Jessica C., who tells a tale of romance.

NOTES

[1] Parts of this chapter appear in McAdams, D. P. Intimacy motivation. In A. J. Stewart (Ed.), *Motivation and society*. San Francisco: Jossey-Bass, 1982. Parts also appear in McAdams, D. P. Human motives and personal relationships. In V. Derlega (Ed.), *Communication, intimacy, and close relationships*. New York: Academic Press, 1984a.

[2] I use the word *Thanatos* here to denote what Freud termed the *death instincts*.

[3] Murray designed the TAT to measure narrative fantasy. In the standard administration of the test, the subject composed stories in response to 20 somewhat ambiguous pictures. The personologist then interpreted the stories in terms of recurrent themes. After World War II, the general method became very popular among clinicians, and today the TAT is one of the three or four most widely used assessment devices in clinical settings.

Though a number of interpretive schemes have been proposed for the TAT, the content analysis systems developed by David McClelland and his colleagues have given rise to the most successful and programmatic line of empirical research employing the measure. Working with John Atkinson at Wesleyan University in the late 1940s, McClelland introduced a number of innovations which rendered the TAT much more suitable for empirical research. McClelland employed the TAT solely as a measure of human motives. The first motive to be studied was the achievement motive (McClelland & Atkinson, 1948; McClelland and others, 1953). New picture cues were chosen as likely elicitors of achievement themes in stories. Rather than telling stories verbally, subjects were to write stories which could be subsequently analyzed for content themes. The picture cues were projected on a screen so that large numbers of subjects could be administered the TAT at the same time. A five-minute time limit was imposed for each story. The test's instructions were standardized. And most important, an objective and reliable coding system for the measurement of achievement motivation was developed and published as a manual designed to teach psychologists how to score for achievement reliably (Atkinson, 1958).

McClelland's scoring system for achievement motivation was derived empirically rather than theoretically. The researchers began with a general sense of the meaning of achievement motivation gleaned from Murray's (1938) writings on the topic. Clearly the motive concerned a desire to be successful and to do well in certain tasks. Next, McClelland and his associates sought to *arouse* this desire in a group of subjects and then test its effects upon their fantasy productions. This was the step of eliciting a particular motivational state and observing its translation into the stories aroused subjects wrote in response to the TAT.

Subjects participated in one of a variety of conditions in McClelland's original studies, but the most important conditions were the *arousal* condition (in which subjects' immediate concerns for being successful and doing well were heightened) and the *neutral* condition (in which achievement concerns were assumed to be at a baseline level). In the arousal condition, subjects were administered seven short paper-and-pencil tests which, they were informed, were designed as measures of general intelligence and leadership potential. The instructions were assumed to induce in the subjects an achievement set—a heightened concern about doing well. After completing the seven tests, the subjects were administered the TAT. In the neutral condition, the same seven paper-and-pencil tests were given to the subjects, but the instructions were varied markedly. In this case, the subjects were told that the tests were experimental and that the researchers were in fact testing the tests and not the students. These instructions were designed to produce a relaxed, relatively neutral atmosphere in which achievement concerns were held to a minimum. As in the arousal group, the seven tests were followed by the TAT.

A subset of stories written during the arousal condition was compared with a subset written by subjects in the neutral condition. The investigators searched for thematic categories which differentiated stories written under the two conditions. The initial differentiating categories served as the first scoring system for the achievement motive. In a second step of *cross-validation*, the remaining stories from the two conditions were scored by scorers unaware of the subjects' classifications—that is, blind to the experimental condition under which each set of stories was written. Those thematic categories which, upon cross-validation, consistently differentiated between stories written under arousal and those written under neutral conditions came to comprise the thematic scoring system for achievement motivation. At this point in the inquiry, the scoring system had been empirically derived through the arousal experiment and then cross-validated. As such, the scoring system existed as a measure of a transient motivational *state:* an artificially heightened concern among students for doing well. In the next step of the inquiry, evidence was garnered for the scoring system's usefulness as a measure of a relatively stable motivational disposition called the achievement motive.

The third step, then, could be termed *construct validation*, in which researchers attempted to relate individual differences in achievement motivation to theoretically predicted behavior. In a typical construct-validation study, the TAT would be administered to a group of subjects under neutral conditions. Subjects scoring relatively high on the achievement motive, as assessed via the previously derived scoring system, were compared with those scoring low on some other variable predicted to be associated with achievement motivation, such as risk taking and job performance. To the extent that individual differences in achievement motivation assessed via content coding of TATs were consistently associated with theoretically predicted outcomes, the measure would garner more and more support as an index of a stable personality disposition having to do with a recurrent preference for achieving. The past 30 years of research on achievement motivation have yielded a rich array of findings documenting the construct validity of the TAT measure (see Atkinson, 1958, 1964, 1981; Atkinson & Birch, 1978; Atkinson & Raynor, 1974; Heckhausen, 1967; Maddi, 1980; McClelland, 1961, 1984; McClelland and others, 1953 for reviews).

Despite impressive construct validity, the TAT scoring system for achievement motivation is not without its detractors (Entwistle, 1972; Klinger, 1966). Most criticisms of the method are based on psychometric grounds. The most damning have asserted that the general method of measuring motives through content analysis of fantasy is not psychometrically reliable or consistent. A person's score on achievement motivation can vary significantly from one testing session to the next—a situation that should not occur if the measure is tapping a relatively stable personality disposition. Defenders of the TAT have argued that low test-retest reliability coefficients are partially due to the fact that when a subject takes the TAT a second time, it is phenomenologically no longer the same test. Further, subjects who remember the pictures to which they wrote stories in a previous TAT session will most likely write different stories the second time, not wishing to repeat themselves. Indeed, Winter and Stewart (1977) and Lundy (1980) have shown that when subjects are told they may, if they wish, write stories similar or identical to ones they have written in previous TAT sessions, test-retest coefficients rise to psychometrically respectable levels.

The controversy over the psychometric reliability of the TAT as a measure of human motives is extremely complex and beyond the scope of this book. Though there is little doubt that the TAT is more subject to the vagaries of random, extraneous effects (e.g., mood, level of fatigue) than are highly structured questionnaires in which subjects choose given responses rather than generating their own, the impressive array of findings supporting the construct validity of TAT measures of achievement, power, and intimacy motivation suggests that content analysis of narrative fantasy can be an extremely sensitive and valuable method of personality assessment. McClelland (1980, 1981, 1984) provides thoughtful analyses of the relative merits and limitations of thematic apperceptive methods of motive assessment. Atkinson (1981, 1982) has also considered in detail the controversy and has proposed a sophisticated theoretical model, termed the *dynamics of action*, to explain why traditional psychometric indexes of test-retest reliability cannot be logically applied to open-ended assessment devices such as the TAT.

[4] I began the process of deriving and validating the thematic coding system for intimacy motivation (McAdams, 1980) in an attempt to revamp the older measure for the *need for affiliation* (Atkinson, Heyns, & Veroff, 1954; Heyns, Veroff, & Atkinson, 1958; Shipley & Veroff, 1952). By 1977, 25 years of research with the TAT coding system for affiliation appeared to have yielded little consistent evidence for the construct validity of the measure (Boyatzis, 1973; McAdams, 1979). Conceptualized and developed in light of a drive-reduction model of human motivation, the scoring system for the affiliation motive appeared to tap into an instrumental, goal-directed striving to establish, maintain, and restore friendly relations with others, which suggested more a fear of rejection than a positive hope for warmth and closeness, an avoidance rather than an approach motive (Boyzatzis, 1973; McClelland, 1984). Originally, therefore, this revamping was to emphasize the more positive and less instrumental aspect of interpersonal relations as described by such theorists as Maslow (1968) in B-Love, Buber (1970) in the I-Thou encounter, Sullivan (1953) in the need for interpersonal intimacy, and Bakan (1966) in communion. In the process of deriving and cross-validating scoring categories reflecting this new theoretical orientation, I began to realize that the emerg-

ing construct was conceptually and empirically different enough from affiliation motivation to warrant a new name. To indicate that the new construct is focused on a preference for a particular *quality* of interpersonal interaction rather than a general striving to have and maintain relationships regardless of their quality, I termed it the *intimacy motive*.

Recent studies employing the TAT coding systems for intimacy and affiliation reveal moderate and positive correlations between the two motives, typically ranging between .25 and .55 (McAdams, 1982a). With respect to differences in the ways in which the two motives relate to other measures of behavior and experience, two general distinctions have been observed. First, when the two motives have been compared in the prediction of the same thing (say, the prediction of warm and communicative behavior in an interpersonal setting), the intimacy motive has generally proven to be the stronger predictor. Second, when the two have revealed different correlates, the intimacy motive appears to connect more closely to interpersonal behavior indicative of a more passive and communal orientation, whereas the affiliation motive has been associated with a more active and assertive approach to relationships (McAdams, 1982a; McAdams & Powers, 1981). Whereas the affiliation motive appears to highlight *doing* (striving to have relationships), the intimacy motive seems to reflect, both in its theoretical underpinnings and in its empirical correlates, an emphasis on *being*, communing with another in a relationship over seeking the other in order to have a relationship.

[5] The derivation of the intimacy motive scoring system for the TAT (McAdams, 1980) follows closely the general procedure of arousal, cross-validation, and construct validation established by McClelland with respect to the achievement motive. Four different arousal studies were conducted. In the first, fraternity men and sorority women attending initiation ceremonies which typically aroused feelings of interpersonal closeness and warmth wrote TAT stories. In the second, college students reporting that they were "having a good time" at a campus party were administered the TAT. Stories written by students in arousal conditions 1 (sorority/fraternity initiation) and 2 (party) were compared with those of similar students administered the TAT under neutral classroom conditions. In the third study, dating heterosexual couples in which both members scored high on a questionnaire measure of intensity of love felt toward the partner (Rubin, 1973) wrote TAT stories which were compared with those written by a comparison sample of men and women similar in age and educational background under neutral conditions. Finally, study 4 compared stories written before to those written after a two-hour psychodrama session designed to facilitate closeness and communication in a group of volunteer subjects who were strangers. The stories written after the session were considered in the arousal condition, whereas those written before were considered in the neutral condition. The methodological details of the arousal studies have been fully described by McAdams (1980, 1982a) and McClelland (1984).

The resultant scoring system which emerged from repeated cross-validation in the four studies is composed of 10 thematic categories. To score TAT stories for intimacy motivation, the psychologist determines whether each of the 10 thematic categories is present or absent in a given story. If the category is present, it receives a score of 1. If it is absent, it receives a 0. The scoring rules for assessing intimacy motivation in TAT stories are described fully in the scoring manual for intimacy motivation (McAdams, 1984c). Complete with 210 practice stories and numerous examples of scoring categories, the manual is designed to teach the researcher or clinician to score TAT stories for intimacy motivation at high levels of accuracy.

[6] Like the intimacy system, the derivation of the power-motive scoring system for the TAT (Winter, 1973) follows closely the general procedure of arousal, cross-validation, and construct validation established by McClelland and his associates with respect to the achievement motive. The power-motive scoring system, in fact, has

developed through a number of stages over the past 25 years as psychologists have experimented with various methods of arousing the motive (Steele, 1977; Stewart & Winter, 1976; Uleman, 1966, 1972; Veroff, 1957; Winter, 1973). Various arousal studies have sampled TAT stories written by (*a*) candidates for student government office awaiting the results of voting, (*b*) subjects about to enact the powerful role of "psychological experimenter," (*c*) students who had seen a film of John F. Kennedy's inauguration, and (*d*) students who had witnessed a multimedia presentation of inspirational speeches, such as Churchill on Dunkirk and excerpts from Shakespeare's *Henry V*. As in the case of intimacy and achievement motivation, stories written under these arousal conditions were compared with those written under neutral conditions to derive the power-motive scoring categories. The evolution of the power motive measure is fully described in Winter (1973).

The resultant scoring system provided by Winter (1973) is composed of 11 thematic categories, each of whose presence (score + 1) or absence (score 0) is assessed in a given TAT story. The scoring rules appear in Winter's (1973) appendix.

[7] The subjects in Sample B wrote stories in response to six TAT pictures. The six pictures in sequence showed: (*a*) two people sitting on a park bench near a river; (*b*) a man sitting at a desk upon which is placed a photograph of a family; (*c*) a naval officer conversing with another man aboard a ship; (*d*) a man and woman on a trapeze in midair; (*e*) two women working in a laboratory; and (*f*) an older man, younger woman, horses, and dog walking through a field. These pictures compose a standard set, which has proven appropriate in the assessment of intimacy and power motivation in both men and women (McAdams, 1982a).

The TAT stories were scored for intimacy and power motivation by two trained coders whose scoring reliability was well established. Intimacy motivation was scored by a trained coder whose agreement with materials precoded in the scoring manual was .92 (*rho* statistic), with a 91 percent category agreement on the first two categories, which are considered prime tests of intimacy imagery. A different trained scorer coded the TATs for power motivation, showing a .93 (*rho*) correlation with material precoded in the scoring manual (Winter, 1973) and 90 percent category agreement on power imagery. These terms for determining scoring accuracy are adopted from Winter (1973). Category agreement greater than 85 percent and *rho* greater than .85 for agreement with expert scoring of practice materials are considered adequate reliability figures for research purposes.

Raw motive scores were converted to standardized scores (mean = 50, standard deviation = 10) for each of the two motives. Those individuals with intimacy motive scores equal to or greater than 50 were classified as "high intimacy" (26 subjects: 15 female, 11 male), whereas those scoring below 50 were classified as "low intimacy" (24 subjects: 15 female, 9 male). For power motivation, the distribution was split at the standard score of 49 in order to produce approximately the same number of highs and lows. Thus, individuals whose power motive scores were equal to or greater than 49 were classified "high power" (26 subjects: 14 female, 12 male), and those below 49 were classified "low power" (24 subjects: 16 female, 8 male). A comparison of intimacy and power motive scores for males and females yielded no statistically significant sex difference. For power motivation, the average male score was 50.8 (standard deviation = 11.1), and the average female score was 49.4 (standard deviation = 9.5). For intimacy motivation, the average male score was 48.9 (standard deviation = 9.1), and the average female score was 50.8 (standard deviation = 10.7).

[8] For all 50 tapes, interscorer reliability was estimated using *kappa*, a relatively conservative test for association in categorical data. *Kappa* = .67 for ratings on comedy, .73 for romance, .82 for tragedy, and .73 for irony. When the two scorers disagreed on a given rating, the mean of the two ratings was used in the data analysis.

[9] Like all of the subjects' names used in this book, Sandy M. is a pseudonym.

Chapter 4

Narrative Complexity

Structure is the composition of a book, a development of events, one event causing another, a transition from one theme to another, the cunning way characters are brought in, or a new complex of action is started, or the various themes are linked up or used to move the novel forward.

(Vladimir Nabokov, 1980, p. 16)

Every story embodies a certain content, style, and structure. In his course on the masterpieces of world literature, Vladimir Nabokov inspired in his students a deep appreciation for the beauty and the intricacies of these three literary dimensions in the classic works of such writers as Austen, Dickens, Flaubert, and Proust (Updike, 1980). For Nabokov (1980), content refers to the recurrent images and ideas which serve as the raw thematic stuff from which the story is crafted. Content themes are repeated again and again in the novel much as particular tunes reoccur in a fugue. Style, on the other hand, refers to "the manner of the author, his special intonations, his vocabulary, and that something which when confronted with a passage makes a reader cry out that's by Austen, not by Dickens" (p. 16). Third, structure refers to the characteristic organization of the story, the integration of the various characters, settings, events, and happenings into a cohesive and coherent narrative whole. In simple terms, content is the thematic substance of the story; style is the idiosyncratic way in which the story is told; and structure is the formal organization or patterning of the story.

This chapter concerns structure. My wish is to consider the structure or organization of the life stories which humans compose as their identities. A brief comparison of two great stories from literature will set the stage for an inquiry into structure.

Ernest Hemingway's *The Old Man and the Sea* is the story of a Cuban fisherman who battles a giant marlin for three days and nights. The old fisherman, Santiago, is the simple and beautiful hero of a story whose beauty resides, to a large extent, in its simplicity. A man of extremely modest tastes and means, Santiago appears to have three great loves in his life: fishing, Joe DiMaggio, and a young boy in town named Manolin. At the story's outset, Santiago has gone 84 days without catching a fish. His fellow fishermen consider him a pathetic old man who has been stricken with the curse of being unlucky. Only Manolin believes in the old man, and the night before the fateful voyage, Manolin wraps an army blanket around Santiago's shoulders to keep him warm. Before dawn, Santiago begins his journey, rowing far away from the pack of village fishermen, out further than he has ever fished before. At midday, Santiago hooks the marlin, and the battle begins. Though the huge fish actually tows the skiff for at least a day as Santiago hangs desperately on, the old fisherman eventually emerges victorious, only to have his vanquished prey devoured by ravenous sharks. At the end of the story, Santiago deposits the leviathan's skeleton on the beach, walks slowly home, and falls into a deep sleep. The next day, he discusses his adventure with Manolin.

Though Hemingway's masterpiece is a rich and profound saga that can be interpreted on many different levels, it is *structurally* a very *simple* story. There is a single story line about an old man who wins and then loses a huge fish. The central action sequence is bracketed by the opening and closing sections in which Santiago and his young friend engage in simple conversation. The story in fact ends where it begins—with the interaction of two friends—though in the interim the old man wages a monumental battle which, in the final analysis, affirms his manhood. The story is stark, straightforward, and laconic. Hemingway, the virtuoso of economy in storytelling, makes every sentence count. There are no subplots or counterplots; there are no stories embedded within stories.

Fëdor Dostoyevsky's *The Brothers Karamazov* is a tale of four brothers and the murder of their father. Though Dostoyevsky claims that the youngest brother, Alyosha, is the novel's hero, a case could be made for the eldest son as protagonist, the passionate Dmitri who is convicted of murdering the old man and whose wild exploits before the murder and after, at his trial, constitute almost a third of the book. In contrast to *The Old Man and the Sea*, Dostoyevsky's epic is structurally an extremely complex story. There are a number of very prominent characters whose lives are described in great detail by the author: Fyodor Karamazov (the father), Alyosha, Ivan, Dmitri, Smerdyakov (the real murderer and illegitimate son of Fyodor Karamazov and the village idiot, "stinking Lizaveta"), Father Zossima, Grushenka, Katerina, Madame Hohlakov, and Ilusha. There are myriad subplots and stories within stories (within stories). At one point,

Dostoyevsky suspends the action and presents the "The Grand Inquisitor," the famous poem about Christ's insensitivity to humankind authored by Ivan—the intellectual brother—and embedded in a lengthy conversation between Ivan and Alyosha concerning Christianity and the destiny of Russia. At another point, Dostoyevsky inserts "Notes from the Life of the Deceased Priest and Monk, the Elder Zossima, Taken from his own Words," a lengthy discourse on prayer, love, hell, and the significance of the Russian monk written by Alyosha, Father Zossima's protégé. Woven into a complex and intricate tapestry are the separate yet interacting stories of Dmitri's obsession with Grushenka, Alyosha's life as a monk, Alyosha's friendship with the village boys, Lise's love for Alyosha, Ivan's intellectual quest and eventual fall into madness, the life and death of the young Ilusha, and the life, death, and work of Zossima, to name a few.

This is not to imply that *The Brothers Karamazov* is a better (or worse) story than *The Old Man and the Sea*. Indeed, one literary critic wrote that Hemingway's story, for which the author received the Nobel Prize in literature in 1954, was "as nearly faultless as any short novel of our times" (Cowley, 1952). And some scholars consider *The Brothers Karamazov* to be, quite categorically, the greatest novel of the world's greatest novelist (Komroff, 1957). My comparison of the two works, furthermore, is *not* meant to imply that the only or the most significant difference between the two is structural complexity. Indeed, the two classics differ dramatically on the levels of content, style, and structure. Because of their marked difference in length, moreover, some might argue that they represent two distinct literary genres. The intent of this comparison is merely to point to one of a host of dimensions on which stories can be contrasted and compared. In this light, *The Old Man and the Sea* is a virtual paragon of structural simplicity, whereas its much longer counterpart embodies considerable complexity in narrative structure.

Structure and Development

It is within developmental psychology—especially the study of cognitive development—that the idea of structure has found some of its most enthusiastic proponents. A major spokesman for the *structural developmental tradition* in psychology is Lawrence Kohlberg (1969, 1981; Kohlberg & Gilligan, 1971; Kohlberg & Kramer, 1969; Kohlberg & Mayer, 1972). He writes:

> Structure refers to the general characteristics of shape, pattern, or organization of response rather than to the rate or intensity of response or its pairing with particular stimuli. Cognitive structure refers to the rules for processing information or for connecting experi-

enced events. Cognition (as most clearly reflected in thinking) means putting things together or relating events, and this relating is an active connecting process, not a passive connecting of events through external association and repetition. (1969, p. 349)

In this passage, Kohlberg is careful to distinguish structure, as pattern or organization, from ideas concerning the connecting of stimulus and response which come out of the behaviorism tradition in American psychology. In another place, Kohlberg distinguishes between structure and the related concept of content:

Cognitive-developmental stages are stages of structure, not of content. The stages tell us how the child thinks concerning good and bad, truth, love, sex, and so forth. They do not tell us what he thinks about, whether he is preoccupied with morality or sex or achievement. They do not tell us what is on the adolescent's mind. (Kohlberg & Gilligan, 1971, p. 1076)

Thus, in cognition, structure refers to the form of information processing utilized by the individual rather than the specifics of the information to be processed per se. In this sense, structure is abstract and formal; content is relatively concrete.

A dominant force in developmental psychology, the structural developmental tradition, is grounded in the writings of J. M. Baldwin, John Dewey, George Herbert Mead, and especially Jean Piaget. Langer (1969) refers to this tradition as the *organic lamp theory* in developmental psychology. According to this view, human beings are active agents in their own developmental processes, interacting with the environment via dialectical transactions in which the person shapes and is shaped by the environment. As self-constructing, self-organizing beings, humans live by constructing patterns of knowing their world which exist as structured wholes of internal relations. These patterns or structures are products of interaction with the world; they are not templates wired into the central nervous system (the nativistic view) nor blueprints passively received from the environment (the environmentalistic view).

At the heart of the structural developmental approach is the doctrine of stages. Stages are to be understood in terms of the four tenets of *discontinuity, invariant sequence, conflict,* and *hierarchy.* In Kohlberg's structural model of morality, moral development proceeds from the lowest *preconventional* stages (in which the individual's perspective on good and bad, right and wrong is highly egocentric and unidimensional) through the middle *conventional* stages (in which the individual justifies morally relevant action in terms of group or societal standards and mores) to the highest *postconventional* stages (in which moral reasoning is premised on internalized principles of social contract and universal fairness).

Each of the six stages in the sequence is qualitatively different from each of the others. Consequently, movement from one stage to the next involves a *discontinuity* in development in that the emergent stage is different from the former not in terms of degree but in terms of kind. Over the course of development, successive stages are traversed in an *invariant sequence*. In Kohlberg's scheme, the individual ideally moves from the stage of "naive hedonism" (stage 2) to what might be called the stage of "social group" (stage 3) in which the person adopts the moral norms of a small family or peer group of which he or she is a member. From this stage, the individual may eventually move to the stage of "social law" (stage 4) in which the norms and standards to which he or she swears allegiance are delineated according to a larger context, such as that of societal institutions or the state. In Kohlberg's scheme, individuals do not skip stages, nor do they regress from higher to lower stages. Rather, development proceeds through a fixed sequence of universal stages, and the end point of a person's development is the stage from which he or she ceases to progress.

Pushing (or pulling) the individual from lower to high stages is cognitive *conflict*. Stage transitions are the dawning awareness that the structures for knowing the world at a given stage produce inconsistencies and inadequacies (disequilibrium) which can only be reckoned with by a higher, more adequate stage in which conflict is, for the time being, reconciled (equilibration). In Kohlberg's scheme, the adolescent or adult may come to see the limitations of a stage-4 view of morality, in which right and wrong are dictated by generally accepted societal conventions, and subsequently make the transition to the postconventional morality of stage 5, in which moral behavior is guided by self-chosen principles of utility and respect for inalienable rights. As Turiel (1974) points out, stage transitions can be periods of marked conflict and flux in the individual's development as old structures have been discarded but new ones are still in the process of being constructed.

Finally, and perhaps most significantly, structural stages comprise a developmental *hierarchy*. This is to say that later (higher) stages are built upon earlier (lower) stages of development, and that higher stages are reintegrations or reorganizations of their lower forerunners. Kohlberg and Gilligan (1971) write, "Each stage, then, is a better cognitive organization than the one before it, one which takes account of everything present in the previous stage, but making new distinctions and organizing them into a more comprehensive or more equilibrated structure" (p. 1069). Thus, higher stages displace lower ones not via suppression but through reorganization. The process has been compared to a conceptual revolution in science, as described by Kuhn (1962), in which an old paradigm (such as Newtonian physics) is replaced by a new paradigm (Einstein's relativity), revealing the old to be an incomplete manifestation or special case of the new paradigm. Likewise, Kohlberg's stages cast their ontogenetic forerunners in new, more adequate terms. The new stage is thereby seen as better, more mature, and more adequate than the old. Kohlberg adds that the new stage is more *complex*, that is, more differentiated and more hierarchically integrated.

The idea of complexity of structure, introduced at the outset of this chapter through a comparison of two stories, is articulated further in the writings of Heinz Werner (1957). For Werner, development proceeds according to the orthogenetic principle which states that there is an inherent direction in development from states of relative simplicity to those of increasing differentiation and hierarchic integration. In the realm of cognitive development, the individual comes over time to see more and more distinctions in his or her world (greater differentiation) and more and more connections as well (greater integration). Thus, higher structures are more differentiated and more integrated, and integration typically takes the form of hierarchy in which information is embedded in classes which are likewise embedded in larger classes. As Koestler (1979) depicts it, each part of an hierarchically integrated system is Janus-faced—one face aimed outward at the whole of which it is a part and the other aimed inward at the parts that constitute its own wholeness.[1]

A product of the structural developmental tradition in psychology is the highly integrative and neatly operationalized model of ego development presented by Jane Loevinger (1966, 1973, 1976). Through the analysis of responses on a sentence-completion test, psychologists investigating ego development are able to catch a glimpse of a person's process of making sense of self and world and are thus able to determine the extent to which this process is structurally simple or complex. I will consider Loevinger's model and measure of ego development in some depth, for it is this index of structural complexity that is employed in the present inquiry into the life stories which make up human identities.

Structural Complexity and the Ego

Loevinger's View of the Ego

Ever since the seeds of "ego psychology" were sown in Freud's (1920/1955) *Beyond the Pleasure Principle*, psychologists have identified a host of related processes in human functioning which fall under the general rubric of the "ego." These processes include perception, memory, reality testing, defense, dream censorship, and integration, and all of them serve the purpose of facilitating the person's overall adaptation to the world (A. Freud, 1936; Hartmann, 1939; Hartmann, Kris, & Lowenstein, 1964). Ego psychologists tend to de-emphasize classic psychoanalytic concepts of sexual and aggressive energy (such as the libido, cathexis, death instinct, and the economic/hydraulic model of the psyche) in favor of the variegated functions of the ego as a defender against anxiety and threat and a consummate synthesizer of experience. Of all the functions variously ascribed to the ego, it is *synthesis* or *integration*—the putting together of disparate elements into meaningful wholes—that Jane Loevinger (1966, 1973, 1976) has underscored as the essence of ego. She writes, "The organization or the synthetic function is not just another thing the ego does, it is what the ego is" (1976, p. 5). Thus, "the striving to master, to integrate, to make sense of experience is not one ego function among many but the essence of the ego" (1969, p. 85).

Though Loevinger's conception of ego development shares some similarities with those of the ego psychologists who trace their theoretical lineage back to Freud, she is quick to point out that there are many differences as well and that the original impetus for her work resides in early studies of mothers' attitudes about family life rather than in any theory per se (Loevinger, 1983). Indeed, rather than the psychoanalytic theories of the ego put forth by Anna Freud, Hartmann, and others, Loevinger's conception shares a good deal more with Sullivan's view of the "self-system" and Perry's view of ethical and intellectual development.[2] For Loevinger, the ego is the *integrative framework of meaning* that the individual subjectively imposes upon experience, an overall frame of reference defining one's customary orientation to self and to world.

In Loevinger's structural developmental model, qualitatively distinct frames of reference or ego stages are arranged on a continuum from extreme globality and simplicity to extreme differentiation and hierarchic integration. The stages specify not only different levels of development across the life span, but also individual differences within an age cohort. Loevinger's scheme, therefore, is a developmental typology, and in adulthood, one's stage of ego development is a major individual-differences dimension of personality.

Loevinger conceives of the ego as a multifaceted abstraction which nevertheless implies an underlying wholeness or integrity. During the course of ego development, what changes is a "complexly interwoven fabric of impulse control, character, interpersonal relations, conscious preoccupations, and cognitive complexity, among other things" (Loevinger, 1976, p. 26). Loevinger points out that there are various ways of looking at ego development, one of which is "to look at it as a series of achievements, or as a succession of increasingly complex views of the world" (1976, p. 75). With respect to structural complexity, then, Loevinger argues that the early and relatively immature stages in her hierarchic model of development bespeak simplistic, global, and egocentric frameworks of meaning in which issues and concepts are apprehended in black-and-white terms and one's orientation is toward self-protection or banal conformity. At higher stages, however, one comes to question the simple dictates of convention, and one's understanding of a range of issues and concepts becomes more highly differentiated and integrated so that contradiction and ambiguity eventually become tolerable and the individuality of others and their own systems of belief and value is accepted, or even "cherished" (Loevinger, 1976, p. 25).

Stages of Ego Development

Loevinger's stages of ego development may be correlated with chronological age, but they are defined independently of age. Each stage is a structured whole with its own internal logic and coherence. Each stage builds on its predecessor and lays a foundation for its successor. Over the course of development, no stage can be skipped, though individuals stop developing, with respect to ego, at various points making for the developmental typology. Each stage is given a code number beginning with the letter *I*.

The first stage of ego development is the undifferentiated stage of infancy (I-1) in which the infant comes to form an attachment bond to the caregiver. The primitive, nonverbal quality of this earliest stage of meaning-making defies measurement on Loevinger's sentence-completion test. Thus, the first *measurable* ego stage is I-2.

With the development of language, the child enters the *impulsive* stage (I-2). The child's own impulses help him or her to affirm a separate sense of self. The orientation of the impulsive stage is egocentric. The world is seen as a concrete setting for the satisfaction of physical needs. The child is demanding and dependent in interpersonal relationships. Morality is Kohlberg's stage 1 (premoral) at which the child understands good behavior to be that which is rewarded and bad that which is punished.

The impulsive stage as a frame of reference is structurally rather simple. The child's classification of people into the general categories of good versus bad is a global value judgment rather than an articulated moral judgment per se. Good and bad may be confounded with "nice to me" and "mean to me" or with "clean" and "dirty," recalling what Ferenczi (1925) called the "sphincter morality" of young children. Though emotional experiences may be very intense in this stage, the individual's descriptions of these stages are relatively crude and global, limited to such terms as *mad, upset, sick, turned on,* and *high*. The impulsive individual's orientation is primarily toward the present rather than past or future. Loevinger states that the child who remains too long at this stage may be seen by others as "uncontrollable" or "incorrigible" (1976, p. 16).

In the *self-protective* stage (Delta), the child shifts from an immediate frame of reference to one in which he or she is able to anticipate short-term rewards and punishments. Delay of gratification becomes a salient individual-difference variable. Rules appear for the first time, but "getting caught" breaking the rules defines what is wrong, not the rules themselves. The good life is the easy life. Friendships may be seen as nice things, to be collected, much like money. An older child or adult who stagnates at the Delta stage may become opportunistic, deceptive, and Machiavellian in his relations with other people. As Loevinger (1976) puts it, "For such a person, life is a zero-sum game; what one person gains, someone else has to lose" (p. 17).

With the shift from an egocentric frame of reference to an identification of one's own welfare with that of a group, the individual makes a true developmental leap and enters the *conformist* stage (I-3) of ego development. Morality becomes conventional (Kohlberg stages 3 and 4) and is defined strictly by the rules and norms of the group (be it a small-scale social group or society as a whole). People, as well, are essentially defined according to their group allegiances. This may lead to stereotyping, a cognitive hallmark of the conformist stage. As others come to be classified primarily according to external criteria such as sex, age, race, nationality, or the size of the family car, the resultant stereotypes are virtually impervious to any consideration of individual differences within groups. The conformist person may, therefore, see most people as being pretty much alike, or at least he/she believes they ought to be. The conformist person values niceness, helpfulness, and cooperation with others, a contrastingly prosocial orientation vis-à-vis what may be an opportunistic stance of Delta. Interpersonal experience and affective states are described by simple clichés and banal terms, such as *happy, sad, glad, sorrow,* and *love and understanding.*

The first transitional phase—which is sometimes considered a stage in its own right—may arise when one realizes it is impossible to live up to all of the standards of one's defining group. The break with the group and conventional thinking begins slowly with an increasing self-awareness and an appreciation for the multiple possibilities in situations. In this way is ushered in the *conformist/conscientious* transition (I-3/4), an extremely prevalent, perhaps modal, adult form. The individual at I-3/4 is becoming increasingly aware of his or her inner life, but the descriptions of experience are still couched in relatively banal terms. The individual at I-3/4 may speak of relatively vague feelings with some reference to relationships with others using such words as: *lonely, embarrassed, homesick,* and *self-conscious.* Exceptions to stereotypes may be acknowledged, though more complex patterns of attribution await later stages.

At the *conscientious* stage (I-4) of ego development, internalization of rules is complete. The major elements of adult conscience are present: long-term, self-evaluated goals and ideals, differentiated self-criticism, and a sense of responsibility. Mutuality in interpersonal relations is the result of more sophisticated forms of perspective taking. Human behavior is seen in terms of internal determinants such as traits and motives. A rich and differentiated inner life is characteristic of individuals at this stage. Only a few persons as young as 13 or 14 reach the conscientious stage.

The increased conceptual complexity manifest in the conscientious stage is evidenced in greater differentiation between, say, moral standards and social manners or between moral and esthetic standards. Loevinger (1976) writes:

> Things are not just classified as "right" or "wrong." A Conscientious person thinks in terms of polarities, but more complex and differentiated ones: trivial versus important, love versus lust, dependent versus independent, inner life versus outward appearances. (p. 21)

The second transitional phase—the *individualistic* level (I-4/5)—is marked by a growing tolerance for others' individuality and a greater awareness of the conflict between heightened individuality and increased emotional dependence. Though the realization that conflict is an inherent part of the human condition awaits I-5, the person at I-4/5 manifests an increased ability to tolerate paradox and contradiction—a sign of greater conceptual complexity. Distinctions are made between inner reality and outward appearances; between psychological and physiological responses; between process and outcome. Psychological causality and psychological development, "which are notions that do not occur spontaneously below the Conscientious Stage, are natural modes of thought" to persons at the individualistic level (Loevinger, 1976, p. 23).

With the development of a capacity to cope adequately with the conflicts of the individualistic level, the *autonomous* (I-5) stage of ego development is ushered in. The individual at this stage reveals toleration for ambiguity and high cognitive complexity. He or she has acquired a respect for the autonomy of others while realizing that emotional interdependence is inevitable. Self-fulfillment partly replaces achievement as a salient conscious preoccupation. The person at this stage expresses his or her feelings vividly and convincingly, including sensual experiences, poignant sorrows, and existential humor intrinsic to paradoxes of life. He or she formulates broad and abstract social ideals and makes moral decisions accordingly (Kohlberg stage 5). This developmental position is rare among adults and virtually unheard of in adolescence.

Rarer still is the fully *integrated* (I-6) individual. This is the most difficult stage to describe. In general, most of what is true for I-5 remains true for I-6 with the added element of what Loevinger terms "consolidation of a sense of identity" (1976, p. 26). At I-5 and I-6, the person is able to transcend, in part, the polarities of earlier stages, seeing reality as complex and multifaceted. Opposites, from the vantage points of lower stages, may be reconciled at the highest stages of ego development, making for what some psychologists have termed "dialectical thinking" (Riegel, 1978). Some of Maslow's (1968) "self-actualizing" individuals may be examples of I-6.

Table 4.1 offers a concise schematization of Loevinger's ego development stages classified in terms of impulse control and character development, interpersonal style, conscious preoccupations, and (most important for our purposes) cognitive complexity. A more detailed explication is available in Loevinger (1976). Loevinger claims, however, that the researcher or clinician seeking to understand ego development must study and "get a feel for" the scoring system used in the measurement of the ego in order to comprehend the tacit meanings of each stage. This scoring system is applied to responses to the Washington University Sentence Completion Test (WUSCT), which is Loevinger's standard measure of ego development.[3]

Research on Ego Development

The growing research literature on Loevinger's model of ego development has been reviewed by Hauser (1976) and Loevinger (1979). Here I wish merely to highlight some representative studies to round out this introduction to the concept and measure.[4]

One of the earliest empirical investigations employing the WUSCT was a study of ego development and conformity undertaken by Hoppe (1972). Hoppe predicted that conformity behavior in adolescent boys should peak within the conformist ranges of ego development (I-3 and I-3/4), rising from relatively low levels in the early impulsive (I-2) and self-protective (Delta) stages and falling to relatively low levels again in the higher stages of conscientious (I-4) and autonomous (I-5). Hoppe administered the WUSCT to 107 adolescent boys and then collected observations of their behavior using a diverse array of techniques: an experimental measure of conformity, peer ratings of reputation, a self-report conformity measure, and school discipline records. Results obtained through all but the experimental technique revealed the predicted curvilinear trend in conformity with maximum conformity behavior at I-3 and I-3/4.

TABLE 4.1 Some Milestones of Ego Development (from Loevinger, 1976, pp. 24–25)

Stage	Code	Character Development, Impulse Control	Interpersonal Style	Conscious Preoccupations	Cognitive Complexity
Presocial			Autistic		
Symbiotic	I-1		Symbiotic	Self vs. nonself	
Impulsive	I-2	Impulsive, fear of retaliation	Receiving, dependent, exploitative	Bodily feelings, especially sex and aggression	Stereotyping, conceptual confusion
Self-protective	Delta	Fear of being caught, externalizing blame, opportunistic	Wary, manipulative, exploitative	Self-protective, trouble, wishes, things, advantages control	
Conformist	I-3	Conformity to external rules, shame, guilt for breaking rules	Belonging, superficial niceness	Appearance, social acceptability, banal feeling and behavior	Conceptual simplicity, stereotypes, clichés
Conscientious/ Conformist	I-3/4	Differentiation of norms, goals	Aware of self in relation to group, helping	Adjustment problems, reasons, opportunities (vague)	Multiplicity

Conscientious	I-4	Self-evaluated standards, self-criticism, guilt for consequences, long-term goals and ideals	Intensive, responsible, mutual, concern for communication	Differentiated feelings, motives for behavior, self-respect, achievement, traits, expression	Conceptual complexity, idea of patterning
Individualistic	I-4/5	Add: Respect for individuality	Add: Dependence as emotional problem	Add: Development, social problems, differentiation of inner life from outer	Distinction of process and outcome
Autonomous	I-5	Add: Coping with conflicting needs, toleration	Add: Respect for autonomy, interdependence	Vividly conveyed feelings, integration of physiological and psychological, psychological causation of behavior, role conception, self-fulfillment, self in social context	Increased conceptual complexity, complex patterns, toleration for ambiguity, broad scope, objectivity
Integrated	I-6	Add: Reconciling inner conflicts, renunciation of unattainable	Add: Cherishing of individuality		

Note: *Add* means in addition to the description applying at the previous level.

A more recent investigation by Rozsnafszky (1981) looked at ego development and individual differences in personality traits theoretically associated with particular ego stages. Employing Q-sort personality ratings of 91 hospitalized male veterans made by nurses, therapists, and the patients themselves, Rosznafszky garnered an impressive collection of findings bolstering the construct validity of the WUSCT. Preconformist (I-2) subjects manifested significantly higher levels of confused thinking, poor socialization, and limited self-awareness. Conformist (I-3 and I-3/4) individuals placed great value on rules, accepted social conventions, material possessions, and physical appearance, and appeared highly stable. Postconformist subjects (I-4 and I-4/5) revealed greater insight into their own personality traits and motivations behind behavior, and expressed concern over interpersonal communication.

McCrae and Costa (1980) found no relationship between ego stage and objective measures of extraversion-introversion and neuroticism in a sample of 240 adult males. However, as hypothesized, ego stage was positively related to 7 of 10 measures of "openness to experience." Rootes, Moras, and Gordon (1980) investigated sociometrically evaluated maturity in 60 college women. After completing the WUSCT, each woman evaluated all others' readiness for mature functioning in each of four adult social roles: career, marriage, parenthood, and community involvement. Positive relationships were obtained between ego stage and rated maturity in the relatively impersonal domains of career and community involvement. Higher ego-stage women were no more likely, however, to score high on indexes relating to intimate interpersonal roles (marriage and parenthood) than were their peers at lower ego stages.

Gold (1980) documented a negative relationship between ego stage and deviance in 150 adolescent males and females. Administering the WUSCT and the Minnesota Multiphasic Personality Inventory (MMPI), Gold also gathered some support for an association between particular ego levels and certain forms of pathology. Elevated scale scores for hypochondriasis were associated with I-2 and Delta. Higher scores on the MMPI hysteria scale tended to go with I-3, and greater obsessive-compulsive and paranoid scores for I-3/4 and above. In an earlier study also concerned with deviance, inner-city girls judged to be delinquents tended to score at the impulsive (I-2) ego stage whereas the nondelinquent girls, also from the inner city, tended to be located one stage higher, at the self-protective (Delta) level (Frank & Quinlain, 1976). In looking at specific behaviors, the authors also found that fighting, running away, and homosexual encounters were all associated with the impulsive stage.

In a study closer to our central topic of complexity, Candee (1974) explored the structure of political reasoning among student leftists at the University of Chicago and its relationship to ego stage. Interestingly, ego stage was found to be unrelated to the specific *content* of political attitudes; that is, it did not distinguish among those who favored revolution, education, or conventional politics as means of social change. However, ego development was strongly related to the type of considerations and reasons used in forming attitudes. Candee found that lower-stage subjects tended to see politics in relatively global and simplistic terms, typically focusing on the physical or emotional effects of politics on themselves. Higher-stage subjects revealed both a perception of political complexity and the positive assertion of human development and mature justice as political values. The study, therefore, provides support for the notion that ego development "is marked by a more differentiated perception of one's self, of the social world, and of the relationship of one's feelings and thoughts to those of others". (Candee, 1974, p. 622)

Ego Development in the Present Study

In the context of the life-story model of identity, ego development plays a role analogous to that played by the social motives of intimacy and power introduced in Chapter 3. One's stage of ego development, like intimacy and power motivation, is seen as a *predictor* of certain features or characteristics of life stories. Whereas intimacy and power motivation inform the quality of *content* in the life stories that comprise our identities, ego stage is hypothesized to connect more closely to story *structure*, more specifically the *complexity* of story structure. In assessing the relative strengths of intimacy and power motivation via the TAT, I suggested in Chapter 3, the researcher or clinician may be able to make fairly well-informed predictions concerning the relative salience of intimacy and power content themes running through the person's identity story. Likewise, assessing ego development may aid in the prediction of structural complexity, the degree of differentiation and integration, in the identity narrative. To return to Hemingway and Dostoyevsky, I would suggest that the identities constructed by individuals at relatively low stages of ego development may resemble, in their structural simplicity, the story of *The Old Man and the Sea*. Higher-stage persons should construct identities at levels of greater complexity such as that manifested in Dostoyevsky's epic, *The Brothers Karamazov*.

Loevinger maintains that ego stage encompasses many different personality dimensions, including impulse control, interpersonal style, conscious preoccupations, and cognitive complexity, all multiple facets of the person's integrative framework of meaning. My use of her construct in this book, however, is essentially limited to the dimension of complexity. College students in Sample A and midlife adults in Sample B were administered an abbreviated form of the WUSCT developed by Holt (1980) and reproduced in Appendix D. The respondents were divided between those of relatively low ego stages (I-3/4 and below) and those high (I-4 and above). Men and women in the low group, it is assumed, manifest relatively simple frameworks of meaning for understanding self and world. The high group, on the other hand, should provide a more complex frame. The difference in complexity should be reflected in the life story.[5]

Mention should be made of a conceptual distinction implicit throughout this book. The distinction is between the ego and identity. Though the two may be easily confused in everyday parlance, they represent markedly different ideas and are operationalized in markedly different ways in the present investigation. In Chapters 1 and 2, identity is conceptualized as a life story which provides an individual with a sense of unity and purpose. Integrating past, present, and an anticipated future, the life story is constructed in late adolescence and adulthood, and it is a *product of the ego*. The ego, however, produces many things. The ego as an integrative framework of meaning provides a frame or template for identity. It establishes, in a sense, rules and guidelines for the construction of identity. In William James' (1890) terms, the ego is like the "I," the executive of the personality; identity is the "me" or "empirical ego," an outcome of the ego's synthesizing work.

An Exploration: Generic Plots

Ego and Plot

In Chapter 2, I introduced Elsbree's (1982) taxonomy of generic plots. Elsbree's plots are universal action sequences observable in a great number of stories regardless of the genre in which the story is couched. The five plots are: (a) establishing, consecrating a home; (b) engaging in a contest, fighting a battle; (c) taking a journey; (d) enduring suffering; and (e) pursuing consummation.

Hemingway's *The Old Man and the Sea* is an elaboration on a single generic plot—engaging in a contest, fighting a battle. The central action of the story is Santiago's heroic struggle with the great marlin. With respect to Elsbree's generic plots, therefore, Hemingway's classic can be said to be relatively undifferentiated—a structurally simple story with a single action line. Dostoyevsky's *The Brothers Karamazov*, in contrast, is structurally a much more complex story involving elaborations on at least four of Elsbree's five plots. One is reminded of Fyodor and Dmitri's deadly *contest* or battle for the love of Grushenka, Ivan's physical *journey* before the murder of his father and his spiritual journey afterwards, the relentless *suffering* of so many characters trapped in webs of self-abnegation or self-aggrandizement, and the pursuit of spiritual *consummation* and transcendence in the lives of Alyosha and Father Zossima. The only generic plot that does not appear in a rich variety of forms is establishing a home, though certain passages concerning Alyosha and Zossima render this assertion debatable. In terms of Elsbree's plots, therefore, Dostoyevsky's classic is a highly differentiated story.

If an individual's stage of ego development is a prime determinant of the degree of structural complexity inherent in his or her life story (and this *is* the chapter's fundamental thesis), then persons at relatively high ego levels should reveal a more differentiated plot structure in identity, which is to say that they should manifest a greater number of Elsbree's generic plots. Persons at relatively low ego levels should construct life stories with fewer of Elsbree's plots, perhaps elaborating on one or two of them again and again.[6]

To test this prediction, the 50 midlife men and women in Sample B were divided into two groups based on the results of an administration of Holt's (1980) short form of Loevinger's WUSCT. Twenty-six of the subjects (11 men and 15 women) scored at either I-3 or I-3/4, constituting the group low in ego development. Twenty-four of the subjects (9 men and 15 women) scored at I-4, I-4/5, or I-5, making up the group high in ego development. A substantial majority (84 percent) of the subjects in Sample B scored at the I-3/4 (conformist/conscientious) or I-4 (conscientious) levels. In this midlife sample, there were no significant sex differences with respect to ego level, and there was no relationship between ego stage and chronological age.

Two independent scorers, blind to all information on the subjects and hypotheses of the study, coded portions of the life-story interviews of Sample B for Elsbree's generic plots. The scorers coded only the person's long response to the first substantive interview question which asked the subject to think of his or her life as if it were a book with chapters and to describe its content. Answers to all subsequent questions, most of which concern the person's plans for the future, were not considered for coding generic plots. The scorers operated according to a very simple and conservative coding scheme in which each interview protocol was judged for the presence (score + 1) or absence (score 0) of an elaboration upon each of the five generic plots. Thus, each subject received a score of 0 or 1 for each of the five plots and a total score, running from 0 to 5, for the five plots combined. The two scorers were trained using practice interviews in order to establish adequate scoring reliability.[7]

For the purposes of scoring the life-story interviews, Elsbree's five generic plots were defined in the following manner.

1. *Establishing, consecrating a home:* The person devotes a substantial portion of his or her life to the building and/or sustaining of a home (apartment, condominium, etc.) or a family (be it a biological family or a tight-knit community of some kind). Simply buying a house or having a family does not in itself qualify. The person must suggest or imply that the establishment of a home was or is the number one life concern during a specific time period.

2. *Engaging in a contest, fighting a battle:* The person engages in some kind of struggle or serious disagreement with a specific adversary. The struggle or disagreement occupies center stage during at least one specific period of his or her life. In order to score for this plot, the life story must include a concrete antagonist. Simply struggling to make enough money, wrestling with a difficult decision, or fighting to climb to the top of the corporate ladder does not in itself qualify. The contest, furthermore, must afford the possibility of there being a winner and a loser, even if it ends in a draw.

3. *Taking a journey:* The person undertakes a physical or psychological (spiritual, philosophical) voyage for an extended period of time. For a physical journey, simply taking a vacation does not in itself qualify because the person is merely taking a break from the main course in his or her life and returning, in a sense, to the same course afterwards. To score for this plot, the person must devote a well-demarcated segment of the life story to a stint of traveling that is more than a vacation. For a psychological journey, the person must explicitly frame major changes in his or her life in terms of a perceived voyage or pilgrimage.

4. *Enduring suffering:* The person has been harmed by another or experienced prolonged depression or disillusionment in the face of a major setback in his or her life, such as the death of a loved one or loss of a job. It is an unfortunate fact of life that everybody sooner or later suffers. In order to score for this plot, however, the person must suggest that he or she has suffered inordinately more often or more intensely than have most others. Reports of transient guilt or anxiety, recurrent fears, or occasional bouts of depression do not in themselves qualify for this plot.

5. *Pursuing consummation:* The subject seeks and/or finds transcendence, liberation, or self-actualization. This plot typically takes the forms of (*a*) artistic or creative expression, (*b*) religious or spiritual enlightenment, (*c*) emancipation from an oppressive situation, or (*d*) a single-minded devotion to a job, cause, activity, or person which, the person maintains, fills his or her life and brings with it fulfillment.

The scores for total number of generic plots ranged from 0 (2 cases) to 4 (2 cases). The average (mean) score was 1.8. The most frequently appearing plots were establishing a home and taking a journey, each appearing in 21 (42 percent) of the life stories. Pursuing consummation was a close third (20 cases or 40 percent), followed by enduring suffering (17 cases or 34 percent) and engaging in a contest (13 cases or 26 percent).

Table 4.2 summarizes the results of the analysis. Supporting

TABLE 4.2. Mean Scores on Generic Plots Broken Down by Ego Stage and Sex

		Generic Plots[b]					
Ego Stage[a]	N	Home	Contest	Journey	Suffering	Consummation	Total
High							
Male	9	.44	.33	.56	.11	.44	1.89
Female	15	.47	.27	.53	.53	.67	2.47
Total	24	.46	.29	.54	.38	.58	2.25
Low							
Male	11	.27	.27	.55	.18	.18	1.45
Female	15	.47	.20	.13	.40	.27	1.47
Total	26	.38	.23	.31	.31	.23	1.46
All subjects							
Male	20	.35	.30	.55	.15	.30	1.65
Female	30	.47	.23	.33	.47	.47	1.97
Total	50	.42	.26	.42	.34	.40	1.84

[a] Ego stage is determined according to Loevinger's (1976) method applied to the Washington University Sentence Completion Test (WUSCT). Stage scores at I-3/4 and below were designated "low" ego stage; scores at I-4 and above were designated "high" ego stage.

[b] Coders determined the presence (score +1) or absence (score 0) of each of Elsbree's (1982) generic plots in the life-story interviews. Total score is the sum of scores on the five separate plots (maximum = 5; minimum = 0).

the prediction, persons scoring at relatively high ego levels (I-4, I-4/5, I-5) manifested a greater number of Elsbree's generic plots in their life stories (mean = 2.25) than did their counterparts scoring at the lower ego stages of I-3 and I-3/4 (mean = 1.46), F (1,46) = 12.70, $p < .001$. The strong relationship between ego stage and generic plots is reflected in each sex subsample. The number of generic plots observed did not differ significantly between males and females, though women more frequently than men reported enduring suffering, F (1,46) = 5.51, $p < .05$.

The results reinforce a structural continuity between ego and identity. A more complex frame for organizing one's experience gives birth to a more complex product of that organizational effort. Higher ego development is thus associated with greater differentiation in identity or a greater variety of plot categories in the life story. Midlife men and women at higher levels of ego development are more likely to combine in their life stories variations on a greater number of generic plots than men and women scoring at lower ego stages. Whereas a major plot line may involve establishing and consecrating a home for a given individual high in ego development, he or she may juxtapose that category of plot with several other plots—enduring suffering, taking a journey, engaging in a contest, and/or pursuing consummation. The person low in ego development, on the other hand, tends to stick with one or two basic plots, focusing on one or two fundamental narrative forms and constructing variations on each.

Ego and Motive

Chapters 3 and 4 report results of two explorations in person-ology, one focused on the content of life stories and the other focused on structure. In Chapter 3, intimacy and power motivation, assessed via the Thematic Apperception Test, were positively associated with the classification of life stories as comedies and romances, re-spectively. In this chapter, higher stages of ego development, as mea-sured via Loevinger's sentence-completion method, were positively associated with greater differentiation in life story structure, assessed in terms of five generic story plots. The remaining chapters of this book will investigate more closely particular aspects of life stories (nuclear episodes, imagoes, ideological settings, and generativity scripts) as they relate to social motives and ego stage and to each other.

Combining the explorations in Chapters 3 and 4, we can now consider incidental findings not predicted ahead of time. For in-stance, is there a statistically significant relationship between ego stage and mythic archetypes? How do generic plots and social mo-tives relate to each other? Are mythic archetypes and generic plots associated in any meaningful way? And are ego stage and social motives of intimacy and power systematically related to each other?

The answer to the first question is generally "no," with one exception. Stages of ego development in midlife men and women were unrelated to the mythic archetypes of comedy, tragedy, and romance, but a significant relationship was obtained between ego stage and irony. Men and women scoring at *low* ego stages showed *higher* scores on irony than did those scoring at high ego stages (means = 1.62 and 1.25, $F (1,46) = 4.67$, $p < .05$). This unexpected finding suggests that individuals with relatively simple and un-differentiated frameworks of meaning are more likely to construct life stories emphasizing the ambiguities and confusions faced in life. Though they adopt more complex perspectives for understanding self and world, individuals at higher ego stages do not appear to appre-hend the complexity as confusion or chaos, at least with respect to their accounts of their life stories. Perhaps, the more differentiated, more integrated, and less egocentric templates for synthesizing hu-man experience—those conscientious and postconscientious stages of ego development—provide for persons who are able to employ them more adequate answers to life mysteries. Yet, philosophical and religious writings from Confucius to Christianity often imply that the more enlightened members of the human community—those adopt-ing the developmentally most mature or actualized perspectives on reality—manifest an appreciation for the mysteries and paradoxes of human existence. Socrates maintained that as one gains more and more wisdom, one comes to realize how little one knows. Perhaps greater irony would appear in the life stories of men and women at the highest ego stages in Loevinger's scheme (I-5 and I-6). In the present sample, the vast majority of "high-ego-stage" adults scored at I-4, the lowest of the "high" stages.

The relationships between generic plots and social motives are displayed in correlational form in Table 4.3. As can be seen, intimacy motivation assessed via the TAT is positively associated with the presence of Elsbree's (1982) first generic plot: establishing, consecrating a home ($r = .36$, $p < .01$). Power motivation is marginally associated with taking a journey ($r = .27$, $p < .06$). All other correlations are nonsignificant.

The analyses revealed no significant nor near-significant relationships between social motives and stages of ego development. Men and women at I-4 and above were no more likely than those at I-3/4 and below to score high or low on power or intimacy motivation. The TAT and the WUSCT thus appear to be independent measures of personality. The power and intimacy *content* manifested in the TAT is in no consistent way associated with the complexity of *structure* in one's framework of meaning tapped in Loevinger's sentence-completion measure of ego development.

Finally, we should ask the question, "Do these variables such as motives, ego stage, and story forms bear any relation to how happy, satisfied, or well-adjusted a person is?" Though this crucial question will be considered again in the chapters to follow, some general findings can be sketched. We asked each of the 50 midlife adults to complete a short life-satisfaction questionnaire (see Appendix E). Essentially the subject rated his or her own career satisfaction, satisfaction with interpersonal relations, and overall life satisfaction at various points in his or her life on seven-point scales, ranging from 1

TABLE 4.3 Correlations[a] Between Social Motives and Generic Plots

	Motive	
Generic Plot	*Intimacy*	*Power*
1. Establishing, consecrating a home	.36†	−.02
2. Engaging in a contest	.04	.06
3. Taking a journey	−.26*	.27*
4. Enduring suffering	−.16	.26*
5. Pursuing consummation	.22	−.17
6. All plots combined (Σ 1–5)	.12	.21

[a] Correlations for the five single generic plots are biserial. In all cases, $N = 50$.
* $p < .10$
† $p < .01$

TABLE 4.4. Correlations between Life Satisfaction Ratings and Variables Considered in Chapters 3 and 4

	Career Satisfaction	Satisfaction with Relationships	Overall Life Satisfaction
Power motivation	−.12	−.04	−.06
Intimacy motivation	.31†	.13	.26*
Mythic archetypes:			
1. Comedy	.39††	.30†	.27*
2. Romance	.01	.06	.12
3. Tragedy	−.26*	−.07	−.06*
4. Irony	−.20	−.24	−.25†
Generic plots:			
1. Establishing, consecrating a home	.12	.06	.14
2. Engaging in a contest	−.04	.06	.06
3. Taking a journey	.06	.14	.18
4. Enduring suffering	−.26*	−.20	−.11
5. Pursuing consummation	.23	.09	.20
6. All generic plots (Σ 1–5)	.07	.09	.26*

$^*p < .10$
$^†p < .05$
$^{††}p < .01$

(very unsatisfied) to 7 (very satisfied). The correlations between the variables considered in Chapters 3 and 4 and *present* career, relationship, and overall life satisfaction are presented in Table 4.4.

As can be seen, intimacy motivation is significantly associated with career satisfaction ($r = .31$, $p < .05$) and marginally associated with overall life satisfaction ($r = .26$, $p < .10$). Comedy is significantly related to both career satisfaction and satisfaction with relationships, and it is marginally associated with overall life satisfaction. Other near-significant relationships are *negative* correlations between tragedy and career satisfaction, between irony and overall life satisfaction, and between enduring suffering and career satisfaction. Number of generic plots reported is marginally associated with overall life satisfaction. In addition, comparisons of adults high and low in ego stage on the measures of career, relationship, and life satisfaction yielded no significant nor near-significant results.

Though none of the reported relationships are particularly robust, it appears that the only positive predictors of satisfaction with career, relationships, and life are the intimacy motive and the mythic archetype of comedy in life stories. The findings for comedy probably reflect a general attitude of optimism detectable in both life story descriptions and self-report satisfaction ratings. The findings for intimacy motivation are consistent with the results of the longitudinal investigation undertaken by McAdams and Vaillant (1982), in which intimacy motive scores obtained from Harvard men at age 30 were positively associated with ratings of psychosocial adjustment (including marital satisfaction and career advancement) made 17 years later. Still, the results are in no way strong enough to indicate that high intimacy motivation is a necessary ingredient for life satisfaction among adults. There are probably a myriad of life paths and life stories which can lead to satisfaction in human lives. Some subjects scoring very low in intimacy motivation but very high in power reported high levels of satisfaction. High satisfaction with life was also reported by individuals scoring low on both motives. Furthermore, self-reports of satisfaction are doubtlessly crude indexes of how well a person's life is going at a given moment in time. Rating scales of satisfaction are surely influenced by response bias in favor of the socially desirable answer of "Yes, I am satisfied." (Indeed, the adults' ratings of satisfaction were skewed towards the positive end, cutting down the score variance and rendering statistical analyses less significant than they might have been if variance in ratings had been higher.) Even without the problem of response bias, ratings of satisfaction with career, relationships, and all of life do not speak *directly* to other issues involved in overall life adjustment: happiness, sense of fulfillment, mastery over life's challenges, and purpose and meaning in life.

Nonetheless, a positive relationship between life satisfaction and themes of intimacy as reflected in both TAT fantasies and lifestory accounts (via comedy) is a potentially useful finding for both theoretical and practical purposes, if indeed it is replicated in other samples and with other measures. Clinicians may wish to take a closer look at the themes of intimacy detectable in the fantasies and life stories of their clients in an attempt to assist them in their search for happiness, wholeness, and meaning in life.

Returning to complexity, the failure to find any significant relationship between level of ego development and satisfaction is in itself a significant result. Though Loevinger (1976) maintains that the higher ego stages are more differentiated and integrated and, we might thereby conclude, more adequate as synthesizing frames for experience, they do not appear to be associated, at least in our small sample, with reports of life satisfaction. Similarly, Costa and McRae (1983) found no relationship between self-reports of "subjective wellbeing" and ego development in a sample of 240 adult men. Our results do indicate that men and women at higher ego stages construct more complex (differentiated) life stories with respect to Elsbree's (1982) generic plots. This is to say, their stories reveal more variety in plot forms, typically integrating a number of disparate action lines. None-theless, such ego complexity does not appear to assure satisfaction in life. And though the number of generic plots reported (indicating greater complexity in life-story structure) was marginally associated with overall life satisfaction ($r = .26$, $p < .10$), the nonsignificant findings for ego stage and satisfaction suggest that the complex life is not necessarily the more satisfying one, though it is not necessarily the less satisfying one, either.

Summary

This chapter began with a comparison of two different stories—Hemingway's *The Old Man and the Sea* and Dostoyevsky's *The Brothers Karamazov*. Though these two different masterpieces differ in a myriad of ways, one particularly noteworthy distinction between the two is structural complexity. Whereas Hemingway's story is a model of structural simplicity, Dostoyevsky's saga is structurally highly com-plex, containing a wide variety of overlapping plots and subplots. Like stories in literature, life stories, too, can differ dramatically with respect to their complexity. Whereas some are organized around a few very basic plots, others are woven into highly complex, even con-voluted, patterns. Simple stories, then, are global and relatively un-differentiated. Complex stories are highly differentiated and inte-grated, manifesting many and various plots.

I introduced the construct of ego development as a measurable personality dimension serving as a significant predictor of structural complexity in life stories. Thus, as motives are to content so is ego development to structure in the life-story model of identity. Whereas the power and the intimacy motives connect to certain thematic lines or content motifs running through the life story, ego development connects to the relative complexity of story structure—higher stages of ego development being associated with greater differentiation and integration in identity. Ego development refers to one's overall frame-work of meaning for understanding self and world. Synthesizing a number of different ego theories within and outside of psychology, Jane Loevinger writes, "The striving to master, to integrate, to make sense of experience is not one ego function among many but the essence of the ego" (1969, p. 85). In Loevinger's theory of ego devel-opment, qualitatively distinct frames of reference or ego stages are arranged on a continuum from extreme globality and simplicity to extreme differentiation and hierarchic integration. The stages not only specify different levels of development, but also individual dif-ferences within an age cohort. Loevinger's scheme, therefore, is a developmental typology, sharing many of the formal features of other developmental typologies which have arisen out of the "struc-tural developmental tradition" in psychology.

Measured via the Washington University Sentence Completion Test (WUSCT), ego development defines one's customary orientation to self and to the world, revealing itself as an interwoven fabric of impulse control, interpersonal style, conscious preoccupations, and cognitive complexity. With respect to cognitive complexity, Loevinger argues that the early and relatively immature stages in her model of development (stages I-2 or "impulsive," Delta or "self-protective," and I-3 or "conformist") bespeak simplistic, global, and egocentric frameworks of meaning in which ideological issues are apprehended in black-and-white terms and one's orientation is toward self-protection or banal conformity. At higher stages (I-4 or "conscientious," I-5 or "autonomous," and I-6 or "integrated"), however, one comes to question simple dictates of convention, and one's understanding of a range of issues becomes more highly differentiated and integrated so that contradiction and ambiguity become tolerable and the individuality of others is accepted, even cherished. Many recent studies have related Loevinger's stages of ego development to a number of behavioral and experiential variables; some of the more noteworthy studies were reviewed.

The relationship between Loevinger's ego and Erikson's identity is analogous to that between William James's self as "I" and his self as "me." In other words, the ego is the executive I of the personality which is able, through its integrative powers, to construct the me, that is, to construct identity. The central thesis of Chapter 4 was that higher stages of ego development—greater complexity in the I—should correlate with greater structural complexity in identity (the me). I tested this general proposition via a second exploration in personology in which scores on Loevinger's sentence-completion test of ego development were related to the number of generic plots in each of the 50 life stories constructed by the midlife adults in Sample B. Applying Elsbree's taxonomy of five generic plots to accounts of life stories, I found that men and women scoring at relatively high ego stages (I-4 and above) constructed life stories containing a greater variety of Elsbree's plots than did men and women scoring at relatively low ego stages (I-3/4 and below). Thus, higher ego development was associated with greater differentiation in identity. Whereas a major plot line may involve "establishing, consecrating a home" for a given individual high in ego development, he or she may juxtapose this category of plot with several other plots—"enduring suffering," "taking a journey," "engaging in a contest," and/or "pursuing consummation." The person low in ego development, on the other hand, may tend to stick with one or two basic plots, focusing on one or two fundamental narrative forms and constructing variations on each.

This chapter concluded with the presentation of a number of miscellaneous findings for Sample B. Ego development was empirically unrelated to power and intimacy motivation, suggesting that the former personality disposition with its emphasis upon structure and the latter two with their emphasis upon content are empirically as well as conceptually independent. There were no sex differences on ego development. Higher ego development was not associated with ratings on three of Frye's four mythic archetypes, but a negative and significant association was obtained between ego development and irony in life stories. Intimacy motivation was positively associated with Elsbree's plot of establishing, consecrating a home. Intimacy motivation was also positively associated with self-ratings of present career satisfaction and marginally associated with overall life satisfaction. Ego development was statistically unrelated to satisfaction with career and with relationships, and was also unrelated to overall life satisfaction.

NOTES

[1] Most of the various stage models which have emerged out of the structural developmental tradition in the past 20 years implicitly endorse Werner's proposition that development proceeds from simplicity to increasing complexity, complexity typically understood in terms of differentiation and hierarchic integration. These include Piaget's theory of overall cognitive development and Kohlberg's theory of moral development as well as Perry's (1970) model of intellectual and ethical development in the college years, Selman's (1980) theory of social understanding and perspective taking, Damon's (1977) model of the understanding of justice, Broughton's (1980) common-sense epistemologies, Kegan's (1982) model of the self, Fowler's (1981) stages of faith, and Loevinger's (1976) theory of ego development. Although recent research in developmental psychology has cast serious doubt upon some of the more revered tenets of the structural developmental tradition, such as the doctrine of invariant sequence (Siegal, 1980), most developmentalists appear highly sympathetic to the idea that development, be it of integrated stages or more specific skills or competencies (Fischer, 1980), proceeds from relative simplicity to increasing organizational complexity (Flavell, 1982).

[2] There are a number of forerunners to Loevinger's theory of the ego. In psychology, psychiatry, psychoanalysis, philosophy, sociology, literature, and religion, a great many authors have described related conceptions either in terms of a developmental-stage sequence or in terms of a characterology or dimension of individual differences. Although these various theories differ in many ways, all approach from slightly different angles a core concept of ego as *a master synthesizer of experience.* In Loevinger's view, ego development includes what others have called moralization (Kohlberg, 1969), ethical development (Perry, 1970), relatability (Isaacs, 1956), self-system (Sullivan, 1953), cognitive complexity (Harvey, Hunt, & Schroder, 1961), desatellization (Ausubel, 1952), sense of reality (Ferenczi, 1913), levels of human existence (Graves, 1966), prejudiced and unprejudiced types (Adorno and others, 1950), and social characterologies (Fromm, 1941).

[3] The WUSCT consists of 36 sentence stems, and the respondent is asked to complete each one. Like the TAT, Loevinger's measure of ego development can be classified as a projective test, or what McClelland (1980) has termed an *operant measure,* in which the individual is given a good deal of leeway to structure an idiosyncratic

response to a relatively ambiguous, open-ended stimulus situation. The assumption behind research employing the WUSCT is that the person will structure his or her responses to the sentence stems in such a way as to reveal a consistent and overall frame of reference (framework of meaning) for understanding self and world.

The scoring rules for the WUSCT are outlined in detail in Loevinger's scoring manuals (Loevinger & Wessler, 1978, and Loevinger, Wessler, & Redmore, 1978, for women; Redmore, Loevinger, & Tamashiro, 1978, for men). The psychologist scoring a sentence-completion protocol for ego development must classify each response as an example of a particular ego stage (I-2 through I-6). Once all responses for a respondent have been scored, the total protocol is given an overall ego-stage rating based on "ogive rules" contained in Loevinger and Wessler (1978). In his review of Loevinger's model and measure of ego development, Hauser (1976) concludes that the WUSCT manual with its self-training exercises is sufficiently clear such that high agreement can be maintained across scorers trained by the manual and scorers trained personally by Loevinger and her associates.

Redmore and Waldman (1975) have investigated the psychometric reliability of the WUSCT. They report split-half reliability correlations of .90 and .85 in two studies. Internal consistency is reported to be equally impressive. Although test-retest coefficients have been moderately high (around .79), retest scores generally drop, sometimes significantly. Redmore and Waldman explain this discrepency in terms of "motivational set," pointing to a drop in general motivational level of the subjects when the test is to be retaken a short time later for "no apparent reason." Retest protocols are often more banal and briefer than WUSCT protocols from an initial administration, and there may be a preponderance of popular responses since the subjects may see the task as less meaningful the second time around. When a specific rationale is given for the second administration of the WUSCT, however, there is little change in quality of the protocols.

Though style, content, and structure of response are all taken into consideration in scoring sentence-completion tests for ego development, a close look at Loevinger's scoring rules suggests that the structural *complexity* of response is a prime determinant of its ego-stage classification. Scoring rules for the stem "At times she worried about" support this (Loevinger and others, 1978, pp. 262–274). Responses classified I-2 for this stem are typically simple, concrete, and unarticulated: "things" or "something." At the middle levels in the ego-stage hierarchy (I-3 and I-3/4), responses are more complex, indicating increased differentiation between fairly rudimentary and concrete concepts. Responses falling into I-3 or I-3/4 take into consideration more facets and issues than those of earlier stages because, in part, the individual is now attempting to match his or her own egocentric perspective with a different perspective of a defining group. Some examples: "her sister's children" (I-3); "being taken out of school" (I-3); "how to get along with men" (I-3/4); "other people's opinions" (I-3/4); and "doing the right thing for Jimmy" (I-3/4). At the highest ego stages (I-5 and I-6), responses reveal a complex and highly articulated framework of meaning in which multiple issues and factors are taken into consideration (differentiation) and intricate relationships between and among various issues and factors are made manifest (integration). With respect to one particular sentence stem, the authors of the scoring manual write:

> Few new themes appear at I-5, but the familiar ones are expressed with more perspective. Many responses classed I-5 encompass contrasting facets of a problem; for instance, worrying about small things and avoiding important ones, or concern about doing the right thing but doing as one planned anyway (Loevinger and others, 1978, p. 273).

Here are four examples of higher-stage responses to the stem "At times she worried about": "the future so much she forgot to enjoy the present" (I-5); "little things that seemed momentous because they were so close to her" (I-5); "school, grades, friends, boys, life, bombs, Russia, Goldwater, sisters, brothers" (I-6); and "a war which destroyed the world before she fulfilled her dreams" (I-6).

[4] Loevinger has delineated four strands of human development: psychosexual, physical, intellectual, and ego. Although each is partially dependent on the others, and in fact indexes of each may correlate significantly with indexes of the others, the four strands are conceptually distinct. Though granting her the conceptual distinction, some observers have expressed concern over the expected empirical correlation between the intellectual and the ego strands. Correlations between intelligence test scores and ego stage have ranged between about .10 and .50 (Hauser, 1976; Loevinger, 1979). The correlation is typically of greater magnitude in samples manifesting a large spread of IQ scores and relatively diminutive in more homogeneous samples. Correlations between ego stage and verbal fluency (scored according to *length* of responses on the WUSCT) have fallen in the approximate same range (Loevinger & Wessler, 1978). Both Hauser (1976) and Loevinger (1979) conclude that the moderate correlations obtained indicate that the WUSCT is not simply measuring intelligence or verbal fluency. Yet the relationship between intellectual and ego development remains a complex one, still to be fully unraveled.

[5] A word should be said about the division of the subjects into two groups based on ego development. The division is justified on theoretical and empirical grounds. Theoretically, the I-4 level in Loevinger's scheme appears to be the first and lowest level at which the individual has articulated a postconformist ego which is clearly differentiated from the dictates of family and society. The individual encounters the first glimmerings of self-awareness in the previous stage, but it is not until I-4 that long-term self-evaluated goals and ideals, differentiated self-criticism, and a pervasive sense of responsibility become salient characteristics of the person. Empirically, the subjects in both samples cluster at I-3/4 and I-4, and to make a division at another point in Loevinger's scheme would render data analysis and interpretation more difficult. Further, the relatively small number of subjects in Sample B argues against dividing the subjects into more than two ego groups. Though the bifurcate division glosses over potentially interesting differences between, say, I-4 and I-5 individuals, an inquiry focused for the most part on complexity should not be seriously harmed. At this point in our investigation, we are most concerned with assessing the general utility of a single, broad distinction in structural complexity of the ego. Further research may explore finer distinctions.

[6] Like Frye's mythic archetypes in Chapter 3, Elsbree's generic plots are employed in this chapter as categories for conceptualizing life stories which are *not* incorporated within the life-story model of identity presented in Chapter 2. As the analysis of the relationship between mythic archetypes and social motives illustrated the utility of using the power and intimacy motives as predictors of thematic lines in identity in Chapter 3, so is this chapter's study utilizing generic plots designed to illustrate the efficacy of ego development as a predictor of narrative complexity in identity.

[7] For the 50 interviews, the correlation between the two scorers' tabulations of total number of generic plots reported per story was considered high enough to indicate reasonable scoring reliability for research purposes: r (48) = .81. Scores from only one of the two scorers were used in the data analysis.

Chapter 5
Nuclear Episodes[1]

[From] *the incalculable number of impressions which meet an individual, he chooses to remember only those which he feels, however darkly, to have a bearing on his situation. Thus, his memories represent his "Story of My Life"; a story he repeats to himself to warn him or comfort him, to keep him concentrated on his goal, and to prepare him by means of past experiences, so that he will meet the future with an already tested style of action.*

Alfred Adler (in Ansbacher & Ansbacher, 1956, p. 351)

The only home run I ever hit in Little League—and it won the championship! . . . The time I was fired from a job for insubordination . . . The first time she told me she loved me . . . The moment I learned my father had died, and the homily delivered at his funeral . . . The time my best friend told me he was gay . . . A picnic on the seashore with my parents, aunt, and uncle; I was 3 or 4 and mostly remember the seashells . . . The afternoon of November 22, 1963. Our lives are punctuated by certain incidents—some of them seemingly critical or formative and others seemingly mundane—which we draw upon to define who we are, who we were, and perhaps who we are to become. As we construct our identities through narrative, we confer upon certain experiences in our lives a salience or centrality which denotes that they are very, very special. These incidents may be highly positive or negative. They may mark perceived transformations of self— identity turning points—or they may affirm perceived continuity and sameness. They may involve things we did or things that were done to us. They may entail private moments or a shared experience with an entire community. We will term these special incidents *nuclear episodes*. They constitute one of four major components of the life story.

Both Henry Murray and Erik Erikson placed significant theoretical emphasis upon the concrete experiences which coalesce to form the plots of lives. Murray (1938, 1951) considered the *proceeding* to be a basic datum of the psychologist. The proceeding is a circumscribed episode in an individual's life which entails "the completion of a dynamically significant pattern of behavior" (1951, p. 269). Murray wrote:

> Our explorations draw attention to two mutually dependent major problems for psychology: the formulation of small units (single episodes of personality) and the formulation of large units (individual lives). The two problems are mutually dependent because to understand a single episode one must know the settled past as well as the anticipated future, and to understand a life history one must be able to formulate the episodes that constitute it. (1938, p. 740)

Echoing Murray, Erikson (1959) states that "in order to find an anchor point for the discussion of the universal genetics of identity, however, it would be well to trace its development through the life histories or through significant life episodes of ordinary individuals" (p. 110). This chapter, then, considers the significant life episodes that, in the narrating mind of the individual, are reconstructed (Bartlett, 1932; Mandler, 1975) to fit into the life story as its most significant scenes.

Significant Human Experiences

Earliest Memories

That one's earliest memories are psychologically more noteworthy, overall, than memories from later years makes intuitive sense to most laypersons and a good many professional psychologists. At least two pioneers in American academic psychology, G. Stanley Hall (1899) and E. B. Titchener (1900), suggested the same, and in the clinical literature interest in early memories goes back at least as far as Freud (1899/1962). Freud viewed memories from the pre-Oedipal and Oedipal periods as "screens" concealing anxiety-provoking experiences having to do with sexuality and aggression. Concerned for the most part with everyday occurrences but recalled in surprisingly rich detail, these early screen memories were distorted and disguised products of the ego's work in compromising between forbidden wishes and defenses against the wishes. As with dreams, symptoms, and slips of the tongue, Freud contended, the latent content of earliest memories could be discovered through free association.

Emphasizing the revealing over the concealing quality of earliest memories, Adler (1931, 1937) offered an alternative view which is today more in keeping with contemporary theories of memory in many psychoanalytic circles and within the sprawling domain of cognitive psychology. Rather than alerting the psychologist to the dynamics of an ontogenetically bygone era, early memories provided information about the present life situation of the rememberer. The individual selects from his or her past those events, real or fantasized, which validate or justify his or her current view of self and world.

Writing at the same time as Adler but coming from experimental psychology, Bartlett (1932) viewed human memory as a constructive process. For Bartlett, an important factor guiding the reconstruction of the past was the individual's attitudes toward certain past experiences, including relevant motives, emotions, and interest patterns. Bartlett conceived personality as a frame of reference and predicted that those experiences that harmonize best with the current frame of reference would be best remembered and most articulately reconstructed. A number of contemporary information-processing approaches to human functioning have adopted Bartlett's construct of the "schema" as a memory structure or complex organization of past reactions and experiences which guides the reconstruction of the past (Cohen, 1981; Fiske & Kinder, 1981; Markus, 1977; Neisser, 1976).

A recent empirical investigation of earliest memories draws from Freud, Bartlett, and the modern cognitive views. Kihlstrom and Harackiewicz (1982) collected earliest memories from 150 high-school and 164 college students. The older students (in college) tended to report recollections of events from an earlier age (mean = 3.24 years of age) than did the younger high-school students (mean = 3.91). Though the memories varied widely in terms of content and associated affect, high-school students tended to report memories with greater traumatic content than did college students. Following Freud (1899), the authors classified as screen memories those earliest recollections which met at least three of the following four criteria identified by Freud: (1) lacking feeling tone, (2) remembered repetitively, (3) predominantly visual memory, and (4) the person seeing himself or herself in the memory image. Sixty-seven percent of the early memories produced by high-school students were classified as screen memories based on these criteria whereas only 27 percent of the college students reported screen memories. Furthermore, scores on a personality inventory designed to measure "Harmavoidance" (the Personality Research Form or PRF) were positively associated with reporting an earliest recollection classified a screen memory.

Though it is always risky to draw conclusions from a single study, Kihlstrom and Harackiewicz's work at minimum suggests two intriguing notions about earliest memories. First, it appears that the date of the earliest event remembered is partially a function of age in that late adolescents and young adults in college recalled earlier events than did their younger adolescent counterparts in high school. This result may be due to the fact that the older college students (who, by the way, attended Harvard University) were more intelligent, introspective, or psychologically minded than high-school students, some of whom will undoubtedly not be attending college. On the other hand, the results are consistent with the idea that in late adolescence and young adulthood individuals become storytellers in search of identity. More likely to be preoccupied, psychosocially, with the "binding together" of personal past, present, and future than younger students, the undergraduates may, overall, be more actively involved in a searching reconstruction of the past in light of an anticipated future. Desiring to trace their identity origins and mesh them with goals and plans, the undergraduates may be more inclined to trace their life histories back to the earliest of events.

A second implication of the results is a partial vindication of Freud. Students scoring high in Harmavoidance, indicating a more fearful and self-protective stance toward the world, tended to report memories with screen qualities. The authors suggest that this "may well reflect repressive tendencies in these subjects" (p. 145).

Peak and Nadir Experiences

Abraham Maslow (1968) proposed the term *peak experience* to designate the most wonderful and fulfilling moments in an individual's life. Basing his understanding, for the most part, on clinical anecdote and his reading of literature and philosophy, Maslow described peak experiences as personal episodes of perceived wholeness, ego transcendence, truth and goodness, heightened sensation, pure delight, completion, and innocence, to name a few from a vast array of superlatives (Maslow, 1968, pp. 74–96). Unlike Bartlett and Adler, Maslow did not consider the memories of peak experiences to be reconstructions, but he did view them as revelations and not disguises of personality functioning. In Maslow's theory, peak experiences are signs of self-actualization or the full realization of one's potential, and the individual who has more peak experiences than another is the more self-actualized of the two.

Thorne (1963) was one of the first empirical psychologists to translate some of Maslow's ideas on the peak experience into research. Thorne asked subjects to report the "highest (best) experience you ever had in your life" and the "worst time you ever had in your life," the latter denoting what he termed *nadir experiences* or life-history low points. His very primitive classification system for the content of peak experiences (four types: sensual, emotional, cognitive, conative) foreshadowed more rigorous factor-analytic taxonomies, such as that reported in Privette and Landsman (1983).

In general, the empirical research into peak and nadir experiences conducted by psychologists in the past 25 years is sparse and not very illuminating (McAdams, 1982b). Allen, Haupt, and Jones (1964) found that the majority of peak experiences reported by college students could be classified in Thorne's conative category, experiences concerned with instrumental striving. The authors also found that males report more overtly sexual and highly emotional experiences than do females. Not surprisingly, other research has shown that psychotics recall fewer peak experiences and more nadir experiences than do normals (Margoshes & Litt, 1966). Rizzo and Vinacke (1975) asked college students and older adults to recall the "most important personal experiences" in their lives and learned that those whose reports were classified "positive," "happy," and "better" tended to score relatively high on a questionnaire measure of self-actualization. Focusing exclusively on nadir experiences, Ebersde (1970) found that 44 percent of the undergraduates sampled said that their nadir experiences resulted in basically positive effects on their lives in the long run, and 39 percent said that their nadir experiences were *more* important to them than their corresponding peak experiences.

Ecstasy and Flow

It is not uncommon that reports of peak experiences have a mystical or religious dimension. Laski (1962) sought to order and classify experiences of this sort in her survey of episodes of "ecstasy." Sampling reports of ecstatic experiences collected from friends and acquaintances and drawing extensively as well on literary sources, Laski characterized ecstasy as including a range of experiences described as being "joyful, transitory, unexpected, rare, valued, and extraordinary to the point of often seeming as if derived from a praeternatural source" (p. 5).

Like William James's (1902) classic schematization of the varieties of relgious experience, Laski's investigation went beyond the surface of doctrinal belief (what James called "overbelief") to explore the phenomenology and perceived psychological significance of these episodes of transcendence. Experiences of ecstasy were conceptualized in terms of the circumstances under which the experiences took place (the "triggers" of the experience) and the phenomenology of the experiences themselves. Triggers included natural scenery, sexual love, childbirth, exercise and movement, religion, art, scientific or technological knowledge, poetic or literary knowledge, creative work, introspection, and beauty. The phenomenology of the experiences was broken down into statements referring to "gain," statements referring to "loss," and "quasi-physical feelings." In the accounts of ecstatic experiences, men and women speaking of loss typically reported perceived loss of one of the following: time, place, limitation, worldliness, desire, sorrow, differences, sin, self, words and/or images, and sense. They reported gains of unity, timelessness, ideal places such as heaven, release, a new life, satisfaction, joy, salvation or perfection, glory, contact, mystical knowledge, and knowledge by identification. Quasi-physical feelings were couched in words denoting upward movement, moving inside from the outside, light and/or heat, enlargement and/or improvement, darkness, pain, calm, and "liquidity."

Laski categorized ecstasy further into withdrawal and intensity experiences. Withdrawal experiences involve a gradual loss of normal perceptions through a retreat from the corporeal world. Intensity experiences, on the other hand, are "tumescent," involving a crescendo of excitation or stimulation, climax, and what Laski termed an "ecstatic afterglow." Intensity experiences are further divided into three kinds: adamic ecstasies, in which the subject experiences feelings of purification and renewal, of life and the world transformed, and of loving-kindness to all; knowledge-contact ecstasies, in which knowledge is gained often via communication with a distant and powerful source; and union ecstasies, which involve feelings of merger with someone or something else. In the motivational terms adopted in this book, knowledge-contact ecstasies bespeak heightened power, union ecstasies involve an increase in intimacy, and adamic ecstasies may involve either power or intimacy.

In perhaps a more terrestrial vein, Csikszentmihalyi (1977, 1982) has explored experiences of "flow." Interviewing rock climbers, chess players, dancers, and surgeons, Csikszentmihalyi has focused on activities which appear to contain rewards within themselves, what he terms "autotelic" activities. When individuals are totally absorbed in an autotelic activity, such as rock climbing or dancing, they report a sense of fluidity, ease, and grace:

> . . . we shall refer to this peculiar dynamic state—the holistic sensation that people feel when they act with total involvement—as flow. In the flow state, action follows upon action according to an internal logic that seems to need no conscious intervention by the actor. He experiences it as a unified flowing from one moment to the next, in which he is in control of his actions, and in which there is little distinction between self and environment, between stimulus and response, or between past, present, and future. (1977, p. 36)

The experience of flow is almost always enjoyable, though it may not be "pleasurable." For Csikszentmihalyi, pleasure is a homeostatic experience following satisfaction of bodily needs. Enjoyment, on the other hand, is typically a product of activity involving the use of skills in response to increasingly complex challenges. The function of pleasure is contentment, but enjoyment brings change and growth.

And whereas the antithesis of pleasure may be pain, enjoyment in the flow experience is in diametric contrast to boredom and anxiety. Csikszentmihalyi suggests that the relationship between flow and the self is seemingly paradoxical. On the one hand, persons report that in flow the sense of self as an active agent (the self as "I") may vanish: "it cannot be found in consciousness" (1982, p. 29). On the other hand, episodes of flow appear to promote the growth and fruition of the self. In this latter sense, it may be helpful to suggest that flow experiences may enrich the self's (self-as-I) understanding of the self (self-as-me), which is to say that flow may articulate identity. Further exploration of the relationship between flow and identity could enrich our understanding of both.

Nuclear Scenes

In his recent formulation of a "script theory" of personality, Sylvan Tomkins (1979) highlights what he terms *nuclear scenes* of the individual human life cycle. Reminiscent of Murray's proceeding, a scene is a happening in the life of a person, "an organized whole that includes persons, place, time, actions, and feelings" (Carlson, 1981, p. 502). Minimally, a scene must involve at least one affect and one object of that affect. Nuclear scenes are those affect-anchored happenings in a person's life that "capture the individual's most urgent and unsolved problems and that continue to grow by recruiting ever more thought, feeling, and action" (Carlson, 1981, pp. 502–503).

Scenes are connected through a process termed *psychological magnification*. Scenes involving positive affect (joy, excitement) are characteristically magnified (brought together in the mind of the rememberer) through the production of *variants*, the detection of differences around the central core of the scene. Thus, individuals tend to accentuate the differences or variations in their positive autobiographical recollections. Scenes involving negative affect (sadness, shame, anger, disgust, fear, guilt) are typically magnified through the production of *analogs*, the detection of similarities in different experiences. In the case of analogs, the individual may accentuate the perceived similarities among various negative scenes from his or her past.

Illustrating the efficacy of Tomkins' theory in the interpretation of a single case, Carlson (1981) shows how an early childhood scene in the life of one Jane W. was subsequently magnified through the generation of a complex web of remote analogs, each analog very different from every other, but reconstructed in such a way as to emphasize the similarities. These analog scenes, typically involving the affects of shame and anger, came to compose a nuclear script or story about a seductive and betraying woman, frequently disoriented in space, withdrawn and inhibited in the face of confusion, and for whom good things typically turn bad. Carlson concludes, "The more powerful the [negative] scene, the more remote should be the analogs, as greater portions of the person's life space become organized by a nuclear script" (p. 505).

In highlighting earliest memories, peak experiences, ecstasy, flow, and nuclear scenes, Adler, Maslow, Laski, Csikszentmihalyi, and Tomkins are approaching from different theoretical and empirical angles the significant concrete episodes or proceedings (Murray, 1951) in the individual life. Of the various approaches surveyed, Tomkins' is the closest to that adopted in this book. Though addressing general personality structure and dynamics rather than identity per se, Tomkins' script theory resembles, in some of its principles and in its primary metaphors, the life-story model of identity articulated in this volume. Tomkins conceives of the individual as a dramatist or storyteller magnifying salient, affect-laden scenes from his or her past in order to compose dramatic scripts which not only help him or her understand self and world but also exert a paramount influence upon daily functioning, especially in periods of stress. Whereas the nuclear scene is the fundamental structural unit in Tomkins' script theory of personality, what I am terming *nuclear episodes* are one of four major ·components of identity in the life-story model, the other three concerning character (imagoes), setting (ideology), and future plot (generativity script). It is now time to take a close look at nuclear episodes in the life stories which make up the identities of college students and men and women at midlife. I will seek to classify these episodes in various ways and to make sense of them in the twin contexts of power and intimacy motivation and stages of ego development.

Continuity and Transformation in Nuclear Episodes

Collecting Episodes

We collected accounts of nuclear episodes in life stories from the 90 college students identified as Sample A and the 50 men and women at midlife making up Sample B. Appendix A provides background information on these two samples. In addition, data collected in a preliminary investigation from a third and fourth sample (McAdams, 1982b) will be briefly described in order to introduce a later section of this chapter entitled "Episodes of Power and Intimacy."

Nuclear episodes were collected via structured questionnaires and a semistructured interview. All participants in Samples A and B, as well as the two samples in the preliminary investigation of McAdams (1982b), were administered questionnaires asking them to describe in detail certain significant events in their lives: a peak experience, nadir experience, positive childhood experience, and negative childhood experience. The college students in Sample A were also asked to describe their earliest memory. For each experience, the participants were asked to write at least one paragraph detailing what happened to produce the experience, who was there, how the experience felt, what they thought about during the experience, and what (if any) effect the experience had on them. Questions designed to elicit reports of peak and nadir experiences required a bit more explanation. For peak experiences, the question read:

> Many people report occasional "peak experiences." These are generally moments or episodes in a person's life in which he or she feels a sense of transcendence, uplifting, and inner joy or peace. Indeed, these experiences vary widely. Some people report them to be associated with religious or mystical experience. Others may find such a "high" in vigorous athletics, reading a good novel, artistic expression, making love, or simply talking with a good friend. These experiences have been characterized as ones of wholeness, perfection, completion, aliveness, richness, beauty, uniqueness, or insight. Please describe in detail (4–5 sentences) something akin to a peak experience that you have experienced sometime in your life. Please be specific. We would like to know what happened, who was there, how it felt, what you were thinking, and how (if at all) the experience changed you.

The nadir experience was described as follows:

> A "nadir" is a low point. A nadir experience, then, is the opposite of a peak experience. Please think about your life. Try to remember a specific experience in which you felt a sense of disillusionment and/ or despair. This would be one of the low points of your life. Even though this memory is undoubtedly an unpleasant one, we would still appreciate very much an attempt on your part to be honest and straightforward here and to provide for us as much detail as you did for the peak experience. Please remember to be specific.

Finally, the life-story interviews of the midlife men and women in Sample B were examined for accounts of significant events that might qualify as nuclear episodes. A trained judge listened to all 50 tapes and transcribed verbatim segments in which the individual described in detail a specific experience in his or her life which stood out as exceptionally important. In order to be transcribed, the episode had to be described in sufficient detail to specify a concrete place and a circumscribed time period (ideally a few minutes to a few hours) in which the experience occurred, specific behaviors of the actors involved, and the individual's thoughts and feelings during the episode. Most of the experiences identified were contained in the early parts of the interview in which the person described his or her life as a book with chapters (see Appendix B). Indeed, some individuals described many concrete episodes in their lives while some others responded in more general ways, highlighting few specific experiences that stood out. The maximum number of such episodes identified in a single interview was 11; the minimum was 0.

Continuity: Origins, Affirmations

Certain nuclear episodes appear to affirm continuity in identity while others suggest instead identity change or transformation. Episodes of continuity connect the present with the past via an implicit narrative line which suggests that the past nuclear episode serves as an explanation for or a foreshadowing of some aspect of one's present life situation. Episodes of continuity, thus, may function as "origin myths" detailing the genesis of a particular value or value system, perceived personality trait, or any other characterological attribution made by the individual with reference to self. Episodes of continuity may also function as encapsuled "affirmations" or "epiphanies" which depict in a narrative nutshell some essential characterological dimension. In a nuclear episode of continuity, an individual may affirm identity by describing an incident in which "I am at my best," "I am most happy," or "I am most fully myself." In providing a pithy illustration of who I am, these episodes affirm perceived continuity in identity by connecting past with present to reinforce an essential sameness.

A 43-year-old Catholic nun in Sample B, whom we will call Sara N., describes in language laden with passion and pathos a diverse array of nuclear episodes in her life which have gone into the making of her identity. One origin myth is an episode experienced in church at age nine which she describes today as both "weird" and "mystical." Sara's parents were "Yankee Baptists," but at age nine and accompanied by friends from grammar school, Sara found her way into a Catholic church and experienced her first mass. The sanctuary was hot and dark, and Sara was keenly aware of the silence pervading all. She was also aware of "my self reflecting back on my self, and thinking, 'Oh! Who is this person here?' " She reports the sensation that there was something mysterious and all-encompassing in the church, a force or being telling her that this is "home" and "you are welcome." "I knew at this point that I would someday be a Catholic," she adds. In subsequent years, Sara repeatedly defied her parents and attended the Catholic church on the sly. In high school (on Valentine's Day), she was baptized Catholic, a second nuclear episode which serves as an affirmation of her Catholic identity and a manifestation of continuity linking childhood and adolescence.

Not all nuclear episodes are rooted in an actual event experienced by the person. Judy M. is a 45-year-old research assistant and former nurse who relates an incident which functions as an origin myth in her family history and which foreshadows her own identity as well. The episode involves her grandfather when he was a very young man. The consummate pioneer, self-sufficient, rugged, individualistic, Judy's grandfather came to Canada from England at age 17, finding his way to Saskatchewan, which was then a desolate land. The ground was frozen, and the young man could not build a log cabin. He found refuge in a makeshift haystack, under which he lived and survived the long Canadian winter. The pioneer legacy has been marked by a number of "firsts" in Judy's family history. Her grandfather was the first Englishman to settle this part of the Saskatchewan prairie. Her parents were among the first citizens of the small town where she was raised. Her family was the first in town to own an automobile. She was the first in her family to go to college. She was the first to get divorced. And she was the first to leave Saskatchewan for the big city (Chicago), a move reinforcing her image of herself as a pioneer built in the mold of her grandfather.

Among the college students in Sample A, episodes of continuity which function as identity origin myths sometimes appear in the guise of the earliest memory. A sophomore woman traces her fascination with medical settings back to an early childhood experience and suggests that the same experience may be repeated in the future with some other little girl playing her original role and she assuming the role of the frightening nurse:

> My earliest memory involves a feeling of panic. I was playing in the living room of our old house and I overheard my mother on the telephone scheduling a doctor's appointment for me. I can remember trying to figure out when the date was and plotting how to avoid going. (I was going to hide in the closet.) I remember starting to cry when my mother came out of the kitchen and refusing to tell her what was wrong. I don't remember why I was so terrified of going to the doctor, but I always have been. What's pretty funny about the whole thing is that I'm in nursing now. Someday some little kid will be scared of me.

Many of the peak experiences reported by midlife adults and the college students in our samples appear to qualify as episodes of continuity affirming sameness over time. Typical are accounts of intimate family gatherings, often during holiday seasons, when one reports feeling completely at ease and behaving in a way with others which in some sense functions as a revelation of one's true self. These experiences often restate some perceived truth that the person believes characterizes his or her life story. Though the aspect of self restated is typically a positive one, some individuals relate nuclear episodes which epitomize truths which may be very disturbing as well. A trenchant nuclear episode articulated by one Martha P., an urbane and introspective housewife married to a college professor, describes Martha's mother teaching Sunday school in Germany during World War II while next door lived an SS trooper. In another nuclear episode, her husband, an intellectual and a pacifist, is brutally beaten by thugs in a subway station in Chicago.

Both episodes affirm a truism at the heart of Martha's very pessimistic view of the modern world and her place in it. Since World War II, the goddess of goodness and learning has been forced to make her bed with the devil, in the guise of German Nazis and American ruffians, who represent evil, ignorance, and banality. Martha's jaded world view is a thread of continuity in her life story, extending backwards to her earliest childhood days under Hitler. Her accounts of some nuclear episodes illustrate this. They are affirmations of continuity and sameness in her life story.

Nuclear episodes functioning as expressions of continuity sometimes take the form of a reawakening of an aspect of self which has lain dormant. A 40-year-old businesswoman describes a peak experience occurring three years previous in which her sense of self as a vibrant and dynamic woman was reawakened via a romantic tryst. Exhausted from overwork and depressed about her personal life, Erica C. embarked upon a short vacation, alone:

> I felt immediate excitement and relief for the first time in memory of doing something entirely for myself without having to consult anyone else's wishes. I chose to go to the island of —————. I stayed at a small motel on a pretty beach where I knew no one and there was no TV. Twice during the week the hotel owner and some of the guests drove into town to go dancing—I love to dance. One guest was a man taking the winter off—After the first night we made love for hours every night. He was an excellent and fiery lover—talked constantly while making love—and had the most remarkable endurance I've ever come across. It was good fun with him at night, but neither of us did more than acknowledge one another during the day. I also made acquaintance with a woman with whom I traveled and talked. The entire vacation was delicious, and I came back in a really happy state of mind with a vibrant sense of physical well-being.

Transformation: Turning Points, Endings

Nuclear episodes suggesting transformation in the life story are often seen by the individual reconstructing his or her past as turning points marking the end of one chapter and the beginning of another.

A rich source of data on life-story turning points are the life-story interviews conducted with the midlife men and women in Sample B. These episodes may be positive or negative; indeed, some of the clearest cases are reported as nadir experiences. College students also report numerous turning-point episodes, many of them characterized as either peak or nadir experiences. Though some of these appear to be induced by common external circumstances (such as high-school graduation, religious confirmation ceremonies, death of a loved one), others appear to follow a more internally articulated blueprint as in the case of religious conversion, career choice, or some other kind of major life decision made by the subject himself or herself.

A professor of music at a university in the midwestern United States, Richard W. reports a number of life turning points encapsuled in concrete nuclear episodes. One junior-high-school incident marks the end of an early chapter in which Richard was seen by others and by himself as a "dummy" and a "klutz" and the beginning of a new chapter proclaiming increased instrumental and interpersonal competence and talent recognized by others. One day in eighth grade, Richard is sent to the principal's office for misbehaving in class. Rather than mete out punishment, the man who was to become Richard's first life-story hero puts Richard in charge of the upcoming PTA talent show. He also suggests that Richard begin thinking about college. Largely due to Richard's superb organizational efforts, the talent show is a raging success. Shortly afterwards, Richard's school grades improve dramatically and throughout high school he is seen by teachers and peers alike as one of the more gifted students. Today Richard wonders if he would have attended college had he not encountered his eighth-grade principal that day.

In the context of the life story which makes up Richard's identity, it is fairly academic whether or not the nuclear episode reported from eighth grade did in some real way make a major difference in his life course. What is important is that Richard, as an identity storyteller, suggests that it may have. In identifying the most significant events in our lives, we attempt to make sense of our past in light of the present and anticipated future. Though our efforts may occasionally appear farfetched as relatively mundane events are remade into virtually apocalyptic ones, the listener must attempt first to understand and appreciate the individual's life story before he or she begins to pass judgment concerning its objective veracity or even its psychological usefulness as a guiding life fiction.

A great majority (82 percent) of men and women in Sample B reported at least one nuclear episode which appeared to function as a life-story turning point.[2] Triggering these episodes are a host of planned and unplanned factors and forces ranging from being fired from a job to meeting the perfect mate accidentally on a cruise ship. I end this section with two verbatim accounts of turning points. The first is reported as a nadir experience, and it describes a failure in love which marked a move for the subject from dependence on others to an almost narcissistic independence:

> About 1½ years ago—I nearly fell for a guy who didn't return my feelings. I wanted him to like me so much—I don't think I've ever felt so intensely about anyone as him. And there was no basis for it in terms of mutuality—we never even dated. It was like an adolescent crush. Yet I became very aggressive—or at least what I considered to be very aggressive for a woman. I asked him to lunch, just sat down with him for coffee, and gave him little presents. Actually, it turned out to be one of the best learning experiences I've ever had—I learned a lot about myself and began changing patterns of behavior—the beginning of falling in love with myself.

This account is more an entire chapter of this person's life story than a specific marker event with a circumscribed setting and time period. The second report is more typical in that it refers to a single event taking place on a given day. It is characterized by the woman as a peak experience. The episode is a somewhat macabre account of a brush with death for the woman's mother and the woman's wish (prayer) that her mother indeed die so as to end the misery. The mother survives, it seems miraculously, and the daughter is left with a newfound feeling of tranquility:

> In the autumn of 1975, I was summoned home early from work; my mother was seriously ill. She'd been sickly most of my young adulthood so I was used to that, but this was different. She had no feelings in her right leg, and it was turning black. My two aunts and my cousins had arrived, and we rushed her to the hospital. They informed us that the blood to her leg had ceased to flow. Amputation was required. Below the knee, they said. Six hours later after she'd gone to the operating room, the doctor approached us. The leg was gangrene and it had spread to the thigh area. All of the time I was praying to the Lord to help her through this, but now I asked him to take her into his bosom for I knew this was the end and she had suffered enough. I cried and prayed and cried until I felt peace within myself and strong to carry on if it meant without her. He saw fit to let her stay with me a little longer. It's been seven years, and I still feel an inner peace within my soul.

Episodes of Power and Intimacy

A Preliminary Investigation

In the life-story model of identity, two thematic lines around which identities are organized are power and intimacy. The relative salience of power and intimacy in an individual's life story is hypothesized to be a direct function of the level of power and intimacy motivation as assessed via thematic coding of the Thematic Apperception Test (TAT). As introduced in Chapter 2, Hypothesis 1 of the present study in identity states that individuals scoring high in power motivation should manifest greater levels of power content in nuclear episodes while those high in intimacy motivation should present nuclear episodes emphasizing intimacy. The first test of this hypothesis was undertaken in a preliminary investigation of motives and autobiographical memory in college students (McAdams, 1982b). I will briefly discuss this investigation as a way of introducing the topic of social motives and nuclear episodes.

McAdams (1982b) collected written reports of autobiographical recollections from two samples of undergraduates: 56 student volunteers at Harvard University (24 male and 32 female) and 86 male summer-school students. The students were first administered the TAT, which was subsequently scored for power and intimacy motivation. The first sample of 56 students described in written form a peak experience from their lives. The second sample of 86 male summer-school students described a peak experience, a "satisfying experience," a "neutral experience," and an "unpleasant experience." The latter was indicated to be an episode of relatively mild dissatisfaction or disappointment rather than a nadir experience. The written responses for both samples were content analyzed according to two rather simple coding schemes. The degree of power content in a given response was estimated by coding the presence or absence of four specific content themes centered around having impact and feeling strong: (*a*) *Physical or psychological strength* (enhanced perception of one's own physical power, newfound knowledge, or heightened virtue); (*b*) *Impact* (exerting a particular influence or control on others); (*c*) *Action* (vigorous physical activity); and (*d*) *Status* (increase in fame or prestige). The level of intimacy content in autobiographical memories was coded in terms of the presence or absence of five intimacy themes: (*a*) *Interpersonal* (person interacts with at least one other person); (*b*) *Friendship/love* (heightened liking or loving or increase in emotional bond between people); (*c*) *communication/sharing* (reciprocal and noninstrumental dialogue, be it verbal or nonverbal, between person and others); (*d*) *Sympathy* (person shows concern for another or another shows concern for person through a helping behavior); and (*e*) *Touch/physical closeness* (reported physical closeness or tender touching such as kissing, hugging, making love, handshaking, caressing).[3]

The main results of the preliminary investigation are presented in correlational form in Table 5.1. In both samples, TAT motive scores on power and intimacy accurately predicted levels of power and intimacy content respectively in recollections of personal experiences

TABLE 5.1. Correlations between Motive
Scores and Content Theme Scores in
Autobiographical Recollections of Peak,
Satisfying, Neutral, and Unpleasant
Experiences (from McAdams, 1982b,
pp. 296, 298)

| Type and Content | Motive | |
of Experience	Power	Intimacy
Peak 1[a]		
Power	.40†	−.21
Intimacy	−.19	.44††
Peak 2[b]		
Power	.51††	−.02
Intimacy	−.11	.49††
Satisfying		
Power	.24*	−.17
Intimacy	−.10	.26*
Neutral		
Power	−.13	−.11
Intimacy	−.19	.18
Unpleasant		
Power	.08	−.05
Intimacy	−.16	.16

[a] First sample: $N = 56$ (24 male, 32 female).
[b] Second sample: $N = 86$ males. Satisfying,
neutral, and unpleasant experiences refer to second
sample.
*$p < .05$
†$p < .01$
††$p < .001$

that were seen by the subjects as particularly meaningful, what I term
in this chapter nuclear episodes. Individuals high in power motivation described autobiographical memories of peak experiences,
and to a lesser extent satisfying experiences, that concerned feelings
of personal strength, increase in knowledge or virtue, having an
impact on others, increase in prestige or recognition, and physically
vigorous activity. No relationship, however, was found between
power motivation and themes of power in neutral and unpleasant
experiences, recollections which do not appear as personally significant or as meaningful as, say, peak experiences. Similarly, individuals
high in intimacy motivation tended to describe peak experiences, and
to a lesser extent satisfying experiences, which concerned interaction
with others, love and friendship, communication or sharing, helping
others and being helped, and tender interpersonal touching or physical closeness. Again, intimacy motivation was not related to themes
of intimacy in neutral and unpleasant experiences.

The results suggest that motives are selectively related to the content of autobiographical memory. One could conclude that individuals high in intimacy motivation find warm, close, and communicative interpersonal exchange to be particularly rewarding and that they bestow upon memories of such exchange a privileged status in a hierarchy of readily remembered personal experiences. Thus, the intimacy motive appears to confer upon particular classes of experience a special meaning or salience that facilitates the relatively efficient processing and ready retrieval of such information in a setting in which the person is asked to recall a particularly meaningful event, that is, a nuclear episode. The setting is especially important. The person high in intimacy motivation is *not* constantly besieged with memories of friendship and love, nor will he or she recall and report such memories in response to any random cue or question. The relationship between the motive and content of autobiographical recollections is not merely a result of a general verbal style. Rather, the motive and the experience appear to connect in a thematic manner *only when the individual is recalling an experience that might be called a nuclear episode.* Other episodes, less essential to one's identity life story, are *not* thematically connected to motives.[4]

Data on nuclear episodes collected from Samples A and B permit a replication and extension of these results and further discussion of their bearing on identity as a life story. I will first consider in more detail the main themes of power and intimacy in nuclear episodes introduced in McAdams (1982b) and investigated further in Samples A and B. Then I will review the overall results for nuclear episodes classified as positive (such as peak experiences) and negative (such as nadir experiences).

Four Main Themes of Power: Strength, Impact, Action, Status

Tom H., a 43-year-old communications worker employed by the police department, describes a peak experience that is a protypical power episode:

> During a particularly exhausting physical training session in military service, I experienced an immensely high sense of unity with a group. While being observed by training officers and high-ranking military officials, several groups were being put through intense exercise routines for the better part of an hour. A strong sense of competitive attitude became apparent between the groups which one by one began to falter and break pattern very obviously due to the pressure and discomfort. My own feelings were mixed ones of resentment against the training officers and a responsibility to the unit coupled with a sense of pride in still being able to keep the pace. All of this was consistently overridden by physical pain. In the final

minutes we seemed to become aware that the other units were fal-
tering and without outside direction we began to function as one
large being, rather than 60 men. I felt, as did the others, a tremendous surge of energy and our precision of movements was faultless.
The bond we had been seeking for so many weeks suddenly was
there and petty differences and jealousies no longer existed.

This experience illustrates three of the four main power themes
we have observed in reports of nuclear episodes. Toward the end of
his account, Tom tells us that he and the others in his group felt "a
tremendous surge of energy" as the "precision of movements was
faultless." This segment is an example of one way in which the theme
of *strength* can be manifested. In this case, the strength takes a physical form. Other people report experiences of mental, spiritual, or
psychological strength. In each, the person reports an enhanced
sense of his or her own potency as a thinking, feeling, intuiting,
sensing, willing, or acting agent. Examples include gaining knowledge or wisdom, spiritual inspiration, superior empathy or moral
power, supersensory or extrasensory perception, and insight.

Tom's peak experience involves vigorous physical *action*, a second major theme of power. The men engage in an intense exercise
routine which is so taxing that many of the groups "began to falter
and break pattern." Some reports of vigorous physical action entail a
testing of power through pain, as in this case, though many do not.
A third power theme of *status* is evidenced in the newfound prestige
the group obtains in the eyes of the training officers and high-ranking
military officials observing the proceedings. To a lesser extent, it is
also evidenced in Tom's "sense of pride in still being able to keep the
pace." The theme of status in nuclear episodes involves the individual's gaining prestige, recognition, or higher status from others because of something he or she has done. Many examples involve winning contests, being promoted, or receiving honors.

A fourth theme of power is *impact:* the person reporting that he
or she exerts a particular influence upon another, controls, persuades,
manipulates, or in some way has an impact on another such that the
other is forced to make some kind of change. The theme of impact is
obvious in this account of a peak experience written by a 24-year-old
woman, a sophomore in Sample A:

Oddly enough, a confrontation with a man I highly respect and ad-
mire resulted ultimately in what you might call a "peak experience."
I am normally intimidated, admittedly self-inflicted, by those whom
I greatly admire. The incident occurred at a school board meeting.
Present were members of the board, a few parents in the audience,
the principal, and our pastor, the man with whom I debated. I had
been working on a parent survey from March through November.
The pastor wanted to completely dismiss the value of the survey

findings purely on the basis of a few points with which he disagreed. We were sitting face to face across a table. As I listened to him tear down months of work, I thought, "I can't let him do this." Then the confrontation began. For approximately 20 minutes we debated and compromised. All the while, I was sure that he would dislike and resent me from that time on, but I had to risk it. I was wrong. In our conversation following the meeting, I learned that his attitude toward me had changed. I had earned *his* respect! I felt both relieved and exhilarated.

Strength, action, and status are central themes in the following nuclear episode reported by a 21-year-old junior. In her last year in high school, she was chosen captain of the school gymnastics team. Early in the account, she describes the vigorous physical *action* which resulted in her being chosen captain:

> Having had no previous experience in the sport, I worked many tiring, sweaty hours to try to perfect the routines. I knew that I had to practice hard and perform my best to set a good example for the teammates.

While performing during an important match, she experiences a physical potency (*strength*) characteristic of many power experiences:

> My specialty was the uneven parallel bars. From the tension of the mount until the flying dismount I put all my power into every move. At these times I felt a sense of strength and ease.

At the end of this stellar performance, her peers, her coach, the crowd, and the judges all endorse her heightened *status* as a preeminent gymnast:

> After my routine, my teammates smiled their approval and patted me on the back. I was stunned to see my score of 9.0. The coach cheered along with the crowd, and I felt a great sense of accomplishment. Today the score still stands as the highest on record.

In a somewhat more private experience, a 21-year-old junior man describes an episode of strength (couched in terms of "freedom") and action (as fast movement):

> My last peak experience was cruising down the Edens Expressway in my Trans Am with _____. The day began as a boring fall Sunday with nothing to do but homework. Then I decided to skip the depression by calling up my girlfriend (or two) and going for an 80-mph ride in my Turbo Trans Am with the top off and music blaring. The girls and I get along great and always have a good time regardless of what we smoke. When we started off, I noticed the cool fall day was beautiful, the girls were great, and the music made a great atmosphere. I got a great sense of freedom in that experience, in freedom from cops, the drains of homework, and my terrible predictions of that day.

Reminiscent of Luther's revelation in the privy, a sophomore woman describes an even more private account of insight (strength) received in the bathtub:

> This may sound strange, but I think most clearly when I am in the bathtub (stop laughing!). Anyway, it was probably two or three years ago and was as if I knew I could make my life work. I had been going through troubles with my boyfriend and wasn't sure about school. It was as if the fog I was in lifted, and I could say where I wanted to go and how to get there. I realized I had the power to achieve what I wanted, and the experience gave me tremendous insight on what I was doing wrong in my life and soon things would be right.

These are but a few of the many nuclear episodes collected from Samples A and B which are laden with themes of power: strength, impact, action, status. In all of them, the individual has expanded himself or herself as an active agent having an effect on the environment. In terms of David Bakan's duality of human existence, power experiences are generally more *agentic* than *communal*, though Tom H.'s account of the military regimen contains traces of both. The activity reported may occur in a public setting (especially when the theme of status is present) or in private (more often associated with strength through insight). The person emerges from the experience triumphant in some manner—triumphant over the physical environment, others, destiny, or sometimes over self. One's power is affirmed as the individual is momentarily transformed into someone larger, wiser, better, smarter, more influential, more esteemed, or more active.

Four Main Themes of Intimacy: Communication/Sharing, Friendship/Love, Sympathy, Touch

A sophomore woman describes a peak experience which illustrates well three of the four major intimacy themes we have observed in accounts of nuclear episodes.[5] The experience, however, is not devoid of power in that the reported coming together of the subject and a loved one leads to a heightened moral strength. The intimacy themes which appear are communication/sharing, friendship/love, and touch:

> In the last month I had the opportunity to experience a true peak experience—an actual "rebirth" of sorts. I have become very close to an individual who has a very high moral system—one which I myself used to have and an innocent beauty I want to recapture. Together we have discussed all the events that have occurred between us and the guilt which hovered over some of our actions. And we

decided to start over in purity. We went walking down the beach after going to Mass one night and it was beautiful! It was a warm night—stars were everywhere. Never before had I felt so close to God and so close to another human. We waded into the water—next thing I knew we were up to our waists in water. We laughed and cried and hugged while the water swirled around us and we promised to each other a new start—a new fidelity to God and to our faith and a promise not to tempt but rather help each other. When we left the lake that night and walked back squishing and dripping we were happy—totally one with each other and with the heavens above. It was absolutely the most wonderful happiness possible.

In *communication/sharing*, the individual exchanges information or tangible objects with another person in a reciprocal, non-instrumental way. In this episode, the subject and a friend "discussed all the events that have occurred between us and the guilt which hovered over some of our actions." In this case, the sharing involves highly personal and delicate information, though this need not be the case. Many examples of communication/sharing in nuclear episodes entail simple and nonrevealing conversations, sometimes even about the weather. As long as the sharing is mutual (reciprocal) and as long as it is not in service of an instrumental goal (as would be the case in, say, an interview or class discussion), an episode of sharing will qualify for this very common theme.

In *friendship/love*, the individual falls more deeply in love with another, becomes a closer friend, comes to like another person, or experiences a sense of community or union (oneness) with others. This undergraduate woman reports feelings of love and oneness vis-à-vis her friend, God, and the "heavens above." The third theme present in her account is *touch*. Experiences of intimacy frequently involve tender physical touching between actors. In this case, there is "hugging." Other examples include kissing, making love, handshaking, and caressing.

The themes of friendship/love and touch are poignantly portrayed in an account of the birth of his daughter written by Dean K., a 36-year-old engineer in Sample B:

A very very special experience that recently happened in my life was the birth of my last child, _____, in October 1978. She was born nine years after the birth of my second child and was the first daughter after two sons and many years of waiting. Perhaps the greatest moment of my life was the time when she was born since, unlike the birth of my two sons, I was able to be in the delivery room at my wife's side while she was being born. Her birth is a moment I will never forget, especially when she was placed on my wife's chest immediately after the birth and she just stared at the two of us without crying. I found myself crying instead, out of pure joy and happiness. Since that day three years ago, _____ has brought boundless love and happiness into my family life and has brought more love out of me than I thought existed.

Illustrating intimacy themes of communication/sharing and friendship/love, the following peak experience described by a freshman woman is representative of a number of nuclear episodes concerning intimacy reported by the college students in Sample A:

> My experience involved a relationship with one of my friends. We had known each other for a short while but there was a certain feeling of being closer, of feeling like you have known this person longer. One day, we were both talking and suddenly we both began telling things each of us had never told anyone before. We were having a completely honest and open conversation with each of us exposing some of ourselves that had never been shown to anyone else. It was just the two of us talking and pouring out our hearts. We both cried. Some of the things I spoke about were painful, but an immediate sense of release and relief came over me after I had opened up. I was thinking of how good it felt to be so open with this friend. Our friendship strengthened as a result of this. We have a strong bond between us, and our friendship is something I cherish. This experience changed my concept of myself. I learned to be more tolerant of my faults. It helped me to feel more alive, more loved than ever before.

The fourth theme of intimacy is *sympathy*. This theme typically involves the subject or another person expressing some kind of concern for the other, often leading to a helping behavior or, in some cases, some kind of sacrifice. The object of sympathy may be a single other (typically a friend or lover) or a larger group of people (as in the cases of humanitarian service to others). One junior man describes the organization of an Easter party for a home for retarded children. A sophomore woman tells of the time her boyfriend was seriously injured playing football and of her dutiful ministering to his ailments. She fed him, took him for walks, and helped him to the bathroom. A number of the students in Sample A and one of the midlife adults in Sample B described long conversations with close friends which served the purpose of helping the friends through traumatic episodes in their lives. Here is an exemplary account of the theme of sympathy in an episode in which a male undergraduate plays the role of therapist for his roommate and the roommate's girlfriend:

> There was one very special moment that happened to me just recently. Last year my roommate got into a fight with his girlfriend whom I had just met that day. She lived a few blocks away from us. When they got into this fight, she left the room crying and started to walk home. Noticing how upset she was, I started after her. I told her that I wanted to be her friend and that I wanted to help her with her problem but I didn't want my roommate mad at me. When we

had finished talking about her problem, I found that the problem was communication. When I decided to help her I went to my roommate and talked to him. I think I helped them solve their problem, and at the same time I made a very beautiful friendship with my roommate's girlfriend. It was a short friendship but very enriching. The peak was that I actually helped someone and made a friend at the same time.

Manifesting themes of communication/sharing, friendship/love, sympathy, and touch, episodes of intimacy in the lives of college students and men and women at midlife are generally more *communal* than *agentic*. In these experiences, the self merges with another, be the other a dear friend or all of humankind. Thus, the focus of the intimacy nuclear episode is on the *relationship* between the individual and his or her interpersonal context rather than the action of the individual over and against the context.

Positive Nuclear Episodes: Overview of the Findings

Accounts of peak experiences and positive childhood experiences recalled by the college students in Sample A and the midlife men and women in Sample B were assumed to display, for the most part, a positive emotional tone and thus were deemed positive nuclear episodes. The procedure for scoring these episodes for themes of power and intimacy was the same as that used in the preliminary investigation (McAdams, 1982b).[6] Two independent coders scored the accounts for the presence or absence of each of the four main themes of power and the four main themes of intimacy.[7]

Sex differences were first examined. In Sample A, the only statistically significant sex difference with respect to content theme scores was for the power theme of action in accounts of positive childhood experiences. Male undergraduates were significantly more likely than females to report a positive childhood experience entailing vigorous action of some kind ($p < .05$). In Sample B, midlife men tended to score higher on total power themes for peak experiences ($p < .05$), total power themes in peak and positive childhood experiences combined ($p < .05$), the power theme of status in childhood positive experiences ($p < .05$), and (surprisingly, perhaps) the intimacy theme of communication/sharing in reports of childhood positive experiences ($p < .01$).

Tables 5.2 and 5.3 present the analysis of the relationships between power and intimacy content scores in positive nuclear episodes and power and intimacy motivation. Replicating the preliminary investigation, the findings provide support for Hypothesis 1 of the present study which predicts a positive correlation between social motives assessed via the TAT and corresponding content theme scores in nuclear episodes. In both samples, power motivation was strongly associated with total power theme scores in peak experiences. Power motivation was also positively related to power themes in childhood positive experiences. The four power themes did not perform equally well, however. It appears that strength and action show the most consistent positive relationships with power motivation, while impact is significantly related to power motivation in Sample A but not B. The theme of status appears the weakest of the four, failing to correlate significantly with power motivation in both samples and for both positive experiences reported. The pattern of findings was consistent across the two sexes in Sample A with the significant relationships obtained for the entire sample holding up well within each sex subsample. Because of Sample B's relatively small size (containing only 20 men), we were not able to determine with any degree

TABLE 5.2.   Correlations between Motive Scores and Content Themes in Positive Nuclear Episodes among College Students in Sample A

Episode	Power Motivation	Intimacy Motivation
1. Peak experience		
a. Power themes total	.53††	.05
(1) Strength	.28†	.12
(2) Impact	.37††	.12
(3) Action	.32†	−.11
(4) Status	.16	−.00
b. Intimacy themes total	.07	.33†
(1) Communication/Sharing	.08	.19
(2) Friendship/Love	.04	.14
(3) Sympathy	.06	.22*
(4) Touch	−.02	.37††
2. Childhood positive experience		
a. Power themes total	.37††	−.08
(1) Strength	.21	.05
(2) Impact	.33†	−.07
(3) Action	.24*	−.30†
(4) Status	.15	.11
b. Intimacy themes total	−.14	.20
(1) Communication/Sharing	.06	.06
(2) Friendship/Love	−.27*	.09
(3) Sympathy	.01	.15
(4) Touch	.02	.17
3. Peak and childhood positive combined		
a. Power themes total	.63††	−.02
b. Intimacy themes total	.01	.40††

Note: N = 90 college undergraduates (57 female, 33 male).
* $p < .05$
† $p < .01$
†† $p < .001$

of assurance the comparability of results across the two sexes for midlife adults.

Though the findings for intimacy were not as substantial as those for power, the pattern of results was similar. Again, accounts of peak experiences reflected well the motivational profiles obtained from the TAT. Intimacy motivation was positively associated with total intimacy theme scores and the single theme of sympathy in peak experiences for both samples and with the theme of touch in peak experiences for Sample A. For childhood positive experiences, intimacy motivation was positively associated with total intimacy theme scores for the midlife subjects, but not among undergraduates. The positive relationship for the midlife sample, however, was due to the very strong correlation between intimacy motivation and the single theme of friendship/love in positive childhood experiences. The

TABLE 5.3. Correlations between Motive Scores and Content Themes in Positive Nuclear Episodes among Midlife Adults in Sample B

Episode	Power Motivation	Intimacy Motivation
1. Peak experience		
a. Power themes total	.50††	−.02
(1) Strength	.51††	.15
(2) Impact	.14	−.02
(3) Action	.31*	−.08
(4) Status	.08	−.14
b. Intimacy themes total	−.01	.33*
(1) Communication/Sharing	−.10	.21
(2) Friendship/Love	.07	.20
(3) Sympathy	.08	.32*
(4) Touch	−.08	−.14
2. Childhood positive experience		
a. Power themes total	.40†	−.09
(1) Strength	.35*	.36*
(2) Impact	.00	.00
(3) Action	.31*	−.22
(4) Status	.14	−.18
b. Intimacy themes total	−.22	.43†
(1) Communication/Sharing	−.15	.02
(2) Friendship/Love	−.19	.61††
(3) Sympathy	.00	.02
(4) Touch	.01	.01
3. Peak and childhood positive combined		
a. Power themes total	.53††	−.07
b. Intimacy themes total	−.10	.49††

Note: N = 50 (30 female, 20 male).
* $p < .05$
† $p < .01$
†† $p < .001$

other three intimacy themes were unrelated to intimacy motivation among the midlife adults. As in the case of power, the pattern of results for intimacy was consistent across the two sexes in Sample A.

Negative Nuclear Episodes: Overview of the Findings

The examination of the content of negative nuclear episodes—nadir experiences and childhood negative experiences—was more exploratory. An initial reading of the accounts indicated that the four main themes for power and intimacy did not appear relevant for the coding of these episodes, even when the positive aspect of the theme was changed to the negative as in the case of friendship/love being changed to failure to engage in friendship or love relations or loss of such a relationship. Blind to the motive scores of the subjects but now familiar with the overall content of these responses, my associates and I settled inductively on four new themes for each of the two content categories of power and intimacy. In some cases, the new themes bear some resemblance, typically as an opposite, to the original themes used in the analysis of positive nuclear episodes. In other cases, any similarity is lacking.

The four power themes in negative nuclear episodes were defined as follows:

1. *Failure/Weakness*—The person fails in some task or venture. The person is unable to do something that he or she wants to do because of some factor(s) within him or her. Consequently, the person is unable to experience the goal state of feeling strong or powerful.
2. *Losing face*—The person experiences shame (though not necessarily guilt), embarrassment, or humiliation in the presence of others.
3. *Ignorance*—The person is unable to *know* something that he or she desires to know. The person is confused, disoriented, "in the dark." Consequently, he or she is unable to experience mental strength, and he or she regrets this inability.
4. *Conflict*—The negative experience is a direct result of a conflict or disagreement between the person and others. This includes arguments or fights.

The four intimacy themes were

1. *Separation*—The person is separated from friends, family, or lover. This can occur through a variety of means: breakup, circumstances over which nobody has control (moving, going off to school), death, etc. The person must express negative affect about the separation or aloneness per se, that is, the *being apart* from the other.

2. *Rejection*—The subject has been rejected by somebody who has been a friend or lover. The other person wishes to terminate a previously intimate (loving, caring, communicative) relationship. The subject must express negative affect about the rejection per se. This is a completely separate category from the previous, though the two may occasionally co-occur as in the case where the other person explicitly rejects the subject causing a breakup in the relationship, and the subject remarks explicitly that he or she experienced *both* the separation (being apart) and the rejection (the process of initiating the separation) as aversive.

3. *Disillusionment about people*—As a result of an aversive experience, the person remarks that he or she has lost faith in others (either a particular other or a group or even all of humankind) or is feeling disillusionment about people and their worth or goodness. This is often accompanied by a sense of betrayal or a breaking of a trust.

4. *Another's misfortune*—The person experiences vicariously the plight of another. The person is saddened by another's misfortune, pain, or death. A common example is depression experienced over the death of a loved one. If the negative affect in this case were also explicitly connected by the writer to the experience of now being alone or separated, then the example would also score for the first theme of separation.

Two independent coders, blind to subjects' motive scores, coded the nadir experiences and childhood negative experiences for the eight themes indicated above.[8] In the college sample, women tended to score higher than men on total intimacy theme scores for nadir experiences and for the single theme of disillusionment with people in nadir experiences. Among the midlife adults in Sample B, no significant sex differences were observed.

Content theme scores for nadir and childhood negative experiences were correlated with power and intimacy motivation from the TAT. The results of these analyses are summarized in Tables 5.4 and 5.5. Power motivation and power themes were highly correlated for nadir experiences in both samples and for childhood negative experiences among the college students in Sample A. The overall correlation between power motivation and the number of power themes from nadir and childhood negative experiences combined was extremely high for both college students ($r = .55$) and midlife adults ($r = .72$).

The results for intimacy, however, were much more equivocal. Intimacy motivation was positively correlated with total intimacy theme scores among college students but not among the midlife adults. In the college sample, the relationship was fairly strong for childhood negative experiences ($r = .39$) but only marginally signifi-

TABLE 5.4. Correlations between Motive Scores and Content Themes in
Negative Nuclear Episodes among College Students in Sample A

Episode	Power Motivation	Intimacy Motivation
1. Nadir experience		
a. Power themes total	.50††	.06
(1) Weakness/Failure	.28*	.02
(2) Losing face	.44††	.05
(3) Ignorance	.36††	−.03
(4) Conflict	.12	.06
b. Intimacy themes total	−.13	.23*
(1) Separation	.09	.05
(2) Rejection	−.05	.13
(3) Disillusionment about people	−.12	.32†
(4) Another's misfortune	.16	−.08
2. Childhood negative experience		
a. Power themes total	.36††	−.22*
(1) Weakness/Failure	.24*	−.04
(2) Losing face	.02	−.00
(3) Ignorance	.31†	−.23*
(4) Conflict	.23*	−.23*
b. Intimacy themes total	.07	.39††
(1) Separation	.07	.25*
(2) Rejection	−.02	.14
(3) Disillusionment about people	.11	.17
(4) Another's misfortune	.12	.10
3. Nadir and childhood negative combined		
a. Power themes total	.55††	−.10
b. Intimacy themes total	−.04	.38††

Note: N = 90 college undergraduates (57 female, 33 male).
*p < .05
†p < .01
††p < .001

cant for the nadir experiences ($r = .23$). Individual intimacy theme
scores correlated significantly with intimacy motivation in only two
cases: disillusionment about people in nadir experiences and separation in childhood negative experiences, both for college students
only.

In comparing the patterns of results within each of the two sex
subsamples of college students, we found that whereas the pattern is
similar for males and females with respect to power motivation and
power themes, the results for intimacy reveal a major disparity. It
appears that the significant relationships between intimacy motivation on the one hand and intimacy themes in nadir and childhood
negative experiences on the other for Sample A are due solely to the
females, for whom these relationships are strong and positive in both

TABLE 5.5. Correlations between Motive Scores and Content Themes in Negative Nuclear Episodes among Midlife Adults in Sample B

Episode	Power Motivation	Intimacy Motivation
1. Nadir experience		
a. Power themes total	.63††	.05
(1) Weakness/Failure	.62††	−.06
(2) Losing face	.07	.16
(3) Ignorance	.27	.05
(4) Conflict	.40††	.07
b. Intimacy themes total	−.12	.07
(1) Separation	−.09	.17
(2) Rejection	−.06	−.08
(3) Disillusionment about people	−.04	.15
(4) Another's misfortune	−.05	.11
2. Childhood negative experience		
a. Power themes total	.26	.01
(1) Weakness/Failure	.20	.02
(2) Losing face	.12	.06
(3) Ignorance	−.01	−.18
(4) Conflict	.09	.03
b. Intimacy themes total	−.15	.22
(1) Separation	−.18	.11
(2) Rejection	−.15	.01
(3) Disillusionment about people	.00	.00
(4) Another's misfortune	.13	.30
3. Nadir and childhood negative combined		
a. Power themes total	.72††	−.04
b. Intimacy themes total	−.25	.21

Note: N = 50 midlife adults (30 female, 20 male).
* *p* < .05
† *p* < .01
†† *p* < .001

cases ($r = .27$, $p < .05$ for nadir experiences; and $r = .53$, $p < .001$ for childhood negative experiences). Among the men, however, the relationships simply do not exist ($r = -.10$ for nadir experiences, and $r = -.07$ for childhood negative experiences). Thus, the hypothesized significant relationship between intimacy motivation and themes of intimacy in negative nuclear episodes is supported only in the case of college women.[9]

Overall, the analysis of social motives and nuclear episodes indicates that some discrete proceedings or events recalled by an individual in reconstructing his or her life story can be fruitfully characterized in terms of power and intimacy content themes. Especially valuable are episodes with a strong positive or negative emotional tone, such as peak and nadir experiences. In general, these experiences manifested a good deal of power and intimacy content. Further, the content scores obtained from these episodes were significantly correlated, in many cases, with TAT motivational scores in a manner offering substantial support for Hypothesis 1, first presented in Chapter 2. The results illustrate a thematic continuity in lives—a mirroring of salient motivational themes in accounts of significant life episodes. The most salient underlying motives in our lives appear to color our recollections of the past by underscoring particular content themes in the especially critical episodes of the stories we tell ourselves in order to live.[10]

Complexity and Nuclear Episodes

In Chapter 4, I introduced the topic of complexity in the life story. Complex identities are those life stories which manifest considerable differentiation and integration in structure. In the life-story model of identity, stage of ego development (Loevinger, 1976) is hypothesized to be a major predictor of the degree of complexity in an individual's life story. Those persons scoring at relatively high ego stages, such as the postconformist stages of I-4 and above, should bring to the understanding of self frames of reference which can potentially accommodate substantial narrative complexity. They should make more distinctions among events and ideas in their life stories (greater differentiation) and should construct more connections among the disparate parts as well (greater integration). The exploration of ego stage and generic plots in Chapter 4 provided initial support for this proposition. Midlife men and women in Sample B who scored at I-4 or above on Loevinger's sentence-completion measure of ego development manifested greater complexity in plot structure than did those men and women scoring at I-3/4 and below. Those scoring at the higher stages constructed identity stories which contained a greater number of Elsbree's (1982) generic plots, compared to their counterparts scoring lower in ego development.

The predicted relationship between ego stage and nuclear episodes is set forth in Hypothesis 2 from Chapter 2. Quite simply, persons at high stages of ego development should report a greater number of nuclear episodes than should those scoring low in ego development. Complex life stories should have a greater number of significant story scenes, such as turning points, origin myths, and affirmations. Relatively simple life stories, on the other hand, should contain fewer such scenes as the narratives should unfold in a relatively straightforward, even linear, manner, reminiscent of Hemingway's *The Old Man and the Sea*. Thus, narrative complexity should be manifested in generally greater differentiation at the level of nuclear episodes.

The life-story interviews conducted with the midlife men and women in Sample B provide some data which speak to Hypothesis 2 concerning the relationship between ego stage and nuclear episodes. A trained judge listened to the interview tapes and transcribed verbatim accounts of significant life episodes which were set in a particular time and place and involved specific behaviors of the actors taking part and accompanying thoughts and feelings reported by the respondent.[11] The number of nuclear episodes reported per interview ranged from 0 to 11. The average number was 4.0 (standard deviation = 2.4).

As in the exploration of generic plots, the distribution of ego stage scores was broken between I-3/4 and I-4 with the 26 adults scoring at I-3/4 or below constituting the group low in ego development and the 24 with scores at I-4 and above making up the group high in ego development. When the adults high in ego development were compared to those scoring low, no statistically significant difference was obtained for number of nuclear episodes in the interview. The mean number of episodes reported by subjects at low ego stages was 3.7; at high ego stages the mean was 4.3. The small difference was not statistically sufficient to support Hypothesis 2. In addition, no sex difference was obtained. The mean number of episodes for females was 4.2, and for males it was 3.7, again a nonsignificant difference.

Upon reading the judge's transcripts, however, my associates and I were struck by a difference in the perceived quality of the nuclear episodes reported by adults high in ego development versus those scoring at the lower stages. It appeared to us that higher-stage men and women at midlife tended to describe more incidents which led to perceived changes in their lives than did midlife men and women low in ego development. In other words, the significant scenes which adults high in ego development highlighted in their life stories were often of the type I have described as "transformations," indicating some kind of turning point in identity. To test our hunch, we had a second and third judge, blind to all information on the subjects, read the transcripts of nuclear episodes produced by the first judge and classify each episode as either a turning point or "something else."[12] For an episode to be classified a turning point, the individual had to indicate in an explicit manner a significant life change which resulted from the episode. As mentioned above, a majority (82 percent) of the midlife subjects reported at least one nuclear episode which qualified as a turning point in their lives. Overall, 42.5 percent of the nuclear episodes recorded by the first judge were determined to be life-story turning points. The number of turning points reported by each subject ranged from 0 to 5, mean = 1.7, and standard deviation = 1.3. As expected, number of turning points was positively correlated with number of nuclear episodes ($r = .75$, $p < .001$).

A second analysis of the data provides support for the validity of this serendipitous observation. Adults scoring at I-4 and above revealed a significantly greater number of nuclear episodes classified as life-story turning points (mean = 2.1) than did adults scoring at the lower stages of I-3/4 and below (mean = 1.3), F (1,46) = 4.84, p < .04. Males did not differ from females with respect to turning points (means = 1.4 and 1.9, respectively).

The meaning and significance of this finding are far from clear-cut. The result is essentially the product of an inductive observation rather than a deductive testing of an hypothesis set forth ahead of time. As such, this significant relationship between ego stage and the number of turning points reported in life-story interviews awaits cross-validation with a different, and perhaps larger, sample of men and women. My interpretation of the finding, therefore, is tentative and highly speculative.

Early in the chapter, I made a distinction between episodes of continuity and episodes of transformation. Episodes of continuity, such as origin myths and affirmations, reinforce the sameness of identity over time, whereas episodes of transformation, such as turning points, mark relatively discontinuous changes in the life story. The data suggest that it is these nuclear episodes of the latter persuasion which tend to be structured in such a way as to be commensurate with Hypothesis 2. Men and women at conscientious and post-conscientious ego stages appear to reveal significantly greater differentiation with respect to episodes of transformation in identity than do their counterparts at the preconscientious stages. The relationship breaks down, however, when all nuclear episodes, be they turning points or something else, are taken into consideration. In other words, some evidence supports a significant association between the more complex frameworks of meaning employed by subjects high in ego development and greater complexity, as differentiation, in reported nuclear episodes dealing with transformation. As originally stated, therefore, Hypothesis 2 may be too general in that it includes under its consideration a great variety of reported incidents which appear to meet the criteria for nuclear episodes. Ego stage is not related to the number of nuclear episodes as generally defined but does relate significantly to the number of incidents classified in one particular category—life-story turning points.

That men and women at higher stages of ego development should report a greater number of life-story turning points is consistent with Loevinger's (1976) conceptualization of the ego stage hierarchy. At I-4 and beyond, the individual has theoretically broken from conventional standards, values, and orientations inculcated in the conformist (I-3) stage and established a more personalized, individuated perspective on self and on the world. In so doing, the individual has assumedly progressed through a number of changes in ego (the framework of meaning for synthesizing experience) which may be paralleled by life changes marking the transformations. Thus, the person at the higher ego stages may be more likely than his or her counterpart at I-3/4 and below to view his or her life story as a dynamic narrative of change, a story which includes numerous references to who I was, how I am now different from that, and how I may in the future be different than who I am now. The change may be conceived as personal growth. Persons at lower ego stages, having gone through fewer ego stage changes, may tend to see their lives as exemplifying continuity and stability over time: "I am pretty much the same person today as I was 10 or 20 years ago." At the conformist (I-3) and conscientious/conformist (I-3/4) stages in Loevinger's ego scheme, a view of oneself as a creature of change may be relatively incompatible, in fact, with a framework of meaning for self and world which emphasizes conformity, societal convention, and a simple harmony between self and others. To undergo perceived transformations in identity may, in some cases, imply a nonconformist break from the past and from others. Thus, the life episodes which stand out in bold print in the text of the identity story may, for the person at lower ego stages (I-3 and I-3/4), emphasize continuity rather than transformation and stability rather than change.

Nuclear Episodes and the Quality of Life

The content and the organization of our nuclear episodes should reflect the quality of our lives. For Adler, the earliest memories of the neurotic mirrored a defective life fiction—the dysfunctional myth for the future which was at the root of the neurotic's debilitating anxiety. For Maslow, self-actualization was a direct function of the number and quality of an individual's peak experiences. The fully functioning, psychosocially healthy, mature, and authentic human being tended to experience more moments of ecstasy and wonderment than did the common man or woman mired in psychological mediocrity. Neurotics and psychotics were assumed to have even fewer peak experiences. In describing incidents of flow in work and play, Csikszentmihalyi argues for a psychology of optimal human experience. Flow indicates that the individual and the environment are, for the duration of the flow experience, ideally matched or engaged, sympatico. The antithesis of flow is a malaise—boredom and anxiety—which creeps into our lives when we are unable to engage our environments in creative and spontaneous ways, that is, when we are *alienated* from others and from our world.

To say, however, that life's most significant episodes in some way reflect the quality of life is to say something fairly vague. Indeed, it is difficult to be more precise. Most clinicians and theorists speak at a very general level in delineating the ways in which specific incidents in a person's life—those especially salient events which assume an exalted status in biography—are related to such things as adjustment, happiness, satisfaction, and the quality of life. Research is sparse and equally ambiguous. Rizzo and Vinacke (1975) discovered that emotionally positive nuclear episodes (accounts of the "most important personal experiences" in subjects' lives) were positively associated with self-actualization as assessed via a questionnaire. Margoshes and Litt (1966) found that psychotics recalled fewer peak experiences and more nadir experiences than did normals. More recently, psychologists have studied relationships between the number and intensity of stressful life events (such as death of a spouse, loss of a job, change of residence) and a person's overall coping abilities and adjustment (Kobassa, 1979, 1982; Vinokur & Selzer, 1975). Typically employing such a checklist measure of life events as the Holmes and Rahe (1967) Schedule of Recent Life Events, studies of this sort do not explore, for the most part, the idiosyncratic content and organization of an individual's life episodes. This is to say, most empirical investigations of significant life events fail to consider how the particular event has been *reconstructed* by the subject—what meaning the subject has grafted on to the memory of the event. In the context of identity, this is indeed the central issue.

The statistical analyses of the data collected on the midlife men and women in Sample B do not, unfortunately, shed much light on the general issue of nuclear episodes and the quality of life. As in Chapter 4, I drew upon the ratings of career, relationship, and overall job satisfaction made by the subjects. These were correlated with the various indexes of nuclear episodes employed in the present chapter: intimacy and power content in nuclear episodes, number of nuclear episodes in the interview, and number of turning points. These correlations are shown in Table 5.6. Only one of the 42 correlations computed reached statistical significance: Life satisfaction was positively related to intimacy content in peak and positive childhood experiences combined ($r = .30$, $p < .05$). In general, correlations between intimacy theme scores and satisfaction ratings were low and positive, and correlations between power theme scores and satisfaction were low and negative. It does not appear, therefore, that global ratings of present satisfaction with life, career, and relationships bear any consistent and straightforward statistical relation to the indexes of content and complexity in nuclear episodes employed in this chapter.

This does not exhaust the issue, however. The value of a personological investigation of lives resides not only in the derivation and evaluation of general (nomothetic) statements but also in the discov-

TABLE 5.6. Correlations between Various Indexes of Nuclear Episodes and Ratings of Present Satisfaction with Life, Career, and Relationships

	Present Satisfaction		
Nuclear Episodes	*Life*	*Career*	*Relationships*
Intimacy content			
Peak experience	.22	.11	.12
Positive childhood experience	.17	.24	.27*
Peak and positive childhood combined	.30†	.23	.26*
Negative childhood experience	.24	.14	.16
Nadir experience	.01	.13	.11
Negative childhood and nadir combined	.13	.21	.17
Power content			
Peak experience	.06	−.14	.06
Positive childhood experience	−.05	−.12	−.20
Peak and positive childhood combined	.06	−.12	−.01
Negative childhood experience	−.01	−.08	−.23
Nadir experience	−.11	−.15	−.12
Negative childhood and nadir combined	−.06	−.16	−.14
Number of nuclear episodes in interview	.20	.08	.09
Number of nuclear episodes in interview classified as "turning points."	.15	.01	.00

Note: N = 50 (30 women, 20 men) midlife adults.
* $p < .10$
† $p < .05$

ery of more idiographic propositions grounded in the single case. A nuclear episode in the life story of Julie McP. is a classic example. Julie is a 39-year-old market analyst, married with no children, who consented to be tested and interviewed for Sample B. She scored extremely low on intimacy motivation and moderately low on power. Her ego stage was I-3/4. Her reported peak and nadir experiences appear somewhat vague and blunted. Little in the way of strong affective reactions is reported, and neither of these experiences contains any intimacy or power content. Her self-ratings on life, career, and relationship satisfaction are all in the moderate range.

At the beginning of the interview, Julie shows very little affect and appears mildly depressed. Her life story is extremely brief, replete with vague generalizations and unarticulated accounts of happenings probably best described as "mundane." Though she appears to warm up as the interview proceeds, it is not until the very end that she reveals to the listener a quick glimpse of the basic motivations in life which appear to structure her identity. This account of a nuclear episode in Julie's life—the only episode in the interview or on ques-

tionnaires which she describes in an animated and detailed fashion—
tells us more about the quality of her life than all of the other data
combined. The account arises most unexpectedly, in response to the
interviewer's final question in which she asks Julie to depict the
"underlying theme" in her life story:

> Well, we talk a lot about stability and stuff like that, or relinquishing
> responsibility: That's my utopia. I want to be taken care of. I will tell
> you a story that will tell you where I want to be when I grow up.
> About two years ago, I was in the hospital for two weeks. I was sick,
> but I wasn't in pain. I was in a room by myself; I was in isolation. I
> couldn't have visitors. I wasn't on medication; there was no discom-
> fort. I was there for two weeks, and I chose my meals off a menu. I
> got up every morning at six o'clock and took a shower, put on a lit-
> tle make-up, put on a clean nightgown, sat down, had my breakfast,
> read the paper, read a book till noon, watched Julia Child at noon,
> turned off the TV, read a book or whatever till five or so, and then
> my husband came to visit me or I had dinner served. That couple I
> talked about would come to visit. Then everybody'd leave. At 10
> o'clock I'd turn off my lights and go to sleep. After two weeks, I
> didn't want to go home. I didn't want to go home and be faced with
> laundry and housecleaning and dogs that had to be taken out and a
> husband that had to be waited on. And that to me was like I was
> taken care of. I didn't have to cook a meal. I told them what I
> wanted. I only had to take care of myself personally, and other than
> that, I went to bed at 10 o'clock; I went to sleep; I didn't have to take
> a pill or anything; I woke up promptly at six, without an alarm. And
> I know I was really upset when I had to go home. That's the theme.

After reconstructing her life in the interview, Julie has arrived at
some conclusions about who she is and who she would like to become. She chooses to convey her conclusions through an account of
a critical episode in her own life. The episode casts her enigmatic
interview, her mundane and nondescript description of peak and
nadir experiences, and her generally nonrevealing stories composed
for the TAT into an illuminating and coherent frame, a personological
portrait which could not have been painted if it were not for the
interview's last question. Julie is a disgruntled and alienated woman
whose life dream is to be released from her daily responsibilities
vis-à-vis her husband, her job, and her dogs. Her life is neither
animated by intimacy nor power. She does not value close relationships, even with her spouse; she does not appear to delight in
any instrumental pursuits which might enable her to have an impact
or make a mark on her world, however small it may be; she does not
wish to entertain new experiences or take up new challenges; she
does not wish to grow in any sense of the word. Julie wants to be
taken care of. In the middle of her life, she wants to remain passive

as others minister to her needs and whims. Her wish was granted for two weeks a few years ago when she entered the hospital for a reason which remains unexplained. There she was catered to and allowed to do pretty much what she pleased. People did not bother her. Her husband and two friends visited only occasionally, and these interactions were perfectly controlled and calibrated: They could see her for only a few hours in the evening, lest the interactions become too aversive.

The emotional flatness of her questionnaire and interview responses is consistent with Julie's expressed wish for a life free from strong emotions, a life of tranquility and ease. A number of other threads in the interview may be tied to the episode. Her craving for passivity evident in the hospital scene is reflected in the numerous examples in her life story of the environment's shaping Julie rather than Julie's shaping her environment. Things are constantly happening to Julie, and she appears to have no control (and to desire little). In deCharms' (1968) terms, she is a *pawn* rather than an *origin* in her own mind, an expendable item buffeted about by external, supervalent forces. Her passivity and emotional flatness may be traced, again in her own mind, to her early years before age eight. Julie mentions very briefly that she came to the United States when she was eight, and that before that she was a "refugee in Europe." She does not elaborate, claiming that her mind "is a blank before the age of eight." In a clinical setting, these refugee years might be explored in great detail as the therapist and client might investigate the origin myth underlying Julie's sense of who she is, who she was, and who she would like to become. One might speculate further that such an investigation might unearth emotionally laden material in Julie's past and that this material might be subsequently worked through to achieve a variety of therapeutic ends.

Personologists in research and in the clinic may unearth a gold mine of nomothetic and idiographic information by mining more conscientiously the terrain of nuclear episodes. The most significant scenes in an individual's life story may present in a narrative nutshell an essential truth (or fiction) which animates that life. In this chapter, I have sampled a variety of episodes considered by their creators to occupy a special place in their biographies. I have distinguished between episodes of continuity and transformation. I have classified nuclear episodes in terms of the content motifs of power and intimacy and have shown that these motifs reflect fundamental motivational dispositions assessed via the TAT. I have made some initial forays into the domain of nuclear episodes and ego complexity, though the results are rather equivocal. And I have commented briefly on the crucial issue of nuclear episodes and the quality of life. The concerted examination of the nature and function of what Murray would term

significant *proceedings* in lives awaits further investigations in personology employing innovative measurement techniques and a variety of
theoretical frames. In trying to make sense of the lives of our clients
and our subjects and in trying to make sense of our own lives as well,
we would do well to review the scenes in life stories that stand out in
bold print. Why have we chosen these few scenes, from the vast array
of episodes that might make up our biographies, for special treatment? And what do these scenes say about who we are, who we were,
and who we may become in the future?

Summary

Nuclear episodes are the most significant single scenes in a person's life story. These are the events, incidents, or happenings which
stand out in bold print in the story's text. Murray referred to them as
the salient *proceedings* in an individual's life. Other psychologists
have examined the form and function of single, significant life proceedings under the headings of earliest memories, peak and nadir
experiences, ecstasy experiences, flow, and nuclear scenes. In this
chapter, I reviewed a number of these contributions and then made
one of my own, presenting data collected from the 90 college students
in Sample A and the 50 midlife adults in Sample B. In questionnaires
and in interviews, these subjects were asked to give accounts of the
episodes in their lives which they deemed particularly significant.
These episodes were classified in a variety of ways and interpreted in
the contexts of power and intimacy motivation and ego development.
When nuclear episodes are seen as key incidents in an evolving
identity saga, they can be broadly classified into two general types:
episodes of continuity and episodes of change. Episodes of continuity
connect the present with the past via an implicit narrative line which
suggests that the past nuclear episode serves as an explanation for or
a foreshadowing of some aspect of one's present life situation. Episodes of continuity, thus, may function as "origin myths" detailing
the genesis of a particular value or value system, perceived personality trait, or any other characterological attribution made by the
individual with reference to the self. Episodes of continuity may also
function as encapsulated "affirmations" which depict in a narrative
nutshell some essential characterological dimension. In this case, the
episode displays a fundamental aspect of the person's view of himself
or herself in an extraordinarily clear and convincing manner. The
individual may consider the episode as "proof from my past" that "I
am what I am."
In episodes of change or transformation, however, the incidents
mark turning points in life stories. These may signal the end of one
chapter and the beginning of another. Episodes of change may be

positive or negative in affective tone, and indeed some of the clearest cases are reported as life-story low points. The individual may speak of "bottoming out" or "turning the corner" in the case of moving from a deteriorating life situation to an improving one. In some other cases, the language suggests the reverse: a "turn for the worse," a "loss of innocence," a "fall from grace."

Another way to classify nuclear episodes is to code the prominence of content themes associated with power and intimacy. In this chapter, a number of different kinds of nuclear episodes—some positive and some negative in affective tone—were scored for themes of power and intimacy. In positive nuclear episodes, four prominent power themes are strength, impact, action, and status, and four prominent intimacy themes are communication/sharing, friendship/ love, sympathy, and touch. In negative nuclear episodes, power themes include weakness/failure, losing face, ignorance, and conflict, and intimacy themes include separation, rejection, disillusionment about people, and witnessing another's misfortune. Hypothesis 1, introduced in Chapter 2, stated that power motivation on the TAT should be positively associated with the number of power themes detected in nuclear episodes while intimacy motivation should be positively associated with intimacy themes. Results from Samples A and B provided a good deal of support for the hypothesis, though not all of the findings were consistent. In general, the relationships between power motivation and power themes in nuclear episodes were stronger than the relationships between intimacy motivation and intimacy themes. Taken as a whole, the results illustrate a thematic continuity in lives, a mirroring of salient motivational themes in accounts of significant life episodes. The most salient underlying motives in our lives appear to color our recollections of the past by underscoring particular content themes in the especially critical episodes of the stories we tell ourselves in order to live.

Hypothesis 2 states that persons at high stages of ego development should report a greater number of nuclear episodes than should those scoring low in ego development. Complex life stories should have a greater number of significant story scenes, such as turning points, affirmations, and origin myths. Relatively simple stories, on the other hand, should contain fewer of these scenes as the narratives should unfold in a relatively straightforward, even linear, manner, reminiscent of Hemingway's *The Old Man and the Sea*. Hypothesis 2 was tested in Sample B by relating ego stage scores to the number of nuclear episodes detected in life-story interviews. The hypothesis was not supported. A second look at the data, however, revealed that whereas adults high in ego development did not report more nuclear episodes in life stories than did those low in ego development, the high-ego men and women *did* report more nuclear episodes classified as "turning points"—that is, episodes of change or transformation.

Thus, the person at the higher ego stages may be more likely than his or her counterpart at I-3/4 and below to view his or her life story as a dynamic *narrative of change*, a story which includes numerous references to who I was, how I am now different from that, and how I may in the future be different than who I am. The change may be conceived as personal growth. Persons at lower ego stages, having gone through fewer ego stage changes, may tend to see their lives as exemplifying stability over time: "I am pretty much the same person today as I was 10 or 20 years ago." At the conformist (I-3) and conscientious/conformist (I-3/4) stages, a view of oneself as a creature of change may be incompatible with a framework of meaning for self and world which emphasizes conformity, societal convention, and a simple harmony between self and others.

The chapter concluded by considering the relationships between nuclear episodes and the quality of life. Correlational results concerning self-reports of life satisfaction and various indexes of nuclear episodes for Sample B were generally disappointing. Intimacy themes, power themes, overall number of nuclear episodes detected, and number of nuclear episodes classified as turning points were not related in any straightforward way to satisfaction ratings on career, relationships, and one's overall life. Yet, nuclear episodes often seem to reflect the overall *quality* of an individual's life, and this point was illustrated with the brief case of Julie McP. Clinicians and researchers would do well to consider in more idiographic detail the form and function of nuclear episodes in the lives of their clients and their subjects. And, indeed, all of us might gain some insight into our own identities by examining the scenes in our life stories which appear to stand out in bold print. Why have we chosen these few scenes for special biographical treatment? And what do these scenes say about who we are, who we were, and who we may become in the future?

NOTES

[1] A small portion of this chapter first appeared in McAdams, D. P. (1982). Experiences of intimacy and power: Relationships between social motives and autobiographical memory. *Journal of Personality and Social Psychology, 42*, 292–302.

[2] Nuclear episodes identified in the life-story interviews were each classified as either a life-story turning point or "something else." Further analyses of these data are reported toward the end of this chapter. Examples of turning points were also gleaned from the written accounts of peak, nadir, positive childhood, and negative childhood experiences produced by subjects in both samples.

[3] Two independent coders scored the peak experiences and satisfying experiences in terms of these content categories, with 4 as the maximum score for power and 5 for intimacy. For the accounts of neutral and unpleasant experiences, however, each of the scoring categories was changed somewhat to accommodate the quality of the experience reported. For the neutral experiences, the changes basically involved broadening the criteria to adjust to the more mundane and affectively neutral content of these experiences. For unpleasant experiences, the changes substituted the subject's reported *failure* to experience the desired state (theme) for the presence of the theme itself.

Content coding reliabilities between the two scorers were quite high. For the first sample in this study ($N = 56$), the correlation between the two coders' independent scores for power content in peak experiences was $r = .83$, and for intimacy content it was $r = .91$. For the second sample ($N = 86$), the correlation for power content in the four experiences was $r = .82$, and for intimacy content it was $r = .88$. When the two coders' scores did not agree for a given memory, the average of the two scores was used in the data analysis.

[4] Data for the second sample in this study ($N = 86$) were also analyzed using analysis of variance (ANOVA). A two-way ANOVA for repeated measures assessing the effects of intimacy motivation (high or low, broken at the median score) and type of experience (peak, satisfying, neutral, unpleasant) on intimacy content in the memories showed a significant main effect for both motive score, $F(1,71) = 16.02$, $p < .001$, and type of experience, $F(3,213) = 6.62$, $p < .001$, as well as a significant interaction of intimacy motivation $\times$ type of experience, $F(3,213) = 3.01$, $p < .03$. Another two-way ANOVA for repeated measures assessing the effect of power motivation (high versus low) and type of experience on power content in memories produced parallel results, with a main effect for both power motive score, $F(1,69) = 10.05$, $p < .01$, and type of experience, $F(3,207) = 6.93$, $p < .001$, and a significant interaction effect of power motive $\times$ type of experience, $F(3,207) = 3.99$, $p < .03$. The significant interaction effects indicate that the effect of a social motive on motive-related thematic content in the memories was most pronounced for the peak and satisfying experiences, a result also reflected in the correlational analysis.

[5] The reader will note that I have switched from the five intimacy themes used in the preliminary investigation (McAdams, 1982b) to four. The theme called interpersonal in McAdams (1982b) has been dropped from the present analysis. I now believe that this theme was indeed too general and common to be of much use in discriminating episodes on the basis of intimacy. Indeed, the same theme could justifiably be used to characterize many power experiences in which the subject has an influence on others (impact) or gains recognition or prestige (status). We are thus left with four themes of intimacy which correspond to intimacy themes 2–5 in McAdams (1982b).

[6] The only difference was that the four intimacy themes (2–5 in McAdams, 1982b) were used instead of five.

[7] Interscorer reliability for power content in positive nuclear episodes (peak and positive childhood experiences) was $r = .81$. For intimacy content, reliability was $r = .85$. When the two coders' scores did not agree for a given memory, the average of the two scores was used in the data analysis.

[8] Interscorer reliability for power content in negative nuclear episodes (nadir and negative childhood experiences) was $r = .82$. For intimacy content, reliability was $r = .90$. When the two coders' scores did not agree for a given memory, the average of the two scores was used in the data analysis.

[9] Accounts of individuals' earliest memories were collected from the college students in Sample A. Unfortunately for the purposes of our analyses, many of these

accounts were rather banal and lacking in feeling tone, reminiscent of Kihlstrom and Harackiewicz's (1982) characterization of screen memories. Because they were framed in terms of experiences charged with positive (peak) or negative (nadir) emotions, our coding categories for power and intimacy content in nuclear episodes did not accommodate well the varieties of content detectable in earliest memories. Consequently, the power and intimacy categories for both positive and negative nuclear episodes were broadened to include events and actions similar, though perhaps not identical, to the original characterizations.

Two independent coders, blind to motive scores, coded the earliest memories according to these broadened criteria for power and intimacy themes. Correlations between these scores and power and intimacy motivation were calculated. The results indicated that little if any relationship between motivational profile on the TAT and power/intimacy content in earliest memories appears to exist. All correlations were statistically insignificant for the entire sample and for the men alone. For the women, only one relationship reached statistical significance: intimacy motivation was positively related ($r = .30$) to friendship/love in earliest memories.

[10] Combining the preliminary investigation (McAdams, 1982b) and the results reported for Samples A and B, substantial empirical relationships between TAT social motives and themes of power and intimacy in peak experiences have now been documented in three college samples and one sample of men and women at midlife. The consistently robust correlations suggest the possibility that the thematic coding of peak experiences, and perhaps accounts of other nuclear episodes as well, might serve as an alternative, adjunct methodology for the direct scoring of power and intimacy motivation. The TAT, as a measure of social motives, has traditionally aroused some criticism among psychometricians and other scientists concerned with the instrument's measurement qualities, especially test–retest reliability and internal consistency (see Entwistle, 1972; Klinger, 1966). Critics of the TAT have argued that the study of social motives is relatively method-bound, anchored too strongly to a single measurement method—the TAT—which is psychometrically suspect and generally uncorrelated with questionnaire measures designed to assess similar, if not identical, personality constructs. Though defenders of the TAT have offered some compelling theoretical and empirical rebuttals (Atkinson, 1981; McClelland, 1981; Winter & Stewart, 1977), most observers would agree that the TAT *should* yield motive scores which correlate with those obtained through *some* other measurement methodology, perhaps another thematic methodology (deCharms & Muir, 1978).

Though we have collected no data which speak directly to this issue, we put forth the possibility that the thematic coding of certain nuclear episodes such as peak experiences might qualify as just such a method. It is indeed possible, moreover, that this kind of motivational assessment would be less subject to the perceived psychometric foibles associated with the TAT. Surely the possibility will remain merely a possibility until empirical research is undertaken on the problem. The most promising line of research might entail some combination or pooling (Epstein, 1979) of intimacy or power motive scores obtained from stories written to certain TAT pictures and accounts of certain nuclear episodes, such as peak experiences. By combining the methods, the psychologist may be able to converge on the crucial topic of human motivation from two complementary angles.

[11] The judge was instructed to record only those incidents in the person's life which resembled Murray's characterization of a proceeding and Tomkins' concept of the scene. This is to say, the episode needed to be well circumscribed in time and place if it were to be transcribed. It had to be a happening, complete with a setting, characters, and action which occurred on a given day or during a relatively short time frame and in a specified geographical place. Longer episodes span longer periods of time and

a variety of places as in the case of, say, a person's account of a beautiful summer spent in northern Maine. These longer, more diffuse episodes seemed to border on life chapters in and of themselves, and thus were excluded from consideration.

[12] "Something else" simply refers to an episode which is not classified as a turning point. These episodes showed a good deal of variety in function and form and were not classified further. Interscorer reliability for turning points was determined through a correlation between the two coders' scores for the number of turning points observed per subject: $r = .89$.

Chapter 6

Imagoes[1]

> *The total archetypal system—what Jung termed 'the Self'—has pro-grammed within it the complete scenario for individual life. As the story unfolds, new archetypal motifs emerge, expressing the point which the ac-tion has reached. Much of the time we pay little attention to this inner theatre, which will never close till the very end of the last act, but occasionally—more often if in analysis—one finds oneself suddenly on stage, committed to a part of the performance. At such moments an arche-type has taken hold and one is transfigured by its numinous intensity.*
>
> (Anthony Stevens, 1983, p. 76)

The stories we tell ourselves in order to live are populated by characters whose roles personify profound identity truths. At the developmental dawn of identity formation, the young George Bernard Shaw presents a cast of at least three prominent characters in beginning a first narrative rendering of his life. Introducing the prob-lem of ego identity and its place in the human life cycle through an identity sketch of Shaw at age 20, Erik Erikson (1959) identifies the three protagonists as "The Snob," "The Noisemaker," and "The Di-abolical One." Like "The Father," "The Son as Mute," and "The Son as Spokesman" in the life story of young Martin Luther (Chapter 2), the three central characters for Shaw are identity fragments whose narrative integration is young Shaw's most pressing psychosocial task. Like characters in literature, the three are conceptualized as *persons* or *personified* entities. Their actions and interactions define the story plot.

Shaw saw himself as a snob raised in a family of snobs. Erikson quotes and comments upon Shaw's autobiography, written as a sep-tuagenarian:

> "As compared with similar English families, we had a power of deri-sive dramatization that made the bones of the Shavian skeletons rat-

tle more loudly." Shaw recognizes this as "family snobbery mitigated by the family sense of humor." On the other hand, "though my mother was not consciously a snob, the divinity which hedged an Irish lady of her period was acceptable to the British suburban parents, all snobs, who were within her reach (as customers for private music lessons)." Shaw had "an enormous contempt for family snobbery," until he found that one of his ancestors was an Earl of Fife: "It was as good as being descended from Shakespeare, whom I had been unconsciously resolved to reincarnate from my cradle". (Erikson, 1959, p. 107)

A remnant of his childhood past, the image of self as The Snob was not to be renounced in adulthood but rather reincorporated into an identity narrative which was to bind together past, present, and an anticipated future reinforcing that sense of sameness and continuity which is the hallmark of identity.

Shaw and his family delighted in making music. They played "trombones and opicleides, violincellos, harps, and tambourines" (Erikson, 1959, p. 107), and they all sang. The music making gave birth to the image of self as The Noisemaker. Shaw taught himself the piano and tormented his mother by banging out his favorite selections from Wagner's Ring. Later, he became a music critic, or as Erikson puts it "one who *writes* about the noise made by others" (p. 108, italics in original). Shaw the music critic wrote under the pseudonym Corno di Bassetto, "actually the name of an instrument which nobody knew and which is so meek in tone that 'not even the devil could make it sparkle' " (p. 108). Bassetto was an occasionally strident critic who made a prodigious amount of noise. Again, Erikson quotes Shaw:

> I cannot deny that Bassetto was occasionally vulgar; but that does not matter if he makes you laugh. Vulgarity is a necessary part of a complete author's equipment; and the clown is sometimes the best part of the circus. (Erikson, 1959, p. 108)

The third character, The Diabolical One, is also traced to Shaw's childhood years. Composing literary prayers for "the entertainment and propitiation of the Almighty" (p. 108, Shaw speaking), the little boy adopted his family's general irreverence vis-à-vis religion and played the "little devil of a child" who might defy and tease the Creator above. Erikson writes that Shaw the child "did not feel identical with himself when he was good: 'Even when I was a good boy, I was so only theatrically, because, as actors say, I saw myself in the character' " (p. 108). The "upgrowing moustaches and eyebrows" and the "sarcastic nostrils" of the young man were, as characterized by Shaw himself, somatic reflections of the attitudes of the Diabolical One, which "I had sung as a child" and "affected in my boyhood" and which were to continue to manifest themselves throughout Shaw's adult years (p. 108).

Erikson describes the identity turmoil of the young George Bernard Shaw who wished simultaneously to separate himself from and discover new connections to his childhood and adolescent past. The crisis was resolved, according to Erikson, when Shaw forged an integration of the three major characters and the numerous other roles he sought to play via a superordinate image of self as an "actor," capable of creating "for myself a fantastic personality fit and apt for dealing with men, and adaptable to the various parts I had to play as author, journalist, orator, politician, committee man, man of the world, and so forth" (p. 109, Shaw speaking). Thus, images of self as The Snob, The Noisemaker, and The Diabolical One are nested within larger images of self—"The Actor"—as identity reveals an hierarchic structure of personified life-story characters. Erikson considers this kind of hierarchic integration of images of self to be a sign of mature identity.

The Snob, The Noisemaker, and The Diabolical One are examples of what I am terming in this chapter *imagoes*. Imagoes are *idealized and personified images of self* which function as *characters* in the life stories which are our identities. This chapter is about an initial exploration into the imagoes I have tried to bring to light in the life stories of men and women at midlife (Sample B). This chapter is indeed the most exploratory and speculative of all the chapters. Imagoes are the most difficult to operationalize of all the constructs thus far set forth. Yet, they are potentially the most revealing of the secrets of human identities. I will begin with a brief theoretical overview of concepts related to the imago. Then, I will record initial observations of imagoes in the life stories of the 50 midlife adults making up Sample B. A coding system for imagoes, based on a taxonomy of gods and goddesses in Greek mythology, is then introduced—a system which arose inductively out of my initial observations. Imagoes of power and of intimacy are described in detail as are images of self which combine both power and intimacy and those which appear to personify neither. Relationships between social motives and ego development and the content and structure of imagoes are examined. Finally, I will take up the critical issue of the integration of imagoes as a sign of maturity in identity.

Theoretical Background

Archetypes

The term *imago* was sometimes used by Carl Jung (1943) when referring to his structural concept better known as the *archetype*. An archetype was a universal thought form charged with emotion. Inhabiting the inherited phylogenetic memory or "collective unconscious" of every human being, archetypes suggested unconscious images corresponding to universal experiences of the human species as it has evolved for thousands of years. Archetypes were inherited templates of universal human experience, and the unconscious images they brought forth were matched by the individual to elements of his or her waking life to produce in each generation the repetition and elaboration of the same experiences. For example, the archetype of the "earth mother" creates an internal image in the young child of a mother figure which is then identified with the actual caregiver. Dreams, mythology, religion, folklore, and art are rich sources of archetypal expression as the creative productions of human beings have, since the dawn of civilization, reflected certain universal images and patterns of experience.

In a theoretical synthesis of Jung and modern ethology, Stevens (1983) characterizes archetypes as inherent neuropsychic systems, analogous to what the ethologists term *innate releasing mechanisms*, which are responsible for certain universal patterns of behavior emitted in the presence of an appropriate member of the same species. Included are many behavior patterns which appear to follow an instinctive, though flexible, goal-corrected blueprint (Bowlby, 1969), such as the zigzag mating dance of certain bees and the development of the mother-infant attachment bond in humans. Archetypes, thus, are instinctive patterns of behaving and experiencing which have evolved over the course of human phylogeny and survived because they confer upon species members a selective advantage in adaptation. They are what the sociobiologist E. O. Wilson (1978) would consider genetically programmed features of human nature, and they promote the universal behaviors and experiences which have enabled the species to survive and flourish. As Stevens describes it, "The archetypal endowment with which each of us is born presupposes the natural life cycle of our species—being mothered, exploring the environment, playing in the peer group, adolescence, being initiated, establishing a place in the social hierarchy, courting, marrying, child rearing, hunting, gathering, fighting, participating in religious rituals, assuming the social responsibilities of advanced maturity, and preparation for death" (p. 40).

Jungians have catalogued a host of archetypes doubly rooted in phylogeny and ontogeny. These include the hero, the wise old man, the earth mother, the demon, the child, birth, rebirth, death, power, and magic. Note that the first five of these are *personified*, but the latter five are more abstract or conceptual. (The earth mother is a person; death is a concept.) Some archetypes have evolved to become separate systems within the personality: the *persona* or that aspect of self which is presented for public viewing; and *anima* or unconscious feminine side of the male; the *animus* or unconscious masculine side of the female; and the *shadow* or embodiment of socially reprehensible thoughts, feelings, and actions rooted in our animal ancestry.

Archetypes are frequently couched in terms of opposites: the anima and animus, the wise old man and the child, the earth mother and the great father. The goal of psychological development, or what Jung termed *individuation*, is the reconciliation of paired opposites. This involves an integration of the conscious and the unconscious and a blending of antithetical archetypal images of self. The mandala was Jung's symbol for the unity of self—an accomplishment usually saved for midlife—in which all dualities were dissolved in psychic harmony.

Internalized Objects

The concept of an *internalized object* appears in a variety of personality theories, especially those emphasizing interpersonal relations. Common to all of these is the idea of semiautonomous parts of the self which are products of the introjection (internalization, incorporation) of personified images derived from relationships with significant others. Personality theories developed by Sullivan, Fairbairn, Winnicott, Jacobson, Kernberg, and Kohut all posit internalized objects which influence behavior and experience in sometimes dramatic ways and which interact with each other in an interpsychic arena just beyond our awareness. Predating all of these is Freud's (1923/1961) characterization of the ego ideal (and the superego), which existed as an internalized image of parents created via identification with the parents (or aspects of the parents) at the close of the Oedipus complex.

In his interpersonal theory of psychiatry, Sullivan (1953) spoke of *personifications* built up in the course of individual development. A personification was conceived as an image that an individual has of himself or herself or of another person, an amalgam of feelings, attitudes, and expectations growing out of childhood experiences of need gratification and struggles with anxiety. Rudimentary elements of the child's evolving self-system, personifications often appear as opposites: "the good mother" (built around experiences of need gratification and pleasure in the presence of the mothering one) and "the bad mother" (a result of experiences of tension and anxiety with the same mothering one). Sometimes personifications appear in threes: "the good me," "the bad me," and "the not me." Though inevitable results of normal as well as abnormal development, personifications are nonveridical images of reality, which is to say that they do not correspond well, in any objective sense, to the persons in the outside world who exist as their sources. As the child grows older, personifications fuse into larger configurations, as is the case when the individual blends the good mother and the bad mother into an integrative representation of mother *in toto*.

Internalized objects are the conceptual centerpieces of theories of personality which fall under the general rubric of *object-relations theories*. One of the more influential theorists in this tradition is Fairbairn (1952). Replacing Freud's id with an object-seeking ego present at birth, Fairbairn proposes that individuals compose, from the first day of life, internal images of persons (objects) in their environments. These internalized objects assume an astounding degree of independence from reality as they enact dramatic scenarios on an unconscious interpsychic stage. Healthy psychological development, according to Fairbairn, is a matter of freeing oneself, to the extent possible, from the distorting and debilitating effect of the internal upon the external—of scenarios enacted by internalized objects at an interpsychic level upon interpersonal relations in the real world. To see external relationships through an objective lens, rather than through the distorted spectacles of internalized objects, is to reach Fairbairn's transcendent developmental level termed *mature dependency*. The antithesis of mature dependency is the schizoid personality, the individual whose ego is rife with deep fissures resulting from traumatic interpersonal experiences which have combined to give birth to a host of internalized bad objects. Narcissistic and delusional, incapable of investing affect in external relationships, the schizoid withdraws from reality and retreats to a fantasy kingdom of internalized objects, a safe haven from the frustration and loss which have haunted past relationships.

In a somewhat different vein, Jacobson (1964) writes of the *wished-for self-image,* which is considered an autonomous part of the ego made up of those valued and admired qualities and attributes that are associated with significant others and that the individual longs to make his or her own. Developmentally, the wished-for self-image arises after the child comes to understand that he (she) and the mother are two and that "magical fusion" is an impossibility. Unlike Freud's notion of the ego ideal, the wished-for self-image contains no moral dimension but rather concerns itself with more primitive issues, such as power and effectiveness. Milrod (1982) writes that behavior guided by the wished-for self-image is

> self-interested and is aimed at strengthening the self representation. Concern for others is not of any importance. The wished-for self-image is supremely narcissistic in this sense. (p. 98)

States and Scripts

The approach to personality and psychotherapy labeled *transactional analysis* presents a number of concepts which bear some resemblance to what I am calling in this chapter imagoes. Proponents of this approach, such as Berne (1972) and Steiner (1974), describe three personified *ego states*—the parent, child, and adult—each associated, in many cases, with characteristic patterns of interaction, gestures, mannerisms, facial expressions, intonations, and verbal utterances. Problems in living frequently involve interpersonal interactions in which an ego state manifested by one person is incompatible with that manifested by another. Personified self-images which are more individualized than ego states include *scripts* that people live. When one behaves according to a script, writes Steiner (1974), one is merely playacting and therefore failing to live life in an authentic and spontaneous manner. Particularly stultifying are the "banal" scripts of men and women. For men, these include "Big Daddy," "Playboy," "Jock," "Intellectual," and "Woman Hater." For women there are more: "Mother Hubbard" (the woman behind the family), "Plastic Woman," "Poor Little Me," "Creeping Beauty," "Nurse," "Fat Woman," "Teacher," "Tough Lady," and "Queen Bee." Like Jung's archetypes, the protagonists of Steiner's scripts typically imply their opposites; that is, scripts are typically joined to counterscripts. The therapist should seek to understand both script and counterscript in attempting to facilitate the client's replacement of scripted behavior with spontaneity.

Similar to the scheme implicit in the writings of Berne and Steiner is the framework for understanding psychotherapy proposed by Horowitz (1979). Corresponding to Berne's ego states are what Horowitz terms simply *states*, "recurrent patterns of experience and of behavior that is both verbal and nonverbal" (p. 31). In the course of psychotherapy with one Janice, Horowitz observes six states which appear to manifest themselves in cycles. Two are what he calls "tra-la-la" and "acute self-disgust." The former is a cavalier, cheerful, lighthearted state of mind; the latter is dark, nasty, and cynical. Each state is connected to a particular image of self. In the case of tra-la-la, we have Janice the active, competent, creative, and sexual woman whose interactions with others fly by with ease. For acute self-disgust, the image of self is a version of Janice's mother: the defective, fat, lazy, and egocentric woman, disgusting to others and to herself. The therapist's task is to identify the particular states and corresponding self-images of the client, to evaluate their assets and liabilities, and to assist in the construction of mature self-images to replace more primitive and dysfunctional ones.

Conclusion

My concept of the imago is at the same time more general and more specific than these other concepts. Unlike Jung's structural components of the collective unconscious, life-story imagoes are by definition personified and exist not as part of a phylogenetic col-

lectivity but rather as highly personalized, idiosyncratic images defining how a person is different from others as well as similar to them.
Like characters in good fiction, imagoes are carefully crafted by the
author—the person constructing identity—to be highly individualized. Unlike Sullivan's personifications, imagoes refer solely to images of self, though images of others may be incorporated into images
of self. The writings of Fairbairn, Jacobson, Berne, and Horowitz all
set forth specific propositions concerning the development of various
personified images (internalized objects, wished-for self-images, ego
states, scripts) and concerning their structure and function which are
not essential to my conceptualization of the imagoes in life stories. At
present, I do not know how imagoes develop. They are structured as
personified and idealized images of self, highly individualized and
created to play roles in specific life stories. Their function is that of
character in narrative.

Certain other themes in the writings of these theorists, however,
are quite consistent with this chapter's view and will be echoed in the
data later described. For Jung, Sullivan, and Berne, personified self-
images are typically arranged in pairs of opposites. For Jung and
Sullivan, the merging of these opposites is a hallmark of psychological maturity. Jacobson, too, speaks of the integration of various
wished-for self-images into more complex and coherent wholes as the
child matures. We will see that imagoes can be very usefully comprehended as pairs of opposites, dialectically related as thesis and antithesis. The integration of opposites (synthesis) is witnessed in the best
of life stories—the most mature identities.

Imagoes at Midlife

Initial Observations

I will consider data from Sample B only.[2] This is the midlife
sample of 30 women and 20 men who were administered a number of
psychological tests and interviewed on the topic of their life stories
(see Appendix B for the interview questions). It was in the life-story
interviews that my associates and I hoped we might gain some insight
into the dominant images of self populating our subjects' identities.
Thus, we conducted our initial observations without having access to
information on the participants obtained outside the interview, such
as motive scores and stage of ego development.

We began by listening to 25 of the 50 taped interviews and
recording detailed summaries of the factual information provided by
the subjects. In our first run through the tapes, we sought merely to
encapsule in four to seven typed pages each the face-value information provided by each interviewee, eschewing for the time being all

interpretation. In a second listening, we added any factual information we might have missed the first time through and then composed,
for each interview, a one- to two-page interpretive essay focusing on
what we perceived to be the one or two dominant images of self that
each story implied. Guided by our reading of Erikson on George
Bernard Shaw as well as the other theorists reviewed above, we
sought to identify personified and idealized images of self which
appeared to connect a wide variety of statements made in the interview, such as reported aspirations in the past and for the future,
significant biographical events, attitudes and beliefs, central commitments, significant others, and interpretive reflections of the subject
himself or herself. In most, but not all, of the interviews, we were able
to come up with at least one dominant image of self for which we
could garner substantial life-story evidence.[3]

Listening to the interviews, we were initially struck by the fairly
common appearance of two conflicting images of self, or imagoes, in
many of the adults' accounts. Though our sample was made up of
relatively "normal" and well-adjusted men and women, many of
them described their past lives and hopes for the future *as if* they
were inhabited by "multiple personalities" or discordant subselves,
typically two of these posed as opposites on some fundamental dimension. In stories of self that generally revealed little pathology but
marked multiplicity of self-conception, some individuals explicitly or
implicitly connected these divergent imagoes to specific significant
others in their lives (e.g., heroes, role models, friends), specific childhood experiences which seemed to serve as origin myths for personified images of self, and specific biographical epochs in which a particular imago was ascendant in behavior and experience while the
other appeared to lie dormant.

Consider the following brief example of Curt R. A 39-year-old
editor at a publishing house, unmarried, well-traveled, and earning
what he considered a very modest salary (around $15,000 annually),
Curt repeatedly described himself as the "artist." Creative, imaginative, somewhat Bohemian, but always refined, the artist image
integrated a host of expressed values (aesthetics, culture, good taste),
interests (classical music, visual arts, literature, gourmet cooking),
avocations and activities (writing children's literature, teaching arts
and crafts in schools and churches, making beautiful things), role
models and heroes (an older mentor, his mother), and biographical
events illustrating the perceived "birth and growth" of the artist
imago. Yet a second imago had recently manifested itself with a vengeance. Described as an opposite or at least contrary image of self
vis-à-vis the artist, the "successful, worldly, money maker" had of
late assumed a dominant place in Curt's aspirations for the future.
Taking stock of his life in his late 30s, Curt had tentatively decided he

wanted to make money and accumulate material possessions more than he wanted to be the artist. A number of biographical elements could be connected to this second imago. The two images of self, therefore, defined a central conflict or tension in this man's life story, a conflict that might be described as that between art and reality, aesthetics and economics, transcendent beauty and worldly pragmatics. Curt implied that a major goal for the future was to integrate in some way these two discordant imagoes.

As in the case of the artist versus the money maker, we attempted to provide a short label for each imago encountered in the interviews. The names for imagoes that we agreed upon for each of the initial 25 interviews are presented in Figure 6.1.[4] Two characteristics of this presentation are noteworthy. First, for those cases in which we were able to identify two imagoes juxtaposed as opposites on some dimension, the two are separated by a slash (/). In many of these cases, we first identified the imago listed first (the one on the

FIGURE 6.1. A First Ordering of Imago Names Based on Initial Observations of 25 Midlife Subjects

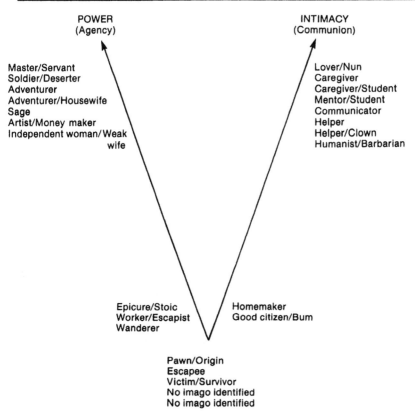

POWER
(Agency)

INTIMACY
(Communion)

Master/Servant
Soldier/Deserter
Adventurer
Adventurer/Housewife
Sage
Artist/Money maker
Independent woman/Weak
    wife

Lover/Nun
Caregiver
Caregiver/Student
Mentor/Student
Communicator
Helper
Helper/Clown
Humanist/Barbarian

Epicure/Stoic
Worker/Escapist
Wanderer

Homemaker
Good citizen/Bum

Pawn/Origin
Escapee
Victim/Survivor
No imago identified
No imago identified

left) and then searched for evidence for some kind of opposite. Indeed, we were motivated to find opposites given our readings of Jung, Sullivan, and Berne. Second, the initial imago names in Figure 6.1 are arranged into three clusters along two vectors—a vector denoting power (or Bakan's agency) and one denoting intimacy (Bakan's communion). Names of imagoes in the upper left cluster, therefore, bespeak power—images of self as a strong, effective, forceful agent—whereas those located in the upper right cluster suggest intimacy. Those in the lower center cluster suggest neither power nor intimacy.

A Taxonomy of Imagoes

Our next step was to make more explicit what we had implicitly been doing in our initial analyses of the 25 cases. We attempted to formulate a list of criteria for the identification of an imago, minimum conditions that an imago must meet. Our case discussions led us to the conclusion that no single criterion nor single combination of criteria would cover all of the 25 cases reviewed so far. Therefore, we settled on a list of conditions that would apply to the "ideal" imago—a perfect prototype. We agreed that the prototypical imago was an idealized and personified image of self reflected in the following features of the life-story interview:

1. *An origin myth.* The person should describe a biographical event or series of events which gave birth to the imago, functioning as a biographical explanation for the genesis of a particular self-image.

2. *A significant other.* The imago should be incarnate in at least one other significant person in the individual's life. This person may have served as a role model, mentor, or object of identification for the subject.

3. *Associated personality traits.* The imago should be characterized by a set of personality traits which it exemplifies.

4. *Associated wishes, aspirations, goals, occupational or interpersonal strivings.* The imago should be reflected in what the person would like to accomplish during his or her life; who the person would like to become.

5. *Associated behaviors.* The imago should be reflected in numerous incidents in which the person behaves in a way that is commensurate with the imago.

6. *Philosophy of life.* The imago should be consistent with some aspect of the person's expressed philosophy of life or with some part of his or her answer to the question concerning the underlying theme in the life story. (See the interview questions reproduced in Appendix B.)

7. *An antiimago.* The imago should be dialectically connected to an opposite image of self for which the six criteria above are applicable. The imago and antiimago define a central conflict in the person's life story.

No single imago identified in the 25 interviews met all seven criteria, but all of them (except the two cases in which no imago could be identified) appeared to meet at least two of the criteria. Still, whether or not an imago identified by one listener adequately meets the criteria listed above is a matter of interpretation, of making an argument for a particular point of view. In our case discussions, contrary arguments for the same case were frequently offered, and we attempted for each to reach some kind of tentative consensus, weighing the strong and weak points of each listener's interpretation of the case. Nonetheless, our initial discussions were fairly chaotic because we still lacked a definitive list of the possibilities for labeling imagoes. In other words, the possibilities in coding were infinite as long as the listener might draw upon any imago label he or she saw fit to characterize the case and the supporting evidence. One could add labels to Figure 6.1 till the end of time: The only limitation would be the number of appropriate nouns contained in the English language. We needed a taxonomy of imago labels in order to limit the possibilities and thereby anchor our interpretations to something solid and circumscribed.

Impressed with the rich diversity of personified self-images presented by our midlife subjects, we endeavored to derive a rudimentary classification system within which imagoes might be ordered. We have tentatively settled on a taxonomy grounded in the mythology of Ancient Greece. On one level, the gods and goddesses of the Greek pantheon represent projected personifications of what the Greeks understood as fundamental human propensities and strivings. Larger and more powerful than mortals, the Greek deities made love and war, experienced rage, envy, and joy, and performed acts of heroism and ignominy in ways remarkably human. Each of the major deities, furthermore, personified a distinctive set of personality traits which were repeatedly manifested in the myths and legends in which his or her behavior can be observed. We chose 12 major gods and goddesses as our models for imagoes. Taken together, the group embodies most of the idealized and personified self-images we observed in the initial 25 cases.

The Greek prototypes for imagoes are organized along the two independent thematic lines of power/agency/mastery/conquest and intimacy/communion/care/surrender. Class 1 imagoes are power imagoes: *Zeus*, the omnipotent and omniscient source; *Hermes*, the swift traveler; and *Ares*, the warrior. Class 3 imagoes are intimacy imagoes: *Demeter*, the caregiver; *Hera*, the friend; *Aphrodite*, the lover. Class 2 imagoes combine power and intimacy: *Apollo*, the healer/artist/ protector; *Athene*, goddess of peace and prudence; and *Prometheus*, the revolutionary. Finally, Class 4 imagoes are "low" in power and intimacy: *Hestia*, the homemaker; *Hephaestus*, the worker; and *Dionysius*, the escapist.[5] Table 6.1 presents a detailed description of our first attempt at a taxonomy of imagoes. We expect that future research will lead to significant modifications in the taxonomy, but for now it is the best we have.

TABLE 6.1. A Taxonomy of Imagoes

Class 1

Class 1 imagoes are personifications of agency (power) and therefore exhibit agency's defining features: self-expansion, self-assertion, self-protection, self-display, mastery, and conquest. They are powerful figures who separate themselves from the environment through physical and/or mental acts of strength.

1A. Zeus—the omnipotent and omniscient source.

Variants:

1. Patriarch/Sovereign/Judge: to rule, to judge, to provide the final authority.
2. Conqueror/Seducer: to overcome, to divide and conquer, to make "mine."
3. Creator/Provider/Source: to father, to provide life, to provide the essentials for life, to initiate, to create.
4. Sage/Wise one: to know all, to gain wisdom, to answer all questions.
5. Celebrity/Star: to be adored, admired; to shine as the brightest of them all.

   Traits (taken from the Adjective Checklist or *ACL* (Gough, 1952)): forceful, dominant, dignified, intelligent, severe, stubborn, sophisticated, wise.

1B: Hermes—the swift traveler.

Variants:

1. Adventurer/Traveler/Explorer: to seek the new, to explore, to keep moving, changing, growing.
2. Trickster/Joker/Thief/Rabble-rouser: to create mischief, to startle, to fool, to jolt the status quo, to laugh at.
3. Persuader/Spokesperson: to speak for, to advocate, to cajole, to lobby, to persuade.
4. Athlete/Game player/Gambler: to master play and sport, to take risks and emerge the victor, to move with grace and speed.
5. Entrepreneur/Capitalist: to make a profit, to master the inanimate world of goods and services.

   Traits (from the ACL): ambitious, clever, enterprising, independent, adventurous, resourceful, restless, shrewd.

1C: Ares—the warrior.

Variant:

1. Fighter/Soldier/Police officer/Strongman: to fight, to exert brute force, to subdue the foe, to display courage.

   Traits (from ACL): aggressive, argumentative, daring, courageous, impulsive, uninhibited, tough, bossy.

TABLE 6.1. (*continued*)

Class 2

Class 2 imagoes are personifications of agency (power) *and* communion (intimacy). They are powerful figures whose actions also promote relationships and the welfare of others. Thus, their actions are designed to benefit both the self and others.

2A: Apollo—the god of light.

Variants:

1. Healer/Doctor/Shaman: to mend, to relieve pain and suffering, to heal, to perform miracles.
2. Prophet/Seer: to foresee the future, to predict destiny.
3. Artist/Musician: to make something beautiful, to move others with beauty.
4. Shepherd/Protector/Vanguard: to protect the flock, to watch over others, to stand guard.
5. Organizer/Legislator: to organize others, to lead others, to mobilize resources in order to effect action.

Traits (from ACL): artistic, clear-thinking, imaginative, foresighted, planful, organized, progressive, rational.

2B: Athene—goddess of peace and prudence.

Variants:

1. Peacemaker/Arbiter: to solve conflict, to make peace, to effect compromises.
2. Counselor/Therapist: to offer advice, to listen and evalute, to promote psychological health and happiness.
3. Teacher/Guide: to teach, to instruct others, to pass on knowledge, to motivate others to seek knowledge.

Traits (from ACL): fair-minded, honest, peaceable, patient, moderate, practical, stable, understanding.

2C: Prometheus—the revolutionary.

Variants:

1. Mentor/Helper/Defender: to come to the aid of others, to guide, to defend the underdog, to support the lowly.
2. Rebel/Revolutionary: to speak and act against authority, to rebel, to challenge establishments.
3. Humanist: to promote humankind, to cultivate and preserve the noblest achievements of men and women.

Traits (from ACL): idealistic, helpful, generous, inventive, persevering, outspoken, rebellious, unconventional.

Class 3

Class 3 imagoes are personifications of communion (intimacy) and therefore exhibit communion's defining features: self-surrender, merger with others, cooperation, openness, contact, union, care. They are intimate figures who connect: relate to their contexts in ways that promote the contexts. They are defined not by their actions, but by their "relatedness."

3A: Demeter—the mother of all that is natural.

Variants:

1. Mother/Caregiver: to care for, to nurture, to cultivate, to provide warmth and support, to promote growth.

TABLE 6.1. *(concluded)*

2. Sufferer/Martyr: to sacrifice oneself, to suffer for others, to endure hardship because of others, to be deprived in order to be enhanced.

    Traits (from ACL): gentle, kind, modest, moody, natural, self-denying, steady, sympathetic.

3B: Hera—the loyal friend.

Variants:
1. Spouse/Helpmate: to cooperate with a partner, to be loyal to the partner, to stand by the partner in sickness and death.
2. Friend/Chum/Confidante/Sibling: to establish friendship, to interact with others who are seen as equals, to like others.
3. Servant/Subordinate/Assistant: to serve another, to help out in a subordinate role, to be behind the scenes.

    Traits (from ACL): appreciative, cooperative, friendly, loyal, praising, sociable, submissive, trusting.

3C: Aphrodite—the lover.

Variants:
1. Lover: to love in all ways, to form loving and passionate unions, to cleave to others.
2. Charmer/Enchanter/Nymph: to delight others, to charm, to divert, to enchant others.

    Traits (from ACL): affectionate, charming, dependent, emotional, sensitive, sincere, softhearted, warm.

Class 4

Class 4 imagoes exhibit neither agency nor communion. Intimacy and power are not major concerns. Imago may be concerned with more basic issues of survival or what Maslow (1954) terms "security needs."

4A: Hestia—feminine stereotype (banal).

Variant:
   Homemaker/Domestic: to make the home, to assure domestic order and tranquility, to carry out rituals.

4B: Hephaestus—masculine stereotype (banal).

Variant:
   Hard worker/Wage earner: to work and to keep working, to make a decent living, to provide resources in order to pay the bills and, perhaps, to have a little left over.

4C: Dionysius—escapist.

Variant:
   Pleasure seeker/Hedonist/Epicure: to play, to regress, to make merry, to forget and escape responsibility, to find pleasure in diversion.

4D: Other

Variants:
1. The origin(versus the pawn)/Survivor: to survive on one's own, to overcome controlling forces, to gain a modicum of autonomy, to exert some control.
2. Unclassified: subjects for whom no imago can be identified.

A second set of coders was trained to use the Greek taxonomy presented in Table 6.1 to code the life-story interviews of all 50 subjects for imagoes. For each interview, the coders wrote an objective and detailed summary of the information provided by the subject. Next, the coders listened to the interview a second time in order to classify the dominant self-image presented by the subject into one of the 12 types. Once a primary imago was identified, the coder listened for evidence of a second self-image which was posed in some way as an opposite of the first. This second self-image was termed an *antiimago*. For each primary imago identified, the coders completed an imago-description sheet (reproduced in Appendix F) which asked for information pertaining to the seven criteria for an imago described above. The imago-description sheets provide a format for the organization of evidence supporting a particular imago interpretation. Specifying answers for every question on the sheets was not a necessary prerequisite for scoring an imago nor was it necessary to find an antagonistic antiimago. Scorers were instead encouraged to do the best they could in completing the forms, with the understanding that such an inquiry was highly exploratory and therefore required a good deal of flexibility and tolerance for ambiguity.[6]

For our entire sample of 50 adults, primary imagoes were classified as Class 1 in 11 cases (22 percent), Class 2 in 7 cases (14 percent), Class 3 in 12 cases (24 percent), and Class 4 in 20 cases (40 percent). Class 4 included three subjects for whom no imago could be identified. For the men, the distribution was 10 percent Class 1, 30 percent Class 2, 15 percent Class 3, and 45 percent Class 4. For women, 30 percent Class 1, 3 percent Class 2, 30 percent Class 3, and 37 percent Class 4. A contrasting antiimago was identified in 70 percent (35 out of 50) of the cases.

Imagoes of Power

Overview

The purest power imagoes are those personified images of self as the omniscient source (Zeus), the swift traveler (Hermes), and the warrior (Ares). These are what I have termed Class 1 imagoes. Midlife adults whose life stories were marked by the actions and interactions of Class 1 imagoes tended to highlight the overlapping themes of self-assertion, self-expansion, conquest, mastery, and agency.

Unlike Class 2 imagoes (which combine power and intimacy), these pure power imagoes generally demonstrate a sense of agency unmitigated by major concerns for relationships. This is not to say that adults displaying these images of self are ruthless or Machiavellian. Rather, they choose to frame their life stories around significant agentic actions rather than communal relationships with others. As part of Hypothesis 3 in Chapter 2, I predicted that higher power motivation, assessed via the TAT, would be associated with Class 1 as well as Class 2 imagoes. We obtained some empirical support for this hypothesis. Mean power motive scores for adults classified into each of the four imago classes were 59.3 for Class 1, 51.7 for Class 2, 47.5 for Class 3, and 45.6 for Class 4. The mean differences among the four groups were significant ($F(3, 46) = 6.16$, $p < .01$), with subjects showing Class 1 imagoes having significantly higher power motivation than Classes 3 and 4 combined ($p < .001$), and Classes 1 and 2 having higher power motivation than Classes 3 and 4 ($p < .01$).

Zeus

The supreme patriarch of Mount Olympus is the almighty Zeus. As the omnipotent and omniscient source, Zeus personifies unmitigated power in all of its multiform guises. As the final judge in all controversies, his decisions are absolute and irreversible. As the ultimate seducer, his amorous adventures transport him to all parts of the heavens and earth, to lie with both goddesses and mortals, and to father generations of offspring. He is the wisest sage, the most bountiful provider, the greatest celebrity in all creation. The essence of Zeus is captured in the Homeric Hymn sung in his honor:

Zeus
who is the best
god
and the greatest
is who
I will sing
he sees
far he rules
he
finishes things
he converses
wisely
with Themis
at his side
be kind
son of
Cronus
who sees far
you're the most
famous
of all
you're the greatest[7]

An imago of Zeus is dominant in the life story of June A., a 44-year-old director of a nursing school at a major university. June is unmarried. She has held several offices in professional nursing organizations, was on the board of directors of a local college, is presently on the board of directors of an adoption agency, and is treasurer and Sunday-school teacher at her church. As June tells it, early in elementary school she overcame her shyness and began to assert herself as a masterful agent in studies and relationships with others. An early episode in which she taught herself to diagram sentences, much to the amazement of her teacher, illustrates her early mastery. She proceeded to be amazingly successful in school despite the fact that she does not consider herself a scholar but rather an organizer and leader of others. After obtaining a BS and nursing certification, June's career skyrocketed such that by age 29 she was able to assume the extremely powerful and prestigious office of director of a university nursing program. After "coasting for a few years," she has of late come to desire more influence and has decided that her paramount goal for the future is to be a college president. She believes that she can do it. Reinforced by the exemplar of her aunt (who could "do anything"—"she was perfect; I felt so betrayed when she got married"), June does many things extremely well. Not only is she the consummate leader of others, but she also makes her own clothes and dabbles, quite seriously it seems, in photography.

The Zeus imago entails major sacrifices, especially in the interpersonal realm. June appears to have little time or inclination to invest herself heavily in any particular relationships, especially romantic ones. Believing that she is supremely competent in a number of areas of life, June does not suffer well the idiocy of fools. She claims that she is relatively intolerant of views which disagree with her own, though this is seen as a serious personality flaw to be corrected in the future. Part of the solution may lie in an antiimago June appears to have cultivated as a means of taming the tyrant within. This is the antiimago of the *servant*, and it is exemplified in (*a*) her belief that she occasionally serves her students as a mentor and (*b*) (more important) her relationship with God. This relationship provides stability in her life, she claims. She is God's servant in her work and in her activities at church and in the community. "God has kept me from doing some drastic things," she states. "I'd be a terrible force if it weren't for this."[8]

Hermes

One of the more complex gods in the Greek pantheon is the versatile Hermes. From the many sides of his demeanor and from his many exploits recorded in myth (see Brown, 1947; McClelland, 1961),

I have taken those which exemplify power and agency. These include Hermes the traveling messenger of the gods, Hermes the trickster and thief, Hermes the advocate and persuader of others, and Hermes the master of play and sport. Born the illegitimate son of Maia and Zeus, the precocious Hermes stole Apollo's cattle, invented the lyre, and kindled the first fire, all during his first day out of the womb. The frenetic activity was not an ephemeral quirk: Hermes became the fleet-footed messenger of the gods and the escort of souls to the underworld. Throughout all of Greek mythology, Hermes is constantly *on the move.*

In the life story of Rebecca K., the central character is the *swift traveler* (adventurer/explorer/pioneer). Rebecca is a 38-year-old, divorced social worker who has traveled the world over. Structured in an episodic style reminiscent of the picaresque novel, Rebecca's life story reads like a romantic adventure in which the heroine's incessant search for new places, new experiences, and new people defines the major plot lines. In describing her philosophy of life, Rebecca states, "It is the journey that matters, not the arrival. I will not stop running; I refuse until I'm in a wheelchair." The nuclear episodes in her life are frequently set in exotic, faraway places, like Mexico and the Orient. There are illicit love affairs, experiments with drugs, tempestuous relations with lovers and friends, strange foods, strange customs, and captivating conversations. The imago of Hermes arises early in the life story when Rebecca finds she is continually "moving against" the nuns in her Catholic elementary school. Though the nuns don't appear to appreciate her endless questioning and frequent explorations into the forbidden, Rebecca continues to cultivate the new-formed imago, reinforced by her mother who insists that she not be intimidated by the nuns and Rebecca's aunt (one of her heroines) who "believed in trying new things."

Rebecca left for Mexico shortly after high-school graduation—a move that she, in retrospect, describes as "running away." This is by no means the last instance of running away. Though she has held the same job for the past eight years, Rebecca continues to travel, regularly visiting Latin America where she has some very dear friends. In Rebecca's life story, physical travel mirrors the psychological/spiritual journey she perceives. In her eyes, she is ever-expanding, ever-growing, ever-changing. Stasis breeds boredom and ennui. With adventure and constant movement comes sophisticated in-the-world wisdom which she contrasts to the idealistic abstractions of her adolescence and early adult years. This contrast hints at what we saw as the central antiimago in Rebecca's life story—the *naive idealist* who as a very young child (before the nuns) played the role of the good little girl and who as an adolescent sought to "save the world." Indeed, the antiimago survives in Rebecca's efforts "to do some good for a few people" in her role as social worker. Yet, in the next breath, she states that she would love to scrap all of that and take off again for Mexico, this time without returning.

Ares

Ares is the god of war, of blind and brutal courage, of bloody rage and carnage. A furious and impetuous god, Ares duels repeatedly with Athene (who frequently outwits him) and is the illicit lover of the beautiful Aphrodite. He is handsome and agile but loses many battles because of poor judgment. I have characterized the Ares imago as the fighter/soldier/police officer/strongman. His central attribute is courage.

Already familiar to the reader for his power peak experience described in Chapter 5, Tom H. is a 43-year-old communications worker employed by the police department whose life story speaks a language of Ares, the noble warrior. Growing up in a southeast side Chicago neighborhood during World War II, Tom recalls a number of significant events in his very early years associated with war, death, and authority. His earliest memories concern the air raid sirens and the childhood fear of "imminent invasion" in the regular air raid drills organized by Chicago neighborhoods. The unexpected death of his grandmother and his dog, the latter killed by a speeding automobile, were two early events associated with a feeling of rage vis-à-vis those who were larger, stronger, and in authority. In 1943, Tom's family moved to a farm community outside Chicago which, Tom reports, resulted in considerable stress. The major conflict in Tom's new community, as he saw it, was between the "farm kids" and the displaced "city kids." He describes his role in the conflict as that of diplomat: "I was like Henry Kissinger doing shuttle diplomacy," negotiating fragile peace treaties between warring factions. Tom found himself assuming a similar role in the wake of family arguments.

All of Tom's heroes in childhood were war heroes. Quick to link his own life history to contemporaneous world events (the beginning of the Korean War, the construction of the Berlin Wall, the assassination of John F. Kennedy), Tom describes the glory years of high school when he attended a military academy and his subsequent "first big failure" at Notre Dame University where he repeatedly battled a host of authority figures, unwittingly cultivating the role of the "rebel." Soon after dropping out of college, Tom enlisted in the Air Force and began another glory chapter as the good soldier. His life story since then is a roller-coaster ride from periods of glory when he is being the noble warrior (as a "good citizen," dedicated politician) to times of depravity and shame when he fails to live up to an implicit warrior code—a regimen of conformity, impulse control, and spartan austerity—and falls into heavy drinking and generally irresponsible behavior. The latter refers to an antiimago which, in keeping with the martial tone of the story, might be termed the *deserter* or the *traitor.* This antiimago is the main character in Tom's chapters of failure— Notre Dame, drinking, his divorce, periods of unemployment.[9] In sum, Tom's life story is a saga of warfare in which the noble soldier is victorious when he is strong enough to keep the internal forces of dereliction and depravity under wraps while channeling aggressive impulses into the arts of preparing for war, negotiating treaties between warring factions (Henry Kissinger), and sometimes making war so as to keep the peace. The noble warrior is the vanguard of domestic tranquility whose work and life promote peace through strength.

Imagoes of Intimacy

Overview

The purest intimacy imagoes are those personified images of self as caregiver (Demeter), friend (Hera), and lover (Aphrodite). These are what I have called Class 3 imagoes. They are indeed the most interpersonal of imagoes in that they are defined in terms of intimate relationships with others. Midlife adults whose life stories were marked by the actions and interactions of Class 3 imagoes tended to frame their narratives in relational terms, often structuring their life chapters around the most significant interpersonal relationships in their lives rather than, say, around life accomplishments or instrumental pursuits. Class 2 imagoes also emphasize intimacy/ communion/care/surrender, but these images of self are also marked by a theme of power/agency/mastery/conquest.

As part of Hypothesis 3 in Chapter 2, I predicted that higher intimacy motivation, assessed via the TAT, would be associated with Class 3 and 2 imagoes. The data provided some support for this prediction. Mean intimacy motive scores for adults classified into each of the four imago classes were 57.9 for Class 3, 53.1 for Class 2, 47.8 for Class 1 (pure power imagoes), and 45.6 for Class 4 (low intimacy, low power). The mean differences among the four groups were significant ($F(3, 46) = 5.31$, $p < .01$), with persons displaying Class 3 imagoes having significantly higher intimacy motivation than Class 1 and 4 combined $p < .001$), and the two classes of intimacy imagoes (Classes 2 and 3) scoring higher than the two classes of imagoes not emphasizing intimacy (Classes 1 and 4) ($p < .01$).

Demeter

Demeter is the bereaved mother who mourns the loss of her daughter Persephone. She is the joyous mother who is reunited with her daughter when she is freed—but only for a time—from her underworld prison. Demeter the goddess of the fertile and cultivated soil—the earth's caregiver, in this agricultural sense—is stricken with grief to learn that her daughter, the lovely but naive Persephone, has been abducted by Hades and transported to the underworld to be his queen. Disconsolate and vengeful, Demeter curses the ground and its fruits. A terrible famine ensues, terrible enough to motivate Zeus to arrange a return of the daughter to the mother. Their reunion is pure ecstasy, but later both learn that Persephone must return for one season of each year to the underworld, this because she ate a sweet pomegranate seed given her by Hades. During that season (winter), the earth will remain barren, but when the beloved daughter returns every spring, the fields will blossom and bloom.

Demeter is the devoted caregiver, ready to sacrifice herself and her domain (the earth's fertility) to save her offspring. As Robert May (1980) depicts it, she is the all-giving martyr who must first experience deprivation (separation, grief, winter, going down under) in order to become enhanced (reunion, joy, spring, rising from above). Though May suggests that the Demeter-Persephone myth epitomizes a recurrent fantasy and even a way of life characteristic of women through the ages, I prefer to consider Demeter as a personification of caregiving qualities as they manifest themselves in the life stories of both men and women.[10] Indeed, the best example of the Demeter imago in our midlife data is a case of a man.

Dean K. tells a life story in which the major personified image of self is the caregiver. A 36-year-old engineer with a wife and three children, Dean has lived his entire life in a southwest-side Chicago neighborhood. It is the same neighborhood in which his parents and their parents before them have lived their entire lives. Dean describes the neighborhood as working-class and extremely stable, an extended but close-knit network of friends, family, and families of friends, most of whom were born and most of whom will probably die on the same city block. This neighborhood was the setting for what Dean reconstructs as the idyllic chapter of his childhood and youth: a time of happiness, close family, and many friends. As an adult, he has sought to nurture a family life which recaptures the warmth and closeness of his childhood. With respect to his children, he believes that he has been successful. But his relationship with his wife has been less smooth, and he now acknowledges that he would have left her long ago if he were not completely devoted to his children.

In Dean's life story, the caregiver imago is kind, modest, sympathetic, caring, and somewhat self-effacing. It is reflected in Dean's reports of the greatest moments in his life (the birth of his children, especially his daughter who is "the jewel of my life"), his greatest aspirations for the future (to "make my marriage work" in order to "save the children"; to have another child), and his present involvement as scoutmaster and manager of a little league baseball team. The caregiver speaks most clearly in Dean's answer to the question, "What is the major theme of your life story?" He responded, "To be there for others." And the imago is also reflected in Dean's statements that it is his children and friends who provide for his life the most satisfaction. In Dean's life story, the caregiver imago appears to be placed in opposition to a somewhat suppressed anti-imago which we described as the *drifter* or the *wanderer*. This is the part of Dean, as it were, which would love to leave his southwest-side neighborhood behind and escape to the mountains where he could devote his life to photography. It is the children, Dean concludes, that keep him from going.

Hera

Hera is the queen of Olympus—the wife of Zeus, his immediate subordinate, and probably his best friend. A goddess of somewhat severe beauty whose domain includes marriage and maternity, Hera is distinguished among most of the gods and goddesses in her complete loyalty to her mate. I have chosen to accent this quality in Hera and to characterize the Hera imago as the loyal friend, the helpmate who sometimes assumes a subordinate role to the other, be it a friend or mate or both.

Marty N. is a 41-year-old mother of two who is enrolled full-time in a doctoral level program in counseling psychology. At the beginning of every new chapter in her life story, Marty highlights the status of the most important relationships in her life during that period. Following a happy and relatively uneventful first 11 years, Marty moved to a different part of the city in sixth grade and began to "feel really popular for the first time." Through high school, her friendships with other girls were numerous and lasting, though relationships with boys remained awkward until the middle of college. After college, she married a man 16 years her senior, he a Lutheran and she a Jew. The relationship has been extremely rocky ever since, but she remains faithful to him, committed to making the relationship work no matter how frustrated she feels. Raising two children entailed more sacrifices than she had expected as she felt compelled to give up full-time employment until the children became teenagers. Nonetheless, a couple of part-time jobs as an interviewer for market research buoyed her self-esteem and convinced her that she has a genuine talent for working with people and listening to their concerns.

In 1979, Marty enrolled in the counseling psychology program at a major university. Instrumental in her decision to go back to school were her sessions with a therapist who serves as the most significant exemplar for the Hera imago in her life. Like her therapist, Marty hopes she can be an effective and caring friend to others in her career as a counselor. Her two major goals for the future are to become a counselor and to "have lasting and caring relationships."

Aphrodite

The most beautiful of goddesses and the most enchanting is Aphrodite. She is the goddess of passionate love in both its noblest and most degraded forms. She is the inspiration for the amours of deities and mortals alike. And though she married the ugly Hephaestus, she too is a captive of her own passion, lying with lovers as famous as Hermes and Ares. The dearest object of her affections, however, is probably the mortal Anchises, father of Aeneas. Lucretius said that the heavens are overwhelmed with the beauty of Aphrodite and the sea casts its smile upon her. She is the mistress of playful and seductive repartee, of gracious laughter and the sweet deceits and delicious delights of love.

It is surely an irony of considerable magnitude that the best incarnation of the passionate and erotic Aphrodite in our midlife sample is a nun. The reader has already been introduced to Sara N. whose nuclear episodes of intimacy were described in Chapter 5. Sara tells a beautiful life story in which two ostensibly antagonistic images of self—the passionate lover and the ascetic nun—arise very early and subsequently fuse in her adult years into an image of self as the passionate, loving woman of God. A foreshadowing of the integration of these two—an event which Sara deems highly symbolic—was her conversion in preadolescence to the Catholic faith. She states that she became a Catholic on Valentine's Day.

The lover imago has its roots in Sara's relationship with her grandmother before the age of nine. Never very close to either of her parents (both of whom were fundamentalist Protestants), Sara considered her grandmother her first heroine. She was "the perfect human being," states Sara, "loving, independent, feisty, committed to God and to others." After joining the religious order, Sara joined her faith and her passion to become, in the eyes of others as well as her own, the "earthy one"—the nun steeped in the world and people rather than abstractions and the dogma of the church. Sara describes many very close friendships in unabashedly passionate terms and states that these serve as the greatest source of satisfaction in her life. She also found herself involved in romantic relationships in her earlier years, relationships which she describes as laden with passion and pathos. In one case, she fell in love with a priest as he was deciding to leave the religious life. She, on the other hand, had decided to enter the religious life largely because of the example he set for her as a servant of God. Thus, she declined his proposal of marriage and became a nun.

Sara's dream for the distant future is to set up a religious community in Wyoming where people can live in peace with each other and with God. She speaks of ministering to others both in her work as a school counselor and in her play. Summing up, she states, "I see my life as becoming more and more integrated—to be able to be a space for ministry in my work and with friends, and to enable people to grow and be who they are." Her life theme is, in her words: "A lot of living, dying, and loving."

Mixed Imagoes

High Power and High Intimacy

The most complex images of self encountered in our scheme are those which appear to accent both power (agency) and intimacy (communion). These are represented by the three Greek deities listed in Table 6.1 under Class 2: Apollo, Athene, and Prometheus. All three are extremely forceful deities, even by the exalted standards of Olympus, and yet all three frequently use their power to promote interpersonal relationships and the welfare of others. Though Class 2 imagoes were the least frequently identified in our midlife sample (appearing in only 7 cases out of 50), the results of power and intimacy motivation suggest that individuals manifesting these personified images of self tended to score relatively high on both motives, though not as high on power motivation as those persons showing pure power imagoes (Class 1) and not as high on intimacy motivation as those showing the pure intimacy imagoes of Class 3.

Given the few cases in our data exemplifying these images of self, my discussion of Class 2 imagoes will be relatively brief. First to be considered is the ever-so-versatile and multifaceted Apollo—the god of light, music, healing, and divination. The awesome power of Apollo "the Archer," he "who shoots so far," is typically channeled in the direction of constructive human intercourse. Though he is also the god of sudden death and though he is not above occasional cruelty and the petty jealousies of Olympus, Apollo typically exerts a firm but benign influence on mortals. He relieves pain and suffering; he protects the unprotected; he organizes others and leads them in the pursuit of just goals; he predicts the future; he moves others with the melodies of the lyre. Similar in function though somewhat less versatile is Athene, who is the favorite of Zeus. Like Apollo, Athene uses power in generally benevolent ways, as when she watches over the wandering Odysseus and guides Telemachus in his search for his father. Goddess of storms and lightning, Athene is well known for her skills in warfare (she frequently battles Ares and usually wins), but she is equally revered as the goddess of peace and negotiation. Prudent and never bellicose in times of both conflict and tranquility, Athene promotes peace, well-being, and the pursuit of practical knowledge. She is a goddess who mends rifts, effects compromises, and puts things back together again.

Third is a surprise candidate. Prometheus is probably more well known for what he endured rather than what he did, yet his defiant support of lowly mortals qualifies him well as a god who used power to promote the welfare of others. Because he introduced mortals to the holy fire, Prometheus was bound to a cliff for 30 years. Each day a winged monster pecked away at his liver, but every night the liver grew back. We see Prometheus as the great benefactor and advocate for humanity. As the father of arts and sciences, Prometheus inspires the cultivation of humankind's noblest achievements. As the defiant rebel, Prometheus is the champion of the underdog and the enemy of oppressive authority. Yet his well-intentioned actions sometimes do more harm than good. To punish humankind for receiving the gift of fire, Zeus commanded Hephaestus to fashion the beautiful virgin Pandora. The pain and misery unleashed by the opening of Pandora's box was Zeus' revenge on humankind for accepting the aid of Prometheus.

As a representative of the Class 2 imagoes, I will highlight the life story of Ronald C., a 36-year-old army officer, married with two children. Ronald scored moderately high on both power (52.2) and intimacy (53.1) motivation. The major imago for Ronald is aptly described by the phrase "the good citizen." This imago appears to blend Apollo and Athene, bringing together the organizing and legislating qualities of the god of light and the pragmatic teaching and peace-making of the prudent Athene. Ronald is the consummate organizer, the always-pragmatic and forward-looking planner. All of the following are projects for which he is presently making plans and delineating goals: a curriculum for Sunday school; summer activities for the boy scouts; his career transition from military officer to a post in the civilian world (Ronald plans in advance: He has been working on this for two years and will retire from the military in another six!); choosing a good school system for his son in anticipation of being restationed in Hawaii in two years; mending his relationship with his wife; becoming closer to his son; being less goal oriented, making fewer plans, and living life in a more spontaneous fashion in the near future. Planning to make fewer plans suggests that Ronald has at least a dim awareness that his life may be *too* organized. Characteristically, he plans to reorganize it, so as to build in less organization.

I trust the case has been made for Apollo the organizer. Shades of Athene are reflected in Ronald's many efforts to be of service to others as a teacher and leader. As a career military officer, he is proud of having served his country. He is informed on and concerned about a host of world issues, the most prominent of which is the mainte-nance of world peace in the face of a nuclear holocaust. Ronald be-lieves that the United States is "too individualistic." "People need to work together," he adds. His only hero is Gandhi.

Low Power and Low Intimacy

Twenty of the 50 adults (40 percent) presented life stories whose main characters highlighted neither power nor intimacy. These in-cluded three persons for whom no imago could be identified. I have grouped these diverse responses under the heterogeneous rubric of Class 4 imagoes. These are the idealized and personified images of self that do not fit well into the power/intimacy scheme. Interestingly, these persons tended to score relatively low on both power and in-timacy motivation as assessed via the TAT.

The overall impression of the coders who listened to the inter-view tapes was that Class 4 imagoes were in some sense less "heroic" than the other three classes. Midlife adults presenting these imagoes bereft of power and intimacy seemed to construct the more mundane and pedestrian life stories. Sometimes their stories were downright boring, and one found it difficult to stay with the narrative line over the course of the interview tape. "It may sound a little dull, but this is my life," remarked one woman. "And I kind of like it that way."

I have identified three types of class 4 imagoes—Hestia, He-phaestus, and Dionysius—and have lumped those individuals whose imagoes do not fit into one of these or for whom no imago can be identified into an "Other" category within Class 4. In three cases, the "other" imago appeared to take the form of "the origin/survivor," the person who manages to overcome tremendous odds in order to gain a modicum of control over his or her life. The antithesis of this would be the person who succumbs—the pawn who is controlled by insur-mountable outside forces.

In the case of Hestia and Hephaestus, Class 4 imagoes empha-size stability and security over the risks inherent in the pursuit of power or intimacy. Hestia is the keeper of the house, the guardian of domestic order and tranquility. In most myths, her role is confined to carrying out domestic rituals. The crafty Hephaestus is the tireless laborer who spends most of his day making things. He is much enamoured with the idea of accumulating wealth. In the case of Dionysius, the imago emphasizes diversion, an escape from the humdrum world of Hestia and Hephaestus. Dionysius revels in the corporeal pleasure of the feast, the dance, and the vine.

Hestia plays the leading role in the life story of Constance M., a 44-year-old Irish mental health worker who has never been married. Constance's very happy childhood years were spent in the family home in a rural community outside Milwaukee, Wisconsin. The all-powerful figure in the household was her father, a hard worker whose comfort was the overriding concern of his wife and all the children when he arrived home every evening from work. Moving away from home to attend college ushered in a negative chapter in Constance's story. Though there was little question that Constance would attend college after high school, she took no initiative in choosing a university, rarely thinking about the future at this time in her life. Her mother chose the school, and Constance struggled through four very trying years at a competitive, private, liberal arts college, graduating with a mediocre academic record. Having little idea concerning what to do next, Constance set out to enjoy a leisurely summer immediately after graduation and then followed her boyfriend to Chicago in the fall where she attended secretarial school. When she was 25, her mother died, and shortly thereafter she broke up with the boyfriend.

Around her 30th birthday, Constance moved to Mexico where she learned Spanish and lived for four years with a Mexican family. She dated a Cuban man who subsequently moved to Miami. She followed him and lived in the Hispanic section of Miami for five years. When her father died, she broke up with the Cuban and moved back to the Midwestern United States, where she now resides. She does not want to leave again. "I hate moving," remarks Constance. "I like being in one place for a long time."

Constance has a fairly specific dream for the future. She plans to find a higher-paying job so that she can purchase her sister's share of their family home near Milwaukee and then live in the house where she grew up. Constance believes that her Irish blood predisposes her to love the land and the country life. Living in the country, taking care of the house of her childhood, making a home where she can find happiness and security—these represent a fulfillment of her self-created personal destiny. Until the time Constance is financially able to realize her dream, she lives life day-to-day. "I don't think I have a philosophy of life," she states, "but I do like order, symmetry, and making my own decisions." And, "I very much want to be comfortable."

Imagoes, Complexity, and the Maturation of Identity

Integration of Imagoes

I believe there to be a significant dimension of complexity in the organization of imagoes in life stories. Whereas complexity is translated into *differentiation* in the analysis of nuclear episodes in Chapter 5, imagoes are probably better understood in terms of complexity as *integration*—the coming together of antithetical images of self in mature identity. Hypothesis 4 from Chapter 2 states that one's stage of ego development should be a significant predictor of the relative integration of imagoes in life stories. Integration of imagoes should be more characteristic of the life stories constructed by men and women scoring at relatively high stages of ego development—in our sample, stage I-4 (the conscientious stage in Loevinger's scheme) and above. Imagoes should be less well-integrated at the lower ego stages of I-3/4 and below. Thus, individuals adopting the more complex and multidimensional frameworks of meaning which characterize the higher ego stages should be more aware of their discordant self-images and of the possibilities for reconciling these images in identity. Individuals at lower ego stages should be less aware of contradictory self-images or, if they are aware of them, should be less able to synthesize opposites in the construction of identity through narrative.

That the reconciliation of opposites is a cardinal hallmark of mature identity (or the Self) is a theme which may find its most eloquent expression in Jung. It is not until midlife, argues Jung, that the individual is capable of blending the yin and yang of personality. This is to say, the center of the personality moves from the conscious ego, in Jung's terms, to a position midway between ego and the unconscious. This is the position of the Self, and its elevation to the status of the constellating center is nothing short of a Copernican shift in development. With consciousness dethroned at midlife, the individual resurrects the heretofore hidden parts of the personality, the anima in the man, for instance, and the animus in the woman. Thus, the fully individuated human being in the second half of his or her life cycle accepts what has previously been suppressed. Unconscious aspects of the personality are reintegrated into a more complex and a more actualized sense of Self.

Jung's conception is inherently dialectical. In simple terms, the conscious and the unconscious exist as *thesis* and *antithesis* in the first half of life—opposing forces at loggerheads, one manifest (the conscious) and one largely latent (the unconscious). The fully individuated Self at midlife is the creative *synthesis* which reconciles opposites and renders the person whole. The concept of the imago introduced in this chapter is likewise dialectical. In the hypothetically ideal case, two idealized and personified images of self exist as opposites on a particular dimension—thesis and antithesis or imago and antiimago. In the more mature life story, it is proposed, the two are transformed through a creative rapprochement.

There appear to be, therefore, at least four separate possibilities in the organization of imagoes in the life story. In the first, no imago is identified in the life story. In the second, only one imago is identified, and no antiimago appears to manifest itself. In the third, two imagoes manifest themselves—the primary imago and the antiimago—but they remain unintegrated. The fourth possibility is an imago and antiimago integrated in a fashion that permits the actualization of both. In the midlife interviews, these four possibilities receive complexity scores of 0, 1, 2, and 3, respectively.

The most primitive cases are those receiving the score of 0. For three of the adults in the midlife sample (all men), no single image of self could be consistently identified. Two of the men appear to be in the midst of major identity turmoil, and their life stories are so scattered that it was impossible to detect the presence of any consistent image of self, not even an old image discarded in the search for something better. In the third case, a 37-year-old man describes himself as essentially "Irish, Democrat, and South Side" (from the south side of Chicago). As he sees it, this *is* his identity in a nutshell. Try as the interviewer might, she could not stimulate in this man a line of responses which effectively differentiates who he is from who everybody else is in what he describes as a highly homogeneous environment.

Receiving scores of 1 are the 12 adults out of 50 for whom an imago but not an antiimago could be identified. In these life stories, a single image of self speaks loudly and clearly, and there is no dissenting voice. Generally bereft of any major life conflicts, these life stories may occasionally seem monotonous to the psychologist enamoured with notions of personality transformation and crisis. Events unfold in a predictable fashion. There are few surprises and fewer periods of self-doubt and identity questioning.

Most prevalent in our data are life stories containing an imago and antiimago which are not integrated (scoring 2 on the complexity scale). Twenty-three (46 percent) of our subjects fall into this category. We found that in most of these cases the subordinate antiimago is subject to either *frustration* or *suppression*. In the former, the full expression of the antiimago is stifled by circumstances over which the individual believes he or she has little control. In the latter, the antiimago is not recognized by the individual as a legitimate part of self but rather is projected onto others in the life story. Adopting the terminology of Sullivan (1953), the frustrated antiimago is akin to the "bad me," that part of self which my environment does not support or condone. The suppressed antiimago is the "not me," a dissociated part of self.

Ralph K. relates a life story which illustrates well the frustration of an antiimago. I have characterized the major conflict in the life story of Ralph to be that between the man of leisure (classified Dionysius) and the man of principle. Ralph maintains that his environment reinforces the first of these and undermines the second. Each of these two very complex imagoes integrates a number of separate elements of Ralph's life story. The man of leisure is an epicure who tries many different things but commits himself to nothing. He is the carefree dilettante who dabbles in photography, visits museums, and regularly attends the theatre. Like Ralph's father who represents the most prominent model of the man of leisure in this story, the primary imago is gentle and relatively passive, removed from the grubby world of making a buck and putting food on the table. The man of principle, on the other hand, follows a Spartan course. He is serious, pragmatic, and in the world. Because of his sincere commitments to certain critical issues and significant others, the man of principle enjoys little leisure time. He is embroiled in numerous earthly pursuits, including the making of money, yet he retains his integrity. Ralph's model for the antiimago is Lech Walesa, his only contemporary hero. Ralph's wife also functions as a model for the man of principle.

It is fascinating to note that whereas Ralph sees himself today as the man of leisure, he very much wants to be the man of principle. A first attempt to actualize the antiimago may have been Ralph's desire to become a priest. Motivated by his acquaintance with a priest who had dedicated his life to serving the poor in South America, Ralph attended seminary directly out of high school, but soon dropped out. It seems that this setting, like all other settings in Ralph's story, failed to offer that critical something (a cause, a belief) or somebody (a constituency to serve) to which Ralph could make a categorical commitment. In fact, the seminary appears to have nourished the epicure while leaving the man of principle hungry. What Ralph recalls most fondly about the seminary was the incredible physical beauty of the place, set along the shores of Lake Michigan.

Today, Ralph's life is fraught with ambivalence. It is so easy to be the man of leisure—to sit back, watch, listen, and read as his wife continues to earn more and more money. And there is no doubt that being the man of leisure is fun. But Ralph still longs for a different life in which, like Lech Walesa, he could make a commitment as a man of principle. As he gets older, this different life appears less and less feasible. The man of principle remains frustrated as the epicure continues on top. For Ralph at this time, the two imagoes remain irreconcilable.

Suppression of an antiimago is illustrated in the life story of Ruth P. The leading part in Ruth's story is played by the caregiver (Demeter), epitomized in the life of Ruth's mother who serves as her only role model and mentor. Ruth remarks that she is very much like her mother and always believed that she would grow up to be that way. The family comes first, for Ruth, and daily life appears to revolve around the children. There is little to indicate that Ruth is not satisfied with this imago. A sign of a strongly suppressed antiimago, however, appears in a nuclear episode from college in which Ruth was outraged when a professor insisted that women should not enroll in his chemistry class, seeing that they were all destined to be mothers and not chemists, anyway. As one of the most intelligent students in the class, Ruth refused to withdraw and eventually received an "A" in the course. The incident suggests an antiimago at odds with the caregiver, an image of self as independent and highly competent in a man's world. Ruth gave consideration to being a "career woman" (her words) at one point but decided she "didn't have the personality for it." The antiimago appears to be projected onto her brother and her sons. Her brother "had problems" when he was younger, but is now considered a "genius" in the family after receiving a PhD from a major university. Ruth predicts that her sons will attend college and probably professional or graduate school after that. Like her brother, they should be very successful.

Only 12 of the adults (24 percent) present two contrasting imagoes which are integrated. These cases received complexity scores of 3. It is difficult to make generalizations about these life stories. In each case, the integration of imagoes is accomplished in a different way. One woman integrates a friend/servant imago (Hera) with an image of self as a strong and masterful agent through her role as a psychotherapist. In providing psychological services to others, she is able to fulfill a strong need to be a friend to those who are less fortunate than she while mastering an intellectually challenging field of inquiry. A professor integrates a teacher/guide imago (Athene) with that of the student/follower in going back to school to get an MBA while continuing his teaching at the university. He maintains that only when he has a mentor in his life can he be a mentor to others. For this man, life involves the transmission of knowledge down through a great chain of teachers and students. One is constantly learning while teaching.

One of the best examples of integration in imagoes is Jessica C. Jessica's life story was introduced in Chapter 3 as an example of a romance. The reader may recall that Jessica was preoccupied from a very early age with the question of where she stood in the world. The question sprung from a central duality in her life which she claims to have perceived as a child. This is the duality between the Sicilian (her father) and the German (her mother), and it translates into a conflict between the imago of the artist (Apollo) and an image of self as a realist. The artist transforms reality through imagination, but the realist is better able to get along in the day-to-day world because of her more pragmatic and systematic mode of operation. The artist is corporeal: She uses her body (hands) to form physical matter into something beautiful. The realist is more cognitive: She uses her mind to manipulate abstractions so as to solve problems. In Jessica's narrative, the artist and the realist are the hot-blooded Sicilian and the rational German, respectively. Throughout her life, the two have existed in a dialectical tension of thesis and antithesis.

After failing to make a decent living as an independent artist, Jessica has moved into the business world and is presently working toward an MBA. She is very happy about the switch. In her work, she now relies on her German rationality—her ability to use her mind in a systematic and effective manner. Yet, the artist imago has blossomed anew in an attitude toward her own life as a kind of artistic endeavor in itself. Jessica is herself the creation and the creator. She works on her own personal development the way the artist works on a masterpiece. She sees herself as continually changing—forever an unfinished work of art. At present, the artist and realist appear temporarily reconciled—in balance. "Humans need to search for balance in their lives," states Jessica. Jessica believes that her preoccupation with the question of where she stands in the world has urged her to identify the conflicting parts of her self and to attempt to integrate them. She points out, finally, that integration is an ephemeral thing, here in one chapter of one's life and gone in the next. The truth of the matter is, in her words, that "conflict is inevitable, and we have to accept it."

Findings

We now return to Hypothesis 4. Are individuals at higher ego stages more likely than those at lower ego stages to express greater maturity in identity through an integration of conflicting images of self? To test the hypothesis, we drew upon the imago complexity scores described above. A score of 0 indicated no imagoes identified; 1 indicated a single imago; 2 indicated an imago and antiimago in conflict; and a 3 indicated integration of imago and antiimago. A first comparison of complexity scores for individuals at I-4 and above versus those at I-3/4 and below provided no support for the hypothesis. The mean imago complexity score for the subjects low in ego development (1.8) was not significantly different from the mean for subjects high in ego development (2.0). Further, males and females did not differ significantly with respect to complexity scores.

A second look at the data, however, revealed some peculiarities. The great majority (17 of 23 or 74 percent) of the subjects who received complexity scores of 2 were in the low-ego-stage group, whereas most of the subjects receiving scores of 1 (8 of 12 or 67 percent) or 3 (9 of 12 or 75 percent) scored high in ego development. In other words, low-ego subjects tended to construct life stories with two unintegrated imagoes, whereas those scoring at high ego stages tended to reveal either one imago or two imagoes integrated. Eliminating from the analysis the 15 subjects for whom two contrasting imagoes could *not* be identified (those with complexity scores of 0 and 1), we performed a simple 2 × 2 Chi Square test to assess the association between ego stage and integration of imagoes for the 35 subjects presenting two imagoes that might be integrated. In this case, the expected relationship between higher ego stages and a greater likelihood of integration of opposing imagoes was supported, Chi Square = 6.87, $p < .001$.

The meaning of these results is far from clear. In keeping with Hypothesis 4, we expected that subjects adopting the more differentiated and integrated frameworks of meaning associated with higher ego stages would construct life stories whose imago organization would be more complex. Employing a four-point complexity scale running from 0 for life stories with no identifiable imagoes to 3 for those with two imagoes reconciled, we were unable to confirm our expectation. On the other hand, including in the analysis only those 35 adults who presented two opposing imagoes yielded a significant relationship between ego stage and integration as complexity. It appears that for life stories which pose conflicting images of self, ego development is a good predictor of the degree of imago integration. In conflicted life stories, higher ego development brings with it greater reconciliation of opposites, a hallmark of mature identity. But a sizable number (15 of 50) of the life stories sampled demonstrated little conflict. For these, ego stage does not relate to integration of imagoes because there are no opposing imagoes to integrate. Let us say that Hypothesis 4 receives some equivocal support in a reduced sample.

Our inquiry into the integration of opposing imagoes raises a new question: Is it that many life stories involve a fundamental conflict between images of self and some others are almost conflict-free? Are there two fundamental classes of life stories—those embodying a central conflict and those eschewing it? If the stories we tell ourselves in order to live can be usefully classified with respect to the degree of conflict in personified self-images, then psychologists may require different interpretive schemes for understanding conflicted life stories than for life stories embodying little conflict. I have suggested in this chapter that imagoes can be usefully conceptualized in terms of dyadic opposites, thesis and antithesis. The dialectical frame may not, however, fit all kinds of life stories equally well. A considerable number of the midlife adults presented only one imago standing unopposed. Whether this indicates a previous integration so complete as to leave no remnants of conflicting images of self or a qualitatively different kind of life story than the relatively conflicted majority remains a mystery. What is clear at this point, however, is that our dialectical view of imagoes as paired opposites lends itself easily to many life stories, but not to all. Identity appears to take a tremendous variety of forms. We are beginning to catalogue some of them, but we remain dazzled by the splendid diversity.[11]

Summary

Imagoes are idealized and personified images of the self which play the role of *characters* in the life story. These characters are "parts" of the self which act and interact to define the major plot lines of identity. Theoretical precursors to my conceptualization of the imago include Jung's archetypes, Sullivan's personifications, Freud's ego ideal, Berne's ego states and scripts, and the concept of the internalized object in object relations theories of personality. Examples of imagoes in the life story of Martin Luther (Chapter 2) are the Father, the Son as Mute, and the Son as Spokesman. In his case study of George Bernard Shaw, Erikson identifies three central characters in Shaw's life story: the Snob, the Noisemaker, and the Diabolical One. Imagoes are oftentimes arranged as perceived opposites in the life story—two contrasting parts of the self, thesis and antithesis, which occasionally battle. The synthesis or integration of the two is a sign of maturity in identity.

This chapter was an exploration of idealized and personified images of the self. The life-story interviews from the midlife men and women in Sample B were analyzed in terms of imagoes. Criteria for the identification of a prototypical imago in a life story included (*a*) an event in the story which gives birth to the imago, (*b*) a significant other person in the subject's life who exemplifies the characteristics of the imago, (*c*) personality traits attributed by the subject to the imago, (*d*) wishes and aspirations associated with the imago, (*e*) typical behaviors associated with the imago, (*f*) values and beliefs personified by the imago, and (*g*) an antiimago, or opposite image of self, serving as the antithesis to the primary imago on some personality dimension deemed significant by the subject. The case study of Curt K., a 39-year-old editor in Sample B, illustrated the working of two imagoes in a life story. In Curt's life story, a personified image of self as the creative, imaginative, and refined "artist" integrates a host of expressed values (aesthetics, culture, good taste), interests (classical music, visual arts, literature, gourmet cooking), avocations and activities (writing children's literature, teaching arts and crafts in the schools and churches, making beautiful things), role models and heroes (an older mentor, Curt's mother), and biographical events documenting the "birth and growth" of the artist imago. A frustrated antiimago of the "successful, worldly money maker" exists in Curt's story as an opposite. The two images of self define a central conflict in Curt's identity, a conflict between art and reality, transcendent beauty and worldly pragmatics.

I presented a taxonomy of imagoes drawn from Greek mythology. The primary imago in an individual's life can be placed into one of four classes in the taxonomy. Class 1 imagoes are pure power characters: Zeus, the omnipotent and omniscient source; Hermes, the swift traveler; and Ares, the courageous and impetuous warrior. Adults whose life stories were marked by actions and interactions of Class 1 imagoes tended to highlight the overlapping themes of self-assertion, self-expansion, conquest, mastery, and agency. Class 3 imagoes are pure intimacy characters: Demeter, the caregiver; Hera, the loyal friend; and Aphrodite, the lover. These are the most interpersonal of imagoes in that they are defined in terms of intimate relations with others. Adults whose life stories were marked by actions and interactions of Class 3 imagoes tended to frame their identities in relational terms, often structuring their life chapters around the most significant interpersonal relationships in their lives rather than, say, life accomplishments or instrumental pursuits. Class 2 imagoes combine power and intimacy: Apollo, the healer/prophet/artist/organizer; Athene, the peacemaker/counselor/teacher; and Prometheus, the revolutionary and champion of the underdog. Class 4 imagoes are "low" in power and intimacy: Hestia, the homemaker; Hephaestus, the worker; Dionysius, the escapist.

Supporting Hypothesis 3 from Chapter 2, power motivation was positively associated with Class 1 imagoes (and to a lesser extent with Class 2 imagoes), and intimacy motivation was positively associated with Class 3 imagoes (and to a lesser extent Class 2 imagoes). Individuals whose life stories emphasized Class 4 imagoes tended to score low on both power and intimacy motivation as assessed on the TAT. Case examples were presented to illustrate manifestations of various types of imagoes from the Greek taxonomy in the life stories of the midlife men and women in Sample B.

Hypothesis 4 stated that high ego development should be associated with greater integration of imagoes in the life story. If the integration of discordant images of self is a sign of maturity in identity, then one would expect that individuals with more mature, differentiated, and integrated frameworks of meaning—that is higher ego development—would construct identities judged to be more "mature." Some equivocal support for this hypothesis was obtained from a reduced sample of the subjects participating in Sample B. Among the 35 subjects for whom two imagoes (that is, a primary imago and an antiimago) could be identified in the life story, higher ego development was positively associated with greater integration or synthesis of the two. These 35 adults appeared to construct identities embodying a good deal of conflict between discordant images of self, and it is among these subjects that ego development appeared to predict integration or reconciliation of the conflict. There were 15 adults in Sample B, however, for whom only one imago or no imago could be identified in the life story. These cases of identity appeared to embody much less conflict. Thus, it seems that a dialectical view of imagoes as antithetical images of the self organizes well the data of some life stories but not others. This suggests that personologists may have to adopt different kinds of interpretive schemes for making sense of different kinds of identities, a prospect that reminds us again of the splendid diversity in human identity.

NOTES

[1] Parts of this chapter also appear in McAdams, D. P. Love, power, and images of the self. In C. Malatesta & C. Izard (Eds.), *Emotion in adult development*. Beverly Hills, Calif: Sage Publications, 1984b.

[2] In the present very rudimentary state of our research, we have been able to identify with some assurance imagoes implicit in the life-story interviews only. The questionnaire data collected on the college students in Sample A are not extensive and detailed enough to permit an exploration of personified self-images. It is also possible that even if we had conducted full interviews with the college students, we would be unable to characterize their lives in terms of imagoes. The imagoes identified in our midlife sample connect within a given life story to a host of narrative elements. They are indeed larger and more integrative than specific instrumental or expressive *roles* assumed by individuals. For example, most American adults at one time or another assume the role of "parent." The corresponding imago of "the caregiver" (modeled after the Greek goddess Demeter which is described in the text) is much more encompassing than this specific role, existing as a central character which cuts across many activities, beliefs, values, and goals in only a select group of life stories. The life stories of most college students, therefore, may not express the degree of differentiation in experience necessary for the creation of imagoes cutting across diverse behavioral and experiential domains. As the young adult comes to assume a greater variety of roles and collect a greater number of experiences in his or her 20s and 30s, imagoes may begin to coalesce and crystallize. We have a hunch, however, that the college years may be a bit too early for the composition of imagoes in life stories. Future research on this possibility is greatly needed.

[3] In two of the first 25 interviews, no imagoes could be consistently identified.

[4] We arrived at these imago characterizations through case discussions of each of the 25 subjects which were modeled after Murray's Diagnostic Councils. The author and three research assistants listened individually to each tape and then discussed their interpretive essays in an attempt to reach consensus. Consensus, however, did not always occur. In Figure 6.1, each imago label represents either a label arrived at via consensual validation or, in the cases of substantial disagreement, the author's label for the case.

[5] Special thanks go to Don Allen and Carol Kirshnit for their assistance in developing the Greek taxonomy.

[6] Two independent coders, blind to all other information on the subjects, scored the 50 life-story interviews for imagoes. Given the substantial interpretive effort required to identify imagoes, it is not surprising that scoring reliability figures were only moderate. For the 50 subjects in the present study, the two coders agreed on the general class (Class 1, 2, 3, or 4) of the primary imago 68 percent of the time (34 out of 50, Cramer's phi = .51). In the case of the 16 disagreements, a third independent scorer listened once to the interview and then decided between the two imago classes.

[7] From Homer. [*The Homeric hymns.*] (C. Boer trans.). Dallas: Spring Publications, 1970, p. 89.

[8] Imagoes are the most diffuse and encompassing of the four life-story components set forth in this book's model of identity. Though nuclear episodes (Chapter 5), ideological settings (Chapter 7), and generativity scripts (Chapter 8) are readily distinguished from one another in our research, imagoes occasionally overlap the other three, finding their reflection in nuclear episodes, ideology, or one's script for future generativity, as well as in numerous other areas. Consequently, the coding of imagoes involves occasional redundancy in that data used to illustrate one life-story component (say, a power nuclear episode) may also be used to illustrate an imago (say, Zeus). This is apparent in some of the cases presented in this chapter. This leads to a methodological problem in the present study in that imagoes are not completely independent of the other three life-story components, though the other three are independent of each other. At present, we do not believe this to be a serious problem because the overlap is only occasional and, as far as we can tell, unavoidable. The overlap, however, does prevent us from calculating meaningful correlations between imagoes and the other three story components. Any significant relationships we would obtain might be due to the scoring artifact of sometimes using the same data to code two life-story constructs.

[9] In reading an earlier draft of sections of this chapter, Carroll Izard asked why all the imagoes listed in the taxonomy are by and large positive—based on positive emotions associated with what are perceived as positive aspects of the self. Tom's antiimago of "the deserter/traitor" is a notable exception. Because our subjects were not in therapy and suffered, as far as we know, from minimal psychological disturbance, they generally accented the positive in their life stories. We as researchers, furthermore, were predisposed to seek out positive self-images in this particular sample. The exploration of negative imagoes based on experiences of failure and loss and associated with emotions such as anger, shame, and sadness would be a fascinating endeavor, especially in clinical populations. Future research may determine if the present Greek taxonomy accommodates well negative imagoes or if a new classification system is required. In the present study, negative imagoes are typically relegated to the status of antiimago, as in the case of Tom H. In addition, Class 4 imagoes (Hestia, Hephaestus, Dionysius) appear to contain some "negative" elements, though this is reflected more in the quasiclinical evaluations of the researchers than in the subjects' views of themselves.

[10] It has probably not escaped the reader's notice that the pure power imagoes have as their representatives male gods (Zeus, Hermes, Ares) and the pure intimacy imagoes correspond to female goddesses (Demeter, Hera, Aphrodite). This is not meant to suggest that, in contemporary American society, power imagoes are "masculine" and intimacy imagoes "feminine." Nor is it meant necessarily to suggest that males are more likely to adopt power imagoes and females to adopt intimacy imagoes. The latter, in fact, is an empirical question which awaits extensive research. The qualities personified in our taxonomy of imagoes are universal dimensions of human experience, though traditionally some are more associated with one sex than the other. We have attempted to describe each of the imagoes in sex-neutral terms, with the exception of Hestia and Hephaestus who represent banal feminine and masculine stereotypes respectively. Nonetheless, even Hestia and Hephaestus need not be confined respectively to females and males. In our data, three males and one female scored Hephaestus, and four females scored Hestia.

[11] Ratings on present life satisfaction, satisfaction with career, and satisfaction with relationships (Appendix E) were compared across the four imago classes. A two-way ANOVA (sex x imago class) for each of the three satisfaction ratings yielded no significant differences.

Chapter 7

Ideological Setting

We will call what young people in their teens and early 20s look for in religion and in other dogmatic systems ideology. At the most it is a militant system with uniformed members and uniform goals; at the least it is a "way of life," or what the Germans call a Weltanschaung, a world view which is consonant with existing theory, available knowledge, and common sense, and yet is significantly more: an utopian outlook, a cosmic mood, or a doctrinal logic, all shared as self-evident beyond any need for demonstration.

(Erik Erikson, 1958, p. 41)

We understand who we are in the context of what we believe to be real, to be true, and to be good. There is an ideological dimension to identity which prods us, in late adolescence and throughout our adult years, to become lay philosophers in search of answers to questions of ultimate concern. As ontologists, we seek to comprehend the mysteries inherent in both ends of Hamlet's timeless question: to be (to exist, to be real) or not to be. As epistemologists, we seek to know what is true and what it means to say that something is "true." As moral philosophers, we wish to distinguish between good and evil— what is virtuous and what is inimical. The stories we tell ourselves in order to live are grounded in certain ontological, epistemological, and ethical suppositions which situate the story within a particular ideological "time and space." I shall consider these suppositions to constitute an *ideological setting* for the individual's life story, a philosophical terrain of belief and value upon which the story's characters work, love, and play, and the plot unfolds.

In its most general sense, ideology means a systematic scheme or coordinated body of ideas and beliefs concerning human life and culture.[1] The scope of the term can range from a relatively circumscribed domain such as a particular political ideology (e.g., New Deal liberalism or contemporary neoconservatism) to an all-encompassing world view (Plamenatz, 1970). As an organized set of ideas, ideology implies an abstract and systematic outlook on the world and the human being's place in it. Thus, the formulation of ideology presupposes the ability to reason in an abstract manner so as to conceive hypothetical systems concerning what is and what ought to be.

Most developmental psychologists would agree that the quality of thinking necessary for the formulation of a personal ideology does not emerge in most human life cycles until adolescence. Before adolescence, the individual's thinking is bound to the concrete and immediate world. The nine-year-old is cognitively classifying and ordering his or her physical environment—a naive Aristotle preoccupied with the inductive systematization of the concrete. The 16-year-old, on the other hand, can step away, in a cognitive sense, from his or her operations upon the world and perform operations upon these operations, engage in analyses of prior analyses—in short, think about thinking. With the movement from what Piaget terms concrete to formal operations, the adolescent's mind expands to consider even its own thought processes. Inductive classification of the concrete is supplemented by hypothetico-deduction in the realm of the formal or abstract. For the first time, the individual is cognitively able to entertain those philosophical issues which require concerted and systematic abstraction and consideration of not only what is but what ought to be. Ideology, thus, emerges as a potential problem demanding a coherent solution in the mind of the adolescent.[2]

As enamored with formal operations as is the one-year-old with the newfound ability to take a step, the adolescent may initially stumble across the unfamiliar landscape of ideological things, clumsily grasping onto simplistic ideals—pat answers to questions that may later reveal themselves to be a good deal more complex. Formal operations paves the way to youthful idealism, ushering in the epoch of the idealistic youth who may appear in the eyes of those considering themselves wiser and more experienced to be hopelessly naive, rigidly doctrinaire, out-of-touch, impractical, and even downright dangerous (Erikson, 1968). Early on, the adolescent may seek perfect solutions to ideological questions in utopian formulations of the ideal life, the ideal community, and a golden rule or maxim by which to live (Elkind, 1981). He or she may be especially drawn to absolute creeds and doctrines which promise clear-cut definitions for what appears ambiguous and indisputable answers to questions shrouded in uncertainty.

Erikson (1963) writes, "It is the ideological outlook of a society that speaks most clearly to the adolescent who is eager to be affirmed by his peers, and is ready to be confirmed by rituals, creeds, and programs which at the same time define what is evil, uncanny, and inimical" (p. 263). At this time in the individual's life, he or she is particularly vulnerable to the false promises of charismatic idealogues and the systems of belief they promulgate. The Hitler Youth are but one testament to the ruthless exploitation of youthful idealism and the young person's yearning for certitude.

As the individual matures and adolescence shades into young adulthood, ideology gradually becomes more differentiated, more subtle, and, in Erikson's ideal psychosocial scenario, both more personalized (unique to the individual) and more affirmative of values shared with a community. Joseph Adelson (1975) has traced this gradual progression in the realm of political ideology. He observes that the 12-year-old's mind typically "runs to Draconian solutions" (Hall, 1980), but that over the course of adolescence, political thinking slowly becomes more complex as ideological systems are constructed and reconstructed to afford greater flexibility and tolerance of human diversity. Authoritarianism typically declines over this period. A more tempered political realism may emerge and with it a tough skepticism concerning the legitimacy of certain forms and figures of authority.

Kohlberg and Gilligan (1971) write that older adolescents or young adults may find themselves ideologically afloat in a *postconventional* world of pervasive relativism. Belief systems articulated in early adolescence and anchored to widely accepted societal conventions may lose their moorings. These former ideologies come to be seen as sorely deficient in the face of philosophical issues of greater and greater complexity. Old answers and old truths no longer work. Indeed, the individual may come to the conclusion that the world contains no truths; no categorically right or good formulations. All is relative, and one person's truth is neither better nor worse than another's. The challenge of the postconventional world, according to Kohlberg and Gilligan, is to fashion a personalized commitment amidst relativism. Their ideological agenda for the older adolescent and the young adult is reminiscent of Erikson's concept of *fidelity* in reference to identity as a whole. Fidelity is "the ability to sustain loyalties freely pledged in spite of the inevitable contradictions of value systems" (Erikson, 1964, p. 125).

Furthermore, Kohlberg and Gilligan (1971) and Erikson (1964) remind us that the establishment of commitment amidst relativism is a psychological mandate peculiar to the modern age and, some would argue, to industrial and postindustrial societies. As identity is the "spiritual problem of our time" (Langbaum, 1982, p. 352), so too does ideology call out for personal and societal solutions which enable individuals and societies to take ontological, epistemological, and ethical stands in the face of ambiguity.

This chapter explores the ways young people formulate personal ideological settings which frame the life stories that define their identities. The chapter explores certain dimensions of content and structure in personal ideologies and relates these to the constructs of intimacy and power motivation as well as ego development. The first section reviews an initial study into the development of religious ideology in a special sample of undergraduates attending a church-affiliated college in the upper-midwestern United States. This study introduces issues of structure and content in ideology which are further examined in the next two sections of the chapter in which data from the college students making up Sample A are described.[3] Finally, the last section of the chapter considers transformation in ideology—what I call the reworking of the ideological setting—as it manifests itself in the lives of adolescents and older adults. We end with a case of identity crisis described by novelist Joan Didion, a profoundly ideological crisis calling out for a radical reformation of value and belief in adulthood.

The Development of Religious Ideology: An Initial Study[4]

Background

The study to be described in this section drew upon a special sample of college undergraduates for whom religion was central in their lives. The study's purpose was to examine relationships between the process of formulating religious belief systems in adolescence and young adulthood and three personality constructs assumed to inform this process: ego development, power motivation, and intimacy motivation. The underlying assumption was that the development of a coherent ideology vis-à-vis religion involves matters both cognitive and affective. The adolescent in Erikson's ideal identity scenario is blessed with the "as if" thinking of formal operations such that he or she can construct hypothetical systems of thought and value to be evaluated by internalized standards of cognitive consistency and comprehensiveness. In this respect, the adolescent functions as both a philosopher (Kohlberg & Gilligan, 1971) and a scientist (Kelly, 1955) who actively constructs theories of living to enable him or her to predict, control, and understand the world in a consistent and coherent manner. Yet, the adolescent in search of ideology is not a cool and dispassionate cognizer. As we observed in young man Luther, the development of a personal ideology can be a highly emotional affair. Therefore, the study sought to tap into both cognitive and affective dimensions of religious ideology employing personality variables which likewise emphasized the cognitive (ego development) and the affective (motives).

The research was carried out at St. Olaf College in Northfield, Minnesota during the spring of 1980 (McAdams, Booth, & Selvik,

1981). Affiliated with the American Lutheran Church, St. Olaf is a small (3,000 students) liberal arts college which draws a predominantly white and middle- to upper-middle-class student body largely from the five-state region of Minnesota, North and South Dakota, Iowa, and Wisconsin. More than half of the students who attend St. Olaf list Lutheran as their religious affiliation, and though participation in religious activities and attendance at church services is not mandatory, a good number are actively involved in at least one of a number of religious groups on campus (Wednesday evening communion group, Fellowship of Christian Athletes, etc.).

Fifty-six students (26 male and 30 female) were recruited from psychology classes and religious groups on campus. As a criterion of inclusion in the study, each student had to score high on a short measure of religious salience, indicating a central position of religion in his or her life. For religious affiliation, 36 students listed Lutheran; 11 other Protestant; 6 Catholic; and 3 other. Freshmen through seniors were represented in approximately equal numbers. All were Caucasian.

In two group sessions, the students were administered the TAT, Loevinger's sentence-completion test (WUSCT), and a series of questionnaires concerning religious belief and religious experiences. The TAT stories were scored for power and intimacy motivation in the usual way. The WUSCT protocols were scored for ego development. The questionnaires explored religious ideology in detail through a variety of open-ended questions, rating scales, and multiple-choice procedures.

Four Ideological Statuses

A key question in the study asked whether or not the student had ever gone through a time of reassessment and reformulation of religious ideology. The question read as follows:

> For some, adolescence is a period of great change and tumult. Teenagers and young adults may question the political, religious, and ideological values they have developed in their earlier years. As a high-school and a college student, you may have found yourself questioning values that until recently had seemed very right, very correct. In fact, the questioning may have been (or is) so intense that you would call this period in your life a kind of "crisis"—a time of serious searching for the answers to such questions as, "How can I live a meaningful life?" or, "What does virtue, courage, honesty, or morality mean to me?" Some of you find answers to these questions. Others may continue looking. And some of you may not have experienced a crisis in values. With respect to religion, then, have you in recent years undergone, or are you presently undergoing, a period

of serious questioning? Yes ____ No ____. If yes, please describe the nature of this religious crisis as best you can. What has been questioned? In what way? What led up to the questioning? Has the questioning been resolved? If yes, how?

In reading the students' responses to this question, we were first struck by the frequency with which such crises in religious ideology were indeed reported and the richness of detail provided. Of the 56 students, 41 admitted to a definite period of serious questioning. A number of students reported that the questioning was over, resolved, or at least put aside for the time being. Others suggested that the questioning had just begun and no end appeared to be in sight. Some seemed to see the questioning as a positive sort of thing, an opportunity for growth. Others seemed more ashamed. For this latter group, the questioning was a regrettable occurrence, something that, to their substantial relief, was finally over.

Drawing partially upon the work of James Marcia on ego identity statuses (described in Chapter 2), we developed a classification system in which each student's response was placed into one of four distinct categories: *foreclosure, moratorium, personalized ideology,* or *restabilization.*[5] Each of the four types of response denotes a particular ideological status—a certain developmental position in the formulation of a religious belief system. Classified foreclosure were the 15 students who answered no to the question, maintaining that they had never experienced anything resembling a religious ideological reassessment. Erikson and Marcia describe foreclosure in adolescence and adulthood as the absence of any crisis or period of serious questioning of the old because of a commitment to early (childhood) beliefs and values that remain fixed as one grows older. In stating that no serious reevaluation of ideology had yet taken place in their lives, the 15 students in this category implied they had foreclosed on the issue of ideology and that religious beliefs and values adopted in childhood had yet to be shaken by experience in later years.

The 17 students classified moratorium were each in the midst of a serious questioning process with respect to religious ideology. Old values and beliefs, conventional dogma and liturgy, previous certainty with respect to right and wrong, meaning and void—all or part of this was presently undergoing reexamination. Definite answers had not been found, although these students occasionally reported tentative formulations that sufficed for the time being. A number of these students reported considerable anxiety over their preoccupation with such ultimate issues as the meaning of life, the existence of good and evil, and the relevance of conventional religion. Here are two verbatim accounts:

I don't know if I can actually call this a serious religious crisis, but many of the courses at St. Olaf (such as Bio, Psy, Religion) tend to make one question their religious beliefs or at least study and reevaluate them. In Religion 19 we are studying such problems as: the problem of good and evil, reason and faith, religion versus science, etc. I wouldn't say that I believe any less than I did before, but I am learning that questioning is *good* and that blind faith, as I have been taught to engage in previously, is actually quite unstable (weak) and useless.

I think most of the serious questioning evolved out of ethical problems—friends aborting fetuses, shady practices at my place of work, etc. Right and wrong were no longer clear—if they ever had been. These single issues were maybe resolved one by one, but greater ones arose. I guess one's appreciation (in the pure sense) of evil increases proportionate to age and experience. I stood at the ovens of Dachau and asked how my Sunday-school-class God could have let it happen. The questioning has not yet been resolved, but nor has it been abandoned. I rejoice in the opportunity to rail like Job against my God.

The third category was the logical extension of the second. Students here had already experienced moratorium and had come out of it with a new and more meaningful perspective on religious belief and commitment. The crisis had, for the time being at least, been resolved. Its resolution, however, was accomplished not by a return to a childhood view but rather through a reconstruction of a more personalized and less conventional religious outlook which connected the student to his or her past as well as an envisioned future. The eight students in this category described their ideological struggles in vivid terms as adventures entailing great risk but even greater opportunities for creativity and fulfillment. Because these students were successful in sculpting their own spiritual lives much as the artist or poet fashions a piece of reality that is uniquely his or her own, we termed this group personalized ideology and held it up as Erikson's ideal of crisis and subsequent commitment in the college years. Here is one young woman's account:

I was brought up in a family that was strictly Catholic. We have always gone to church every Sunday and on most of the Holy Days also. During these masses, there was always a lot of ritual and symbolism used. I began to question my religious beliefs at about the time I began to have a feeling of emptiness every time the more ritualistic parts of the mass were performed. (This was in 7th grade.) At first I felt I was missing something—wasn't trying hard enough to feel what everyone else was. I was sure they were experiencing something mystical. Eventually this led to an argument I had with my mother over whether the host was changed into the body of

Christ. My mother absolutely felt that the host was actually the body of Christ. I said it didn't matter if it was really changed and thought of it more as a reenactment of the event. After this I began to question the validity of the Bible (11th grade). This has developed to my present view that there are some very good things in the Bible, but a lot of it is unhealthy and responsible for the present degraded state of Western man. I do still have a reverence for Jesus—I've always been awed by the figure—but I don't think that it's for the same reason that most Christians do. I don't care if he died on a cross in regards to the "saving" context. People have died in concentration camps too. The Jesus of the prodigal son or the woman caught in adultery is the one I respect.

Finally, a fourth fairly common and fairly puzzling kind of response was encountered. Some students reported a crisis in religious ideology followed by a kind of resolution which seemed qualitatively different than that observed in personalized ideology. For this group of 16 students, religious conventions established in childhood had been questioned through a sort of rebellion which was subsequently discarded. These students described a period of wandering from a straight and righteous path (often by indulging in drugs, excessive alcohol, delinquency, or simply falling away from God through doubt or apathy) followed by a return *to that same path*. It was as if they had "sown their wild oats" for a time being and then settled down. No serious questioning of fundamental beliefs and commitments, however, had actually occurred. These students typically described the resolutions of their ideological struggles less as ones of personalized *creating* and more in terms of conventional *refinding*.

The so-called crisis did not seem to promote genuine growth, and, therefore, we saw these students as much more similar to foreclosure than to either personalized ideology or moratorium. Like the foreclosure group, these students had not yet experienced a thoroughgoing reevaluation of their belief systems but had made commitments (a second time) to old patterns of belief and value. We called this group restabilization. Below is one representative account written by a young man whose faith was initially threatened by divergent ideological views but later reemerged in what appears to be essentially the same form, now impervious to threat:

I search for what is real. At St. O. my previous assumptions concerning the Bible, the nature of God, and my personal beliefs and experiences were questioned and as I perceived it—threatened. The Bible was said to be nonauthoritative, only a book. God was more a concept and an idea that was real and not a friend. My personal experience of conversion and of sensing God was considered to be a subjective emotional experience. I prayed and prayed and read a variety of books presenting a variety of ways of looking at God. My search was led by a sense inside me that said Jesus is real, God is alive, and the Bible is his Word. Looking at people's lives was the main reason for reaccepting my first views. I looked at people and watched their lives to see who was different in a good sense—who really cared and loved others. Then I looked at what they believed and listened to them. They also confirmed my inner yearnings. The academic look at God lacked life and life-giving potential. It was interesting and logical but it didn't have what I was looking for in my life.

Ego Development

We predicted that Loevinger's stages of ego development, as assessed on the WUSCT, would be systematically related to religious ideology status. Specifically, we expected moratorium and personalized ideology to be associated with higher ego stages (I-4 and above) and foreclosure and restabilization to be associated with lower ego stages (I-3/4 and below). According to Loevinger's theory, the conformist (I-3) stage specifies that the self is prescribed by group roles and stereotypes, and values of niceness, helpfulness, and cooperation with others are ardently espoused. The conformist-conscientious (I-3/4) phase may eventually manifest itself when one realizes it is impossible to live up to all of the standards of one's defining group. The break from the group and conventional thinking spurs an increasing self-awareness and an appreciation of multiple possibilities in situations. At the conscientious (I-4) stage of ego development, internalization of rules is complete (Kohlberg's *postconventional* morality) and the major elements of adult conscience are present: long-term evaluated goals and ideas, differentiated self-criticism, and a sense of responsibility. Mutuality in interpersonal relations is enhanced by a greater willingness to take the role of the other; human behavior is conceptualized in terms of inner traits and motives; and a rich and differentiated inner life is conveyed in language no longer so banal as that of the earlier stages. At I-4 and above, it is expected that the individual has worked through, or is presently working through, belief systems inculcated in early years.

At least one other study has linked Loevinger's ego development and Erikson's concept of identity. Adams and Shea (1979) found that higher-ego-stage subjects were more likely to score at identity achievement (Marcia's classification) than were subjects at lower ego stages. Also employing Marcia's identity statuses, Podd (1972) found that individuals scoring at the statuses of identity achievement and moratorium tended to function at Kohlberg's postconventional levels of moral reasoning, while subjects at foreclosure and identity diffusion scored at conventional and preconventional levels. One would expect, therefore, that the transition from the conformist (I-3) to the conscientious (I-4) and higher stages of greater cognitive complexity in Loevinger's scheme would be a necessary (but probably not sufficient) developmental dynamic for the questioning of conventions which underlies the formulation of a personalized ideology through moratorium.

The data supported our expectation. Table 7.1 shows the number of students classified into each of the four religious ideology statuses broken down by ego stage and sex. A highly significant difference was found between religious ideology statuses for students high in ego development (I-4 and above) versus those scoring low (I-3/4 and below). Grouping together moratorium and personalized ideology as "higher" or more mature statuses and foreclosure and restabilization as "lower" and less mature statuses, we found that students at high levels of ego development (I-4 and above) tended to score in the higher two ideology statuses, and students low in ego development tended to score in the lower two statuses, $\chi^2(1) = 16.24$, $p < .001$. Of the 22 students at ego stage I-3/4 and below, 20 (91 percent) were classified, in terms of religious ideology, as either foreclosure or restabilization. Of the 34 students at ego stages I-4 and above, on the other hand, 23 (63 percent) scored at either moratorium or personalized ideology. The patterns of results for the two sexes were highly similar.

TABLE 7.1.[a] Number of Students in Four Religious Ideology Statuses by Ego Stage and Sex

Religious Ideology Status	Ego Stage						
	3	3/4	4	4/5	5	6	Total
1. Foreclosure							
Female	1	4	2	0	0	0	7
Male	1	4	2	0	1	0	8
Total	2	8	4	0	1	0	15
2. Restabilization							
Female	0	5	2	1	0	0	8
Male	1	4	3	0	0	0	8
Total	1	9	5	1	0	0	16
3. Moratorium							
Female	0	2	4	3	1	1	11
Male	0	0	6	0	0	0	6
Total	0	2	10	3	1	1	17
4. Personalized ideology							
Female	0	0	1	3	0	0	4
Male	0	0	2	1	1	0	4
Total	0	0	3	4	1	0	8
Total for all 4 statuses:	3	19	22	8	3	1	56

[a] From McAdams, Booth, & Selvik (1981), p. 231.

The Role of Motives

Whereas Loevinger's stages of ego development emphasize structure and cognition (see Chapter 4), power and intimacy motivation tend to highlight content and affect. Indeed, motives have been conceived as "affectively toned cognitive clusters" (Winter & Stewart, 1978), implying general thematic lines in the content of lives and life stories (Chapter 3). We expected, therefore, that students' scores on power and intimacy motivation would be systematically related to particular content motifs in highly affective experiences instrumental in the development of religious ideology. In his classic treatise on the varieties of religious experience, William James (1902/1958) asserted son...ching similar in concluding that the religious life can be most broadly summarized in terms of three "beliefs" (a spiritual universe beyond earth, possible union with this universe, and the power of prayer or meditation) and two "psychological characteristics":

(1) A new zest which adds itself like a gift to life and takes the form either of lyrical enchantment or of appeal to earnestness and *heroism*.

(2) An assurance of safety and a temper of peace and, in relation to others, a *preponderance of loving affections*. (1958, p. 367, italics mine)

James's two psychological characteristics appear roughly akin to the affectively laden experiences of power and intimacy, respectively, which are thematically central to the two social motives assessed via the TAT.

Adopting the general procedure described in Chapter 5 for the collection and analysis of nuclear episodes, we asked the students to describe a number of personal experiences which were in some way implicated in their own religious development, and then we coded the responses for certain content themes. Two particular questions yielded fruitful results. In one, we asked the students to describe a "particularly meaningful religious experience" that "seems important for your own religious development." The second question concerned a specific church service that was experienced as very enjoyable, moving, or meaningful.

As in Chapter 5, students who were high in intimacy motivation described experiences filled with themes of love and friendship. When they described a "meaningful religious experience," they often spoke of (a) feelings of giving and sharing among people, (b) tender touching (such as handshaking or hugging) as an important part of the experience, (c) participation in a religious ritual (for example, liturgy, prayer, communion) in which they detected a sense of community or togetherness, and/or (*d*) a special feeling of God as a kind of intimate companion, a "friend who walks with me" day to day. Students high in intimacy motivation also revealed a focus on friendship and love in their reports of favorite church services, often describing a particular gathering in which they felt love or a sense of community toward other members of the congregation. One high-intimacy student described the following experience:

> There was a communion service at _____ where I have worked the last _____ summers. The service was only for the staff and was early on a Friday morning. Some people had to leave that day for it was the end of the summer. We shared the wine and the bread with each other as we passed it around the circle. When the service was over we had a group hug, everyone standing in a circle with arms around the next person. We broke down in individual hugs afterwards, and at that point we knew what kind of relationship had been developed over the summer through the common bond of Christ within us. I had seen a group of people totally, or close to being, unknown to each other become a loving and sharing community as we would have it forever.

Students high in power motivation, on the other hand, recalled experiences that were strikingly different. Compare this account of a meaningful religious experience written by a high-power student with the one above.

> The energy in my life was gone. I was apathetic and bored. I lived like I wasn't expecting anything, and nothing was happening to change my attitude. A retreat was being held in _____ and I was going . . . The second night of the retreat I was feeling particularly trapped inside of my apathy. People were starting to worship the Lord, and I couldn't get into it like I normally would. Well the preacher for the evening stood up and started talking about a broken and contrite heart. It really touched me. I began to realize that I had been relying on myself and not seeking God or spending time with him . . . It was hard for me to walk up and ask but I did. And after the man prayed for me I hurt inside even worse than before. Then, it was as if God said, "Look up." I looked up and on the wall was a banner that read, "I will never leave you nor forsake you." It was sweet. God poured out his love on me. I was in his presence . . . The following week I tried to change the world and failed. People noticed my renewed joy . . . Some of my friends were around, but I was by myself most of the weekend.

The reader will note that, unlike the report of the high-intimacy student, this account makes little reference to anything interpersonal. Instead, the writer tells us about a profoundly personal experience in which "I was by myself most of the weekend." Rather than a sense of community and warmth experienced with others, the student reports a feeling of divine inspiration and power: God seems to speak to him directly, actively guiding his behavior and moving him to try "to change the world." Students high in power motivation consistently described meaningful religious experiences that spoke only secondarily of intimacy and primarily of heroism, inspiration, and power from above. In reporting favorite worship services, further, they tended to emphasize the power of God's presence and/or an increase in personal power revealed in greater "wisdom" or "understanding."

Intimacy and power motivation were also related to some of the responses on the self-report rating scales and multiple-choice questions. Students high in intimacy motivation reported that, in choosing a church to attend, the "friendliness of the congregation" and the "number and quality of church-related activities and gatherings held during the week" would be prime considerations. Students high in power motivation were more likely to endorse the idea that a prime function of organized religion is "to spread a religious message to those who have not heard it or accepted it," suggesting a mildly expansive view of the church, whose mission is to take powerful action and to have an impact on the world.

Conclusion

Three general conclusions can be drawn from this initial inquiry into religious ideology among students attending a small midwestern college. The first is not very surprising, given the nature of the sample. At least among these students, religious experience and religious belief are perceived as crucial elements in the building of a personal identity, often giving birth to emotionally charged experiences and thoroughgoing crises in ideology when old values and orientations are abandoned and suitable replacements sought.

The second and third conclusions form a bridge to the subsequent two sections of this chapter. It appears that (*a*) the degree to which an individual has "worked through" ideological issues may relate systematically to his or her level of ego development and (*b*) themes of power and intimacy in ideology may be similarly linked to the power and intimacy motives. In that the "working through" of ideology implies a movement from early and more global forms of belief to later and more complex ideological systems, the findings concerning ego development and the four ideological statuses suggest that the degree of structural complexity—the extent of differentiation and integration—in ideology should be a function of ego development. The thematic relationship between content motifs in accounts of formative religious experiences and the motives of power and intimacy calls for further investigation into the relationships between ideology and motivation. Proceeding from these last two general conclusions, we will now consider in a bit more detail the structure and content of the personal ideologies which serve to situate our life stories within their corresponding settings of personal beliefs and values.

The Structure of Ideological Settings

Stages and Complexity

Many developmental psychologists have conceptualized personal ideologies in terms of ontogenetic stages typically running from early epochs of ideological simplicity and globality to later positions of increasing differentiation and hierarchic integration (Fowler, 1981; Kohlberg, 1969; Perry, 1970). The basic assumptions of these structural developmental approaches to such phenomena as morality, ethical development, and religious faith were reviewed in Chapter 4. The reader is reminded that, according to most of these schemes, stages of functioning exist as integrated wholes arranged in an invariant and hierarchical sequence of qualitatively distinct and progressively more complex developmental structures. Helping to move the individual from one stage to the next in the developmental scheme is cognitive conflict engendered by the dawning realization, toward the "end" of a given stage, that old ways of understanding the world and the self (what are sometimes called schemata) are no longer adequate. More complex schemata, therefore, are constructed to make better sense of a world that now itself appears more complex.

Kohlberg's (1969) model of moral development is probably the best known of the structural developmental schemes for conceptualizing personal ideologies. In Kohlberg's ideal developmental scenario, the structure of an individual's moral reasoning passes through three general levels encompassing six qualitatively distinct stages. At the most primitive preconventional level, the focus of one's moral decision making is egocentric, and the constraints upon individual behavior are understood as residing solely in the external environment. Stage 1 is a punishment-and-obedience orientation to morality in which the individual is most concerned with the physical dimensions of acts and their consequences, while the motivation for moral behavior lies in a fear of punishment meted out by powerful agents in the outside world. At stage 2, the person assumes a stance of naive hedonism in which the prime concern in moral decision making is the instrumental needs of the actor, and the motivation for moral behavior is the obtaining of rewards.

Conventional morality implies a movement away from total egocentrism through the internalization of a set of conventions adhered to by either a familial/peer group (stage 3) or a society at large (stage 4). In both stages 3 and 4, the individual seeks to uphold the standards agreed upon by a larger group (one's family, one's state) to which he or she has pledged an implicit allegiance. At the post-conventional level, moral standards transcend the constraints of convention and become more personalized, revealing a private moral code whose scope is larger than the stage-3 social group or even the nation state of stage 4. At stage 5, the individual makes a commitment to certain abstract principles of utility and those implicit agreements or social contracts which undergird specific moral rules and laws. At stage 6, one's commitment is to abstract moral principles which are universally applicable. At this highest stage in moral development, one's perspective on morality embodies a commitment to categorical fairness coupled with a cognitive capacity for ideal role taking. At stage 6 have vanished all remnants of egocentrism in the making of moral decisions.

A more flexible and somewhat more general stage model of personal ideologies is offered by Perry (1970) who speaks of nine "positions" or "forms" of "ethical and intellectual development." Generating his model from extensive interviews of college students followed longitudinally, Perry argues that one's thinking about the good and the true moves from a rigid dualism (black versus white, right versus wrong, true versus false) at the earliest stages, through a realization of multiplicity culminating in an extreme relativism during the middle stages, to the evolution of commitments amidst relativism at the highest stages. Though Perry makes no claims concerning the structural integrity of his stages and their arrangement into an invariant sequence, he does emphasize that the general forward trend in intellectual and ethical development is away from globality and what he terms *embeddedness* toward differentiation, integration, and the actualization of highly personalized ideological systems.

One of the most intriguing stage models speaking to the issue of personal ideologies is Fowler's (1981) characterization of stages of faith. For Fowler, faith is a person's or a community's way of being in relation to an ultimate environment. Faith is a human universal, and though all human beings are not religious, all have faith, and all live by faith. It is part of human nature, says Fowler, to ascribe some kind of order or pattern to the universe and to live according to that ascription. In this way, human living assumes some sort of faith on the part of every individual human and every human community. Thus, faith involves a *relation* to and an *understanding* of an ultimate environment—what Fowler calls "faith as relating" and "faith as knowing."

The *undifferentiated* and preverbal faith of the infant who forms a trusting disposition towards its world (stage 0) gives way to an *intuitive-projective* faith in early childhood (stage 1) in which one's way of being in relation to an ultimate environment is framed by the fluid thought processes and imaginative fantasies so characteristic of the years three to seven. With the onset of Piaget's concrete operational thinking, asserts Fowler, the child typically advances to a *mythic-literal* faith (stage 2) in which beliefs about an ultimate environment and one's relation to it are couched in one-dimensional symbols to be interpreted quite literally. Whereas the quality of the intuitive-projective faith is what Fowler calls "episodic," mythic-literal faith follows a more linear narrative construction of coherence and meaning. The story (e.g., Biblical stories, myths) becomes the major carrier of a faith message at stage 2.

Fowler's *synthetic-conventional* stage (stage 3) typically emerges in adolescence following the advent of formal operations. At the synthetic-conventional level, the meaning and message of an individual's faith experience are translated into and out of dogmas, creeds, and other conventional systems of belief. It is at this stage that faith first assumes an ideological cast, according to Fowler, as the adolescent attempts to systematize his or her beliefs and values concerning an ultimate environment. With the transition to stage 4 or the *individuative-reflective* stage, the individual's systematization takes on a more personalized and complex form as conventions are seriously scrutinized and frequently rejected, and one accomplishes the task of "demythologizing" faith. Fowler's stage 4 shares many similarities with Kohlberg's postconventional morality.

An intriguing remythologizing seems to occur in the next stage of *conjunctive* faith (stage 5), a stage generally not encountered before midlife. Fowler (1981) describes the paradox of conjunctive faith:

> Conjunctive faith involves the integration into self and outlook of much that was suppressed or unrecognized in the interest of stage 4's self-certainty and conscious cognitive and affective adaptation to reality. This stage develops a "second naivete" (Ricoeur) in which symbolic power is reunited with conceptual meaning. Here there must also be a new reclaiming and reworking of one's past. There must be an opening of the voices to one's "deeper self." Importantly, this involves a critical recognition of one's social unconscious—the myths, ideal images, and prejudices built deeply into the self-system by virtue of one's nurture within a particular social class, religious tradition, ethnic group, or the like.
>
> The new strength of this stage comes in the rise of the ironic imagination—a capacity to see and be in one's or one's group's most powerful meanings, while simultaneously recognizing that they are relative, partial, and inevitably distorting apprehensions of transcendent reality. Its danger lies in the direction of a paralyzing passivity or inaction, giving rise to complacency or cynical withdrawal, due to its paradoxical understanding of truth. (pp. 197–198)

Finally, there is the universalizing faith of stage 6. This is an exceedingly rare and rarefied form of faith. Fowler lists the following men and women as candidates for this stage: Gandhi; Martin Luther King, Jr., in the last years of his life; Mother Teresa of Calcutta; Dag Hammarskjöld; Dietrich Bonhoeffer; Abraham Heschel; and Thomas Merton. Stage 6 is a radical and transformative faith which unites the opposites and transcends the paradoxes of the conjunctive stage. At stage 6, one adopts a perspective upon an ultimate environment which synthesizes contradictions and "unites" humankind. All persons are objects of the individual's all-encompassing love and his or her categorical commitment to perfect justice.

Though the emphasis and scope varies among the three, Kohlberg, Perry, and Fowler all focus attention upon the *structure* of values and beliefs which undergirds our life projects and situates the stories we tell ourselves in order to live. All three agree that as we mature, our ideological structures come to encompass larger and larger domains, taking into consideration a greater number of issues and variables and embedding these within more and more coherent and articulated organizational schemes. Thus, postconventional morality is more complex and encompassing than Kohlberg's third and fourth stages of conventional morality because it takes into consideration issues of fairness and duty with respect to principles behind social conventions. Likewise, conjunctive faith is more complex than Fowler's individuative-reflective faith in that it reincorporates the irrational and mythical elements of one's relation to an ultimate environment into the rational and demythologized framework constructed in stage 4.

Some Findings Concerning Ego Development

Guided by the theoretical and empirical work of Kohlberg, Perry, and Fowler, I have examined the relative complexity of the personal ideologies revealed by the undergraduates in Sample A who responded to an open-ended questionnaire concerning religious beliefs and values. My focus here is on religious ideology only. One would expect, in accordance with Hypothesis 6 of Chapter 2, that individuals at the conscientious level of ego development (I-4) and beyond would manifest greater complexity in the organization of their beliefs, regardless of their content, than would individuals scoring at the conscientious/conformist stage (I-3/4) and below. To test this hypothesis, I asked the students to describe in as much detail as they saw fit their present religious beliefs, including those beliefs shared with others and those which they felt to be unique to them. The question as it appeared in the questionnaire is reproduced in Appendix B.

Each student's response was classified as a whole according to a six-point complexity scale derived from Kohlberg, Perry, and Fowler.[6] The scale specifies six positions of relative complexity in ideology which were observed in the data. The six positions imply no particular stage model of ideological development, though they parallel in places the models described above. And none of the six points along the continuum qualifies as a developmental stage per se. Table 7.2 presents the distribution of the students' scores on ideological complexity.

Only one student scored at the lowest point on the continuum, receiving a score of 0. At point 0, the individual expresses no religious ideology whatsoever and no awareness that religion involves anything beyond a simple belief or disbelief in God. Here is the one verbatim response from the college students which was classified in this category:

> Even though I'm not a churchgoer, I believe that there is a God. I don't practice any beliefs like no meat on Fridays, but I do go to church on religious holidays because my parents will get mad if I don't. I believe that God is everywhere, but he lets us do what we think is right. If people pray, that is a way of making them feel better because we think there is a God. I go on with my life now as is because I really don't have the time to be too religious.

Only six percent of the students (5 out of 78) scored at point 1. Here the focus on ideology is solely upon the appropriate rules of conduct which religion may prescribe. At this point on the continuum, the individual expresses global agreement or disagreement

TABLE 7.2. Distribution of Scores on the Structural Complexity of Religious Ideologies among College Students in Sample A

	Number of Students[a]		
	Female	*Male*	*Total*
Ideological Complexity[b]			
0. No ideology	1	0	1
1. Rules of conduct	4	1	5
2. Vague beliefs	12	7	19
3. Dogma or creed, conventional	20	12	32
4. Personalized system, vague	14	6	20
5. Personalized system, integrated	0	1	1
Total:	51	27	78

[a] Only 78 of the 90 students in Sample A responded to the questions in the identity journal about religious ideology (see Appendix B). Students were not obligated to turn in all assignments for the journal, and, therefore, the response rate for most of the questions included in Appendix B was below 100 percent.

[b] The six points on the ideological complexity scale are described in the text.

with specific rules or norms, derived from institutional religions, concerning good and bad behavior. Thus, religious belief is a matter of adhering to or rejecting *in toto* certain concrete rules about action, such as prohibitions on premarital sex or rules about fasting on Rosh Hashanah. At point 1, the individual fails to address in any explicit fashion issues that go beyond codes of conduct. He or she fails to address the question of an ultimate environment and one's relation to it.

Point 2 introduces the consideration of more transcendent issues, albeit in a very vague and global form. The 19 students (24 percent) scoring at this level appeared to be dealing with relatively abstract religious issues. No longer solely concerned with what persons should and should not *do*, these students discussed *central beliefs* about such things as God's relationship with humans, the meaning of truth, salvation, and the function of religion in society. At point 2, however, these beliefs are relatively diffuse and unorganized, scattered willy-nilly across an ideological landscape unmarked by organized creeds or doctrines. In Fowler's scheme of faith development, this position seems somewhere between the mythic-literal faith of stage 2 and the synthetic-conventional faith of stage 3. Here is one example:

> I believe in God and faithfully attend Roman Catholic Mass. My religious beliefs center around my personal commitment to God and the humanity He created. My beliefs are expressed in what I do and in what I think. I don't believe that one can separate expression of beliefs into time slots. I pray whenever it occurs to me to do so in times of happiness, sadness, and need. Mass attendance is my only ritualistic concession possibly out of habit, but I do feel a certain closeness to God and rejuvenation. My beliefs are simple. Not quite as simple as "do good and avoid evil," but I do seek out the good in myself, in others, and in the world God created.

A whopping 41 percent of the students scored at point 3. This position on the continuum entails a categorical adherence to or rejection of an articulated religious creed or doctrine established by a church or some other external institution. Whether the individual accepts or rejects the doctrine, the point of view is decidedly conventional. When the orientation is one of doctrinal acceptance, we are reminded of Fowler's synthetic-conventional faith (Fowler stage 3) and Kohlberg's law-and-order morality (Kohlberg stage 4). Rejection of the conventional system of belief without the construction of a personalized replacement is not unlike Perry's midpoint of relativism and Kohlberg and Gilligan's (1971) transition between conventional and postconventional morality (sometimes referred to as stage 4½ in Kohlberg's model). At point 3, the individual integrates discrete beliefs about one's relation to an ultimate environment under the organizational umbrella of a conventional system or dogma which is either embraced or rejected.

At points 4 and 5 in the complexity continuum, the individual moves beyond convention to construct a more personalized ideological system reminiscent of what Fowler terms individuative-reflective faith (his stage 4). The difference between points 4 and 5 is integration. At point 4, the personalized beliefs expressed appear relatively unorganized and scattered. At point 5, they are integrated in the context of an explicit and coherent ideological scheme, such as a set of abstract principles. Whereas 26 percent of the college students scored at point 4, only one young man described an integrated system of ideology which merited the highest rating of point 5. I present here his response:

> First I believe that there must be a universally powerful being, a God, or some name, but most importantly something that knows all and cares about all. For me the most powerful source of God's presence is the love and goodness I see in other people, and so though God is universal he is not real to me unless I see Him through another human being. I also believe that our search and belief in God goes beyond church and community, though these are very important. I feel we're all striving at our own levels to attain the level of perfectness that has rarely been reached in history—by Christ, Mohammed and Sidhartha Gutamma, and others. My individual personality of this lifetime is not so important as the level of my spirit which lives on, possibly in future lives (having evolved from past lives), always getting closer to perfectness in knowledge but more importantly, in love.

As in the previous analyses employing Loevinger's measure of ego development, I divided the subjects into those scoring high (I-4 and above) and those scoring low (I-3/4 and below) on the WUSCT. Hypothesis 6 predicts that those students high in ego development should manifest a greater level of complexity in religious ideology than should those scoring low. As is evident in Table 7.3, the data support the hypothesis. The average complexity score of the 43 students classified high in ego development was 3.19 whereas the average score for the 35 classified low in ego development was 2.49, a highly significant difference (F (1,74) = 13.42, p < .001). Gender was unrelated to complexity scores (F (1,74) = 1.99, p = .162).[7]

Coupling this significant result with the findings of the initial study on ego development and periods of ideological change among the students at St. Olaf College (McAdams and others, 1981), we see that higher ego development is associated with (*a*) a greater degree of reformulation and questioning in the course of constructing an ideology and (*b*) greater complexity in the structure of the personal ideology that is constructed. The inquiries have centered thus far on

TABLE 7.3. Mean Scores on the
Structural Complexity of Religious
Ideologies Broken Down by Ego
Classification and Sex

	Ego Development[a]		
Sex	High	Low	Total
Female	3.16	2.26	2.82
Male	3.27	2.75	2.96
Total	3.19	2.49	2.87

[a] Ego development is assessed through Loevinger's sentence-completion test, the WUSCT. Subjects scoring at I-4 and above are classified as high in ego development. Those scoring at I-3/4 and below are classified low.

dimensions of religious ideology. Future research should extend the investigation into ideological realms outside the sphere of religion.

The Content of Ideological Settings

Values, Beliefs, Philosophies of Life

Psychologists who have centered their attention on the content of personal ideologies have cast a wide net around such topics as values, attitudes, beliefs, belief systems, and philosophies of life (Feather, 1980). Their investigations have generally fallen within the domain of social psychology as they have been especially interested in how the individual comes to acquire the fundaments of a personal ideology from the social environment and how those beliefs, values, and attitudes come to influence the individual's behavior in a social context. Though a detailed review of their efforts is beyond our concern here, a very brief and general outline of some of the main approaches employed will help put my inquiry into ideological settings into perspective.

A good place to begin is Bem's (1970) conceptual division of *beliefs, values,* and *attitudes.* Though all three are cognitive units encapsuling information we hold as "true," beliefs are nonevaluative propositions about what is, whereas attitudes and values are evaluative and concern what should be. According to Bem, a specific belief that Minneapolis is colder in January than is San Diego is based on more primitive assumptions, what Bem terms *zero-order beliefs,* such as the assumption that "my senses are correct." In the realm of the evaluative, attitudes are related to values in the same manner as beliefs to zero-order beliefs. Attitudes are relatively specific likes and dislikes directed at certain classes of objects: "I favor prayer in the public schools," or "I oppose an increase in national defense spending." These are derived from more basic values which we adhere to as generally unquestioned and inviolate premises about what is good and desirable. Values typically come in two varieties: values concerning means or modes of conduct (*instrumental* values) and values concerning end states of existence (*terminal* values) (Rokeach, 1973). An example of the former is the value of "honesty"; an example of the latter is a "world at peace." The most popular format for the measurement of instrumental and terminal values is Rokeach's (1973) Value Survey in which the individual rank orders the salience in his or her own value hierarchy of 20 instrumental and 20 terminal values.

At a greater level of complexity than general values and specific attitudes and beliefs are *value systems* (sometimes called *belief systems*, Bem notwithstanding) or what I am considering as personal *ideologies*. These refer to the organization of a number of values, attitudes, and beliefs within a relatively coherent framework. In their most general form, these systems can be conceived as highly abstract philosophies of life and reality. On one level of analysis, the classic study of the authoritarian personality (Adorno and others, 1950) concerned itself with an authoritarian value system adhered to by many Americans and Europeans which emphasized values of ultraconservatism, ethnocentrism, and national defense. This value system was embedded within a larger personological portrait of the authoritarian complete with characteristic personality traits and motives. Allport's Study of Values (Allport, Vernon, & Lindzey, 1951) measured the relative importance of six value clusters corresponding to Spranger's (1928) six "types of men." Morris (1956) developed 13 paragraphs describing 13 possible "ways of living," which appear akin to philosophies of life. Here are four of Morris' ways of living: to "preserve the best that man has attained," "experience festivity and solitude in alternation," "control the self stoically," and "meditate on the inner life." As psychologists have investigated broader and more complex value systems, their inquiries have shaded into adjacent areas of personality structure and functioning, such as character traits, motives, and interests.

Two more recent formulations of the content of personal ideologies walk a line between Rokeach's explorations of particular instrumental and terminal values and the more encompassing approaches of Allport and Morris. Both focus on "ethical ideologies." Forsyth (1980) delineates four distinct ethical perspectives and presents a questionnaire (the Ethics Position Questionnaire or EPQ) designed to measure each. The four ethical ideologies are (*a*) situationism, which advocates a contextual analysis of moral action; (*b*) absolutism, which argues for the reliance upon inviolate, universal principles; (*c*) subjectivism, which emphasizes one's own personal values as central determinants of moral decision making; and (*d*) exceptionalism, which admits that exceptions should be made to moral absolutes. The four ethical ideologies are classified in terms of two general ethical dimensions of idealism and relativism. Situationism is high on idealism and high on relativism; absolutism is high on idealism but low on relativism; subjectivism is low on idealism and high on relativism; and exceptionalism is low on both.

Hogan (1973) highlights Max Weber's distinction between two kinds of ethical ideologies: an ethics of conscience and an ethics of responsibility. Hogan measures the prominence of each via a questionnaire entitled the Survey of Ethical Attitudes (SEA). According to Hogan, an ethics of conscience is a "higher-law" perspective, as we find in the German idealism of Immanuel Kant, which advocates universal prescriptions articulated through one's own private moral vision, internalized absolutes, such as the golden rule or Kant's categorical imperative. The ethics of responsibility, on the other hand, is rooted in British utilitarianism, as we find in Jeremy Bentham and John Stuart Mill, and it emphasizes one's commitment to implicit social contracts bound to particular societies. The ethics of conscience and ethics of responsibility bear some resemblance to Kohlberg's stages 6 and 5, respectively, but Hogan maintains that neither is more "mature" than the other. Indeed, the most mature perspective on ethical issues may be some kind of combination of the two, a proposition supported in one study by Nardi and Tsujimoto (1979).

Two Ideological "Voices"

The formulation of ethical taxonomies as we see in Forsyth and Hogan is a response, in part, to Kohlberg's insistence that personal ideologies are best understood in structural terms and as constituting a single and invariant developmental sequence of progressively more mature (more complex) perspectives. Hogan, for one, has been quite outspoken in his opposition to what he perceives as Kohlberg's theoretical imperialism (Johnson & Hogan, 1981). Others, such as Shweder (1982), have echoed his dissent, arguing that Kohlberg's structural model is inherently biased in the direction of certain ideological *content,* such as an implicit partiality in the direction of liberal over conservative values. Most recently, Gilligan (1982) has critiqued Kohlberg's model from the perspective of sex differences, arguing that Kohlberg's theory of moral development is premised on assumptions that are decidedly masculine. Gilligan's thesis is that many women, and indeed some men, live by a morality that does not fit well into Kohlberg's scheme. There are at least two distinct moral "voices," according to Gilligan. One speaks from what has traditionally been understood as a male viewpoint. The other is the voice of the female.

Gilligan takes issue with a good many theories of development—among them Freud, Erikson, and Kohlberg—which implicitly characterize maturity in terms of separation and individuation. In conceptualizing ontogeny as a movement from the symbiosis of the mother-infant bond to the construction of a unique and independent self, many developmental theories speak a masculine language that cannot be translated, in good faith, into terms which illuminate the development of many women. The male voice in psychological theorizing, and in personal ideologies, prescribes all of the following movements: from attachment to autonomy, from concrete to abstract, from the particular to the general, from the immediate to the universal. In Kohlberg's terms, the paragon of moral maturity is the autonomous individual who, in making a moral decision, transcends the exigencies of the concrete flesh-and-blood moment to arrive at abstract principles of justice which uphold the rights of all persons who might be involved in the given situation at any given time. The individual at stage 6 in Kohlberg's scheme lives according to decontextualized universals—absolute and abstract truths concerning justice and rights. This person's principles are so encompassing and so just as to allow no exceptions.

The alternative voice is rarely heard in psychological theorizing, but Gilligan maintains it rings loud and clear in her own interviews of women who have pondered such flesh-and-blood moral decisions as whether or not to have an abortion. This is a voice of care and responsibility, and it bespeaks an antithetical model of human development in which self and others are continually interlinked throughout the lifespan. In making real-life moral decisions, many mature women and some mature men focus not on abstract universals but rather on the concrete network of human relationships involved in the given dilemma and one's responsibilities to that network. We listen here to Gilligan's own words concerning the second voice:

> The abortion study suggests that women impose a distinctive construction on moral problems, seeing moral dilemmas in terms of conflicting responsibilities. This construction was traced through a sequence of three perspectives, each perspective representing a more complex understanding of the relationship between self and other and each transition involving a critical reinterpretation of the conflict between selfishness and responsibility. The sequence of women's moral judgment proceeds from an initial concern with survival to a focus on goodness and finally to a reflective understanding of care as the most adequate guide to the resolution of conflicts in human relationships. The abortion study demonstrates the centrality of the concepts of responsibility and care in women's constructions of the moral domain, the close tie in women's thinking between concep-

tions of self and of morality, and ultimately the need for an expanded developmental theory that includes, rather than rules out from consideration, the differences in the feminine voice. Such an inclusion seems essential, not only for explaining the development of women but also for understanding in both sexes the characteristics and precursors of an adult moral conception. (1982, p. 105)

Gilligan's (1982) argument for two ideological voices is a compelling synthesis of anecdotal data from personal interviews and the reinterpretation of some of the classic works in developmental psychology. Empirical evidence in support of her contentions, however, is quite scarce. A straightforward and ostensibly testable hypothesis from her work is that the personal ideologies described by undergraduate women should emphasize themes of responsibility and care more so than those constructed by undergraduate men. Likewise, those of men should emphasize laws, principles, and rights more than those of women. I add a second hypothesis about personality differences. Men *and* women scoring high in intimacy motivation—with its communal emphasis upon close and warm relationships, communication and sharing, noninstrumental interaction with others—should focus on responsibility and care in their personal ideologies, which is to say that they should "speak" with Gilligan's feminine voice. Men and women high in power motivation—with its agentic emphasis upon the separation of the self from and the mastery of the self over the environment—should emphasize in their personal ideologies themes of individual rights, laws, and principles. My linkage of motives with Gilligan's two ideological voices constitutes Hypothesis 5 as described in Chapter 2. We now examine relationships among motives, gender, and the content of ideological settings in the group of undergraduates making up Sample A.

Some Findings Concerning Motives

I took a second look at the students' descriptions of their present religious beliefs. Focusing this time on the content rather than the structure of the descriptions, I developed a simple coding scheme based on Gilligan's distinction between an ideology of rights/laws/principles (RLP) and an ideology of compassion/care/responsibility (CCR).

A score of 1 was given for RLP to a response which made explicit reference to at least one of the following ideas:

1. Respect for the individual rights of others.
2. Obedience to rules or laws about what one should *not* do.
3. Adherence to abstract principles of justice or fairness.
4. God as lawmaker, guardian of justice, keeper of the peace.

Responses not containing a reference to one of the above received scores of 0 for RLP.

For CCR, a score of 1 was given to responses making explicit reference to at least one of the following:

1. The importance of loving others or being a friend.
2. Behaving in accordance with responsibilities or duties to other persons.
3. Finding God (salvation, etc.) in interpersonal relationships.
4. God as a good friend.

A score of 0 for CCR was given to responses which did not make reference to one of the above.[8]

Because the domain of religious beliefs encompasses a vast array of possible issues and ideas, many of the students' responses covered material that had little or nothing to do with either of Gilligan's ideological orientations. Unlike Kohlberg's moral dilemmas or Gilligan's interviews, my open-ended question about religious beliefs was not directly targeted for responses about moral decision making. A slim majority (55 percent) of the responses received scores of 0 for both RLP and CCR.

Despite the many scores of 0, the results do provide some suggestive support for Gilligan's thesis concerning sex differences. Whereas 43 percent (22 out of 51) of the women's responses made explicit reference to compassion/care/responsibility, only 19 percent (5 out of 27) of the men's responses did. This difference comes very close to being statistically significant, $\chi^2(1) = 3.70$, $p < .10$. The results for RLP, on the other hand, offer no support for the prediction that men more than women should emphasize content themes of rights/laws/principles in their personal ideologies. For RLP, 20 percent of the women and 22 percent of the men scored 1.

The results concerning motives are less than suggestive. Unfortunately for Hypothesis 5, none of the correlations between motives assessed on the TAT and Gilligan's ideological voices was statistically significant. Thus, intimacy motivation bore no systematic relation to compassion/care/responsibility in the students' responses, and power motivation was likewise unrelated to rights/laws/principles. At this point, therefore, we have been unable to document a meaningful relationship between motives and the content of personal ideologies.

There are doubtlessly many reasons for the failure to support Hypothesis 5. A major problem may be the procedure for measuring RLP and CCR. Though these categories for the content analysis of the students' responses appeared to be logically derived from Gilligan's writings, the specific stimulus for those responses—asking the individual to describe his or her own religious beliefs—may have simply been the wrong stimulus. As I mentioned above, a majority (55 percent) of the students' descriptions showed no signs of either RLP or CCR. A different sort of task or question or the probing for further elaboration may have elicited material more relevant to Gilligan's thesis. Nonetheless, the procedure employed was sensitive enough to produce marginally significant sex differences on CCR in the direction predicted by Gilligan.

A review of the past 30 years of research on human motivation, furthermore, reveals that the search for significant and meaningful associations between certain motives and certain content clusters in human values has never been easy (McClelland, 1951, 1980, 1981). McClelland has argued that values, beliefs, philosophies of life, personal ideologies, and other related concepts fall under the rubric of "schemata" in personality structure; that is, conscious cognitive templates for organizing our experiences. Schemata are qualitatively distinct from motives, which refer to recurrent and partially unconscious preferences. Schemata and motives, furthermore, rarely relate to each other in a straightforward manner. Given the independence of motives and schemata, McClelland (1981, 1984) has advocated combining scores on measures of both in the prediction of human behavior. In the context of our study, McClelland's conclusions suggest that it may have been more fruitful to use motives and content dimensions of personal ideologies as separate-but-equal partners to be combined in the prediction of other qualities of behavior and experience, rather than to seek straightforward relationships between the two.

On Changing the Set

Conversion versus Development

Ideologies are not frozen crystals of belief and value. They are instead dynamic systems subject to flux. My explorations of the structure and content of ideological settings and their relationships to ego development and social motives have concerned themselves with personal ideologies as they exist in the present. I have treated them so far as snapshots of a terrain which may experience an earthquake or volcanic eruption tomorrow, a landscape that may change only gradually or may be transformed overnight in the wake of an ideological cataclysm. I now consider briefly the phenomenon of changing the ideological set—of transforming one's personal ideology to provide one's life story with a new backdrop of belief and value.

It is my belief that profound ideological change after young adulthood is relatively rare. This is not to say that personal ideologies are set in stone during the adolescent years. My reading and experience (as well as the interviews with the midlife men and women in Sample B) suggest that there can be a fair amount of change for some. But this is some people—not all and probably not most people.

In the context of the life-story model of identity, the ideological setting constitutes the most basic component of our self-defining narrative. Like the setting in any story, one's systems of beliefs and values is a fundamental background upon which the characters develop and the plot unfolds. The setting is generally taken for granted. Just as the author establishes the story's setting in the first pages of a text, so does the adolescent or young adult consolidate his or her most fundamental beliefs very early in the course of constructing the life story. Just as the reader will find a story not grounded in a setting to be virtually incomprehensible, so will the man or woman without a personal ideology find his or her own life story a bewildering and disturbing personal saga, a story devoid of ideological place and time. In composing our identities, we are both author and audience, writer and reader, and if we fail to situate the action of our story within a context which makes sense, then we are authors who have failed and listeners who remain confused. Thus, we tend to decide early on a setting, usually in adolescence. Later, as adults, we are very reluctant to change.

A kind of metamorphosis in ideology which frequently occurs in adolescence but less often during the adult years is *conversion*. By conversion, I mean a transformation in the *content* of ideology. The transformation may be gradual or sudden, though it is the latter that generally captures our attention. Though it is most often associated with religion, conversion may refer to any ideological domain. In focusing on religion, William James (1902) writes, "To be converted, to be regenerated, to receive grace, to experience religion, to gain an assurance, are so many phrases which denote the process, gradual or sudden, by which a self hitherto divided, and consciously wrong, inferior, and unhappy, becomes unified and consciously right, superior, and happy, in consequence of its firmer hold upon religious realities" (1902/1958, p. 157). James saw conversion as a natural part of the adolescent's search for something and someone to believe in. Writes James, "Conversion is in its essence a normal adolescent phenomenon, incidental to the passage from the child's small universe to the wider intellectual and spiritual life of maturity" (p. 164).

James' observations on the phenomenon of religious conversion led him to conclude that a radical change in the content of one's personal ideology typically resulted in a "state of assurance" characterized by (*a*) an increased passion for living in a world which now appears to afford peace and harmony, (*b*) a knowledge of new truths, (*c*) an appearance of newness in the world which beautifies every object, and (*d*) a pervasive ecstasy of happiness (pp. 198–206). Such an optimistic view of conversion is reflected in a recent empirical study. Paloutzian (1981) found (*a*) that late-adolescent converts scored very high on a Purpose in Life Test (PIL) immediately following a reported "conversion experience," (*b*) that their scores dropped to a baseline level a month later, and (*c*) that within six months after conversion their scores rebounded and stabilized at intermediately high levels. Compared with late adolescents who had not experienced conversion, the converts scored significantly higher on PIL shortly after conversion and at six months following conversion. Item analysis of the PIL revealed that "fear of death" declined dramatically after conversion and continued to decline over at least a six-month span.

Other psychologists have adopted a less sanguine view of conversion, suggesting that sudden changes in the content of personal ideologies often betoken extremism, dogmatism, and instability. An ethic of moderation in all things may be a deep-seated component of an implicit and pervasive ideology of health and adaptation to which many of us, psychologists and lay persons alike, ascribe. We, therefore, tend to view the extremism and singlemindedness of the recent convert—whether it be the born-again Christian, the former liberal turned neoconservative, or the teenager hooked on Herman Hesse and *Siddhartha*—with a certain amount of dismay, even repugnance. Though the Weathermen of the 1960s may have been self-centered Philistines, and the Moonies of the '70s deluded dupes, their embracing of their respective ideologies signals a universal of human development: We seek to supply the ideological settings of our life narratives with *content* that is acceptable to us and with which we can live. Much of our striving and questioning with respect to things ideological concerns content—*what* to believe and *what* to value. In this sense, each of us is "converted"—either gradually or slowly, either partially or totally—from the content of James's "small universe" to the content of a "wider intellectual and spiritual life of maturity."

There is another way, however, that we can change the setting of our life stories. This is *structural* change: transformation with respect to the organization and pattern of what we believe and value. Fowler's stages of faith define a sequence of structural transformations. Each stage can be filled with a wide variety of content, including what Fowler terms *centers of value* and *images of power*. The content is arranged and organized according to structural rules which define the nature of the given stage. Fowler describes structural change:

> By now it should be clear that this means changes in the *ways* or *operations* of faith knowing, judging, valuing, and committing. A

structural stage change represents a qualitative transformation in the ways faith appropriates the contents of religious or ideological traditions. Because readiness for structural change is in part a function of biological maturation and of psychosocial, cognitive, and moral development, there is a certain degree of predictability—at least of readiness and direction—to it. There are, for example, minimum chronological ages below which it would be highly unlikely for particular stage transitions to have begun. But as we have repeatedly seen, faith-stage transitions are not automatic or inevitable. They may occur more slowly in one person or group than another, and some persons find equilibrium at earlier stages than do others. (1981, p. 275–76, italics in original)

Conversion and structural change may coincide in some lives, "as when a Synthetic-Conventional youth with a bland, humanistic background becomes passionately committed—intellectually and emotionally—to the existentialism of Sartre or Camus, requiring the rethinking of his or her commitments and lifestyle" (Fowler, 1981, p. 285). In others, change in content or structure may occur without the other. Fowler considers structural change to constitute development. The term *development* is rarely used, however, to characterize conversion, unless the change in content is accompanied by a change in structure as well.

I suspect that profound structural change—significant development in the structure of one's beliefs and values—is as rare after the age of, say, 25 as is significant change after 25 in ideological content. In the absence of good data, however, this remains an informed hunch. Indeed, Fowler suggests that those few individuals who attain stages 5 and 6 generally do not do so until midlife or after. Yet, he acknowledges that, in the development of faith, they are the exception and not the rule. Most people appear to reach a structural plateau in Fowler's scheme around stages 3 and 4. From the perspective of this book's thesis, we might say that the arrangement of the setting, as well as the ideological contents to be arranged, is generally consolidated in late adolescence and young adulthood, an early accomplishment in the life story. Those relatively rare transformations in content and structure that may occur later on require that the writer recast the narrative in new terms. I propose that transformations of ideological setting, therefore, are the most profound and unsettling transformations in identity. This relatively uncommon metamorphosis in belief and value may precipitate a full-fledged *identity crisis.*

Crises in Ideology and Identity

Consider the case of Joan Didion, the renowned essayist and novelist who describes the identity crisis she encountered as a mature adult living in America in the late 1960s. I quote in full her very moving account:

We tell ourselves stories in order to live. The princess is caged in the consulate. The man with the candy will lead the children into the sea. The naked woman on the ledge outside the window on the 16th floor is a victim of accidie, or the naked woman is an exhibitionist, and it would be "interesting" to know which. We tell ourselves that it makes some difference whether the naked woman is about to commit a mortal sin or is about to register a political protest or is about to be, the Aristophanic view, snatched back to the human condition by the fireman in priest's clothing just visible in the window behind her, the one smiling at the telephoto lens. We look for the sermon in the suicide, for the social or moral lesson in the murder of five. We interpret what we see, select the most workable of the multiple choices. We live entirely, especially if we are writers, by the imposition of a narrative line upon disparate images, by the "ideas" with which we have learned to freeze the shifting phantasmagoria which is our actual experience.

Or at least we do for a while. I am talking here about a time when I began to doubt the premises of all the stories I had ever told myself, a common condition but one I found troubling. I suppose this period began around 1966 and continued until 1971. During those five years I appeared, on the face of it, a competent enough member of some community or another, a signer of contracts and Air Travel cards, a citizen: I wrote a couple of times a month for one magazine or another, published two books, worked on several motion pictures; participated in the paranoia of the time, in the raising of a small child, and in the entertainment of large numbers of people passing through my house; made gingham curtains for spare bedrooms, remembered to ask agents if any reduction of points would be pari passu with the financing studio, put lentils to soak on Saturday night for lentil soup on Sunday, made quarterly FICA payments and renewed my driver's license on time, missing on the written examination only the question about the financial responsibility of California drivers. It was a time of my life when I was frequently "named." I was named godmother to children. I was named lecturer and panelist, colloquist and conferee. I was even named, in 1968, a Los Angeles Times "Woman of the Year," along with Mrs. Ronald Reagan, the Olympic swimmer Debbie Meyer, and 10 other California women who seemed to keep in touch and do good works. I did no good works but I tried to keep in touch. I was responsible. I recognized my name when I saw it. Once in a while I even answered letters addressed to me, not exactly upon receipt but eventually, particularly if the letters had come from strangers. "During my absence from the country these past 18 months," such replies would begin.

This was an adequate enough performance, as improvisations go. The only problem was that my entire education, everything I had ever been told or had told myself, insisted that the production was

never meant to be improvised: I was supposed to have a script, and
had mislaid it. I was supposed to hear cues, and no longer did. I
was meant to know the plot, but all I knew was what I saw: flash
pictures in variable sequence, images with no "meaning" beyond
their temporary arrangement, not a movie but a cutting room experience. In what would probably be the middle of my life, I wanted
still to believe in the narrative and in the narrative's intelligibility,
but to know that one could change the sense with every cut was
to begin to perceive the experience as rather more electrical than
ethical.

During this period I spent what were for me the usual proportions of time in Los Angeles and New York and Sacramento. I spent
what seemed to many people I knew an eccentric amount of time in
Honolulu, the particular aspect of which lent me the illusion that I
could any minute order from room service a revisionist theory of
my own history, garnished with a vanda orchid. I watched Robert
Kennedy's funeral on a verandah at the Royal Hawaiian Hotel in
Honolulu, and also the first reports from My Lai. I reread all of
George Orwell on the Royal Hawaiian Beach, and I also read, in the
papers that came one day late from the mainland, the story of Betty
Lansdown Fouquet, a 26-year-old woman with faded blond hair who
put her five-year-old daughter out to die on the center divider of
Interstate 5 some miles south of the last Bakersfield exit. The child,
whose fingers had to be pried loose from the cyclone fence when
she was rescued 12 hours later by the California Highway Patrol, reported that she had run after the car carrying her mother and step-
father and brother and sister for "a long time." Certain of these
images did not fit into any narrative I knew. (Didion, 1979, pp. 11–13)

The story Joan Didion told herself in order to live lost its power
and its meaningfulness in the late 1960s as events all around her "did
not fit into any narrative I knew." There was the death of Robert
Kennedy, the tragedy of My Lai, the gruesome tale of Betty Lansdown
Fouquet. There was the creeping uneasiness about a life which appeared an "adequate performance" on the outside but which was
experienced inside as a desperate "improvisation," a flurry of scenes
without a script. Though Didion searched for the "sermon in the
suicide" and the "moral lesson in the murder of five," she began to
realize that much of what she had come to believe to be real, true, and
good about life on earth did not and could not help her understand
the nature of things now. As an ontologist, epistemologist, and moral
philosopher, she was unable to answer the fundamental questions of
ultimate concern. As a storyteller of self, she was unable to supply her
narrative with a setting of beliefs and values which, in content and
structure, might situate her own behavior and that of others in an
ideological time and place appropriate for the characters and plot
involved.

I submit that there are at least two different kinds of identity crises: those concerning beliefs and values and those concerning action and striving. The former is a crisis in ideology, and it is the more serious—especially in later adulthood—because it necessitates a thoroughgoing reworking of the life story's most basic component: the setting. This is the kind of crisis of which Didion writes, and it is the same kind of ideological conflagration described in less dramatic terms by some of Fowler's and Kohlberg's subjects experiencing transition between stages and by the St. Olaf students in moratorium. It is a crisis in the composition of the background of one's life story, and it may involve questions of content ("What do I believe?") or structure ("How am I to believe?") or both. This kind of crisis is relatively common in late adolescence and young adulthood and relatively rare thereafter.

The second kind of identity crisis takes us into the next chapter of this book. This kind of crisis has to do with questions of action: "What am I to do?" and "How am I to do it?" Remember the idle women in T. S. Eliot's *The Waste Land:*

> *What shall I do now? What shall I do?*
> *What shall we do tomorrow?*
> *What shall we ever do?*

Identity encompasses value and action, and though the two may be related, there remains a fundamental difference between the questions "What do I believe in my life?" (ideology—Chapter 7) and, "What am I to do with my life?" (a script for the future—Chapter 8). In adulthood, the latter question may be couched in terms of doing something *that lasts;* generating something that survives (for the next generation) as a legacy of one's life. I am speaking here of what Erikson (1963) terms *generativity.* In the next chapter I will argue that generativity is really part of identity and that many life stories are rounded out by a *generativity script* or plan which extends the narrative line into an envisioned future of action.

Summary

An *ideological setting* is a backdrop of belief and value which situates the action of the life story in a particular ontological, epistemological, and ethical "time and place." In this chapter, I considered Erikson's rather general conceptualization of ideology as a systematic set of ideas about human life and culture which exists as an integral part of identity. Though Erikson never explains the precise relationship between ideology and identity, I suggested in this chapter that if identity were a story, one's personal ideology might serve as a kind of setting for the story, a background or context against or within which the action of the story makes sense. Ideological issues become particularly salient in adolescence because, in part, of the emergence of formal operational thought. In formal operations, the adolescent can step away (in a cognitive sense) from his or her operations upon the world and perform operations upon these operations, engage in analyses of prior analyses and, in short, think about thinking. For the first time in the life cycle, the individual is cognitively able to entertain those philosophical issues which require concerted and systematic abstraction and consideration of not only what is but what ought to be.

Psychologists who have focused their inquiries on the *content* of personal ideologies have cast a wide net around such topics as values, attitudes, beliefs, belief systems, and philosophies of life. They have concerned themselves, for the most part, with *what* an individual believes or values. I surveyed briefly some of their contributions and then discussed in some detail the theory of ideological content proposed by Gilligan. Gilligan argues that there are two separate but equal ideological "voices"—two distinct content clusterings in ideology—with which psychologists should be concerned. One emphasizes issues of justice, rights, and abstract principles; and the other focuses on compassion, care, and concrete responsibilities to others. The first reflects a decidedly masculine point of view, and the second is feminine. Though the two views may exist within both males and females, Gilligan argues that men are more likely to construe ideological issues in terms of rights and principles, reflecting fundamental assumptions of human autonomy; whereas women, basing their beliefs on assumptions of human interdependence, are more likely to construe ideology in terms of compassion and responsibilities to specific others.

Amending Gilligan's thesis, I offered Hypothesis 5 of my investigation: Men *and* women scoring high in intimacy motivation should focus on responsibility and care in their personal ideologies, whereas men and women scoring high in power should emphasize justice and rights. Unfortunately for Hypothesis 5, an analysis of undergraduates' accounts of their religious belief systems did not support the prediction. With respect to sex differences, however, there existed a nonsignificant trend for women to emphasize themes of care and responsibility in personal ideologies more often than men, but no evidence was obtained to indicate that men emphasize justice and rights more than women. Certain methodological problems, however, may have worked against both Hypothesis 5 and Gilligan's thesis on sex differences, and these were briefly discussed.

Most psychologists who have focused their inquiries on the *structure* of personal ideologies have adopted many of the empirical methods and theoretical assumptions of the "structural-developmental tradition," best represented by Piaget and Kohlberg. These psychologists have concerned themselves with *how* individuals make ideological sense of their worlds. A number of their contributions were reviewed. My own approach to the topic was represented in two separate studies. In the first, undergraduates for whom religion was a central part of their lives completed Loevinger's sentence-completion test of ego development and responded to open-ended questionnaires which asked about significant crises in religious belief— periods of profound ideological questioning—which they may have experienced in their lives. Students scoring at higher stages of ego development were more likely to have gone through, or to be going through, a period of serious questioning, constructing, in some cases, highly personalized perspectives on questions of ultimate concern. Those scoring low in ego development, on the other hand, tended not to have gone through a period of serious doubt or to have experienced a "pseudo crisis" in which they fell away from conventional religion for a short period but then went back to their original beliefs, incorporating very little, if any, ideological reformulation.

In that the "working through" of religious ideology implies a movement from early and more global forms of belief to later and more complex ideological systems, these findings suggested that the degree of structural complexity—the extent of differentiation and integration—in ideology should be a function of ego development. This proposition was examined further in a second study utilizing data from the undergraduates in Sample A.

Hypothesis 6, then, stated that higher ego development should be associated with greater complexity in the ideological setting of the life story. Guided by the theoretical and empirical work of Kohlberg, Perry, and Fowler, I designed a coding system for the assessment of structural complexity in religious ideology. Undergraduates' accounts of their religious belief systems were rated on a scale running from 0 to 5. A rating of 0 indicated no ideology whatsoever; 1 referred to an ideology composed solely of rules for proper conduct; 2 suggested an ideology comprised of vague beliefs about questions of ultimate concern; 3 indicated acceptance or rejection of a conventional ideology corresponding to an established religious dogma or creed; 4 indicated a replacement of the conventional with a vague but personalized ideological system; and 5 indicated a replacement of the conventional with an integrated and personalized ideological system. Supporting Hypothesis 6, ego development was strongly related to complexity of religious ideology as measured via this fairly simple coding procedure.

I concluded the chapter with a discussion of transformation in ideology—the enterprise of changing the ideological set. After Fowler, two kinds of transformations were distinguished: transformation in content (conversion) and transformation in structure (development). Though both forms of transformation may be quite common in adolescence, I suggested that they are relatively rare in adulthood. In the context of the life-story model of identity, the ideological setting constitutes the most basic component of our self-defining narrative. Like the setting in any story, one's system of beliefs and values is a fundamental background upon which the characters develop and the plot unfolds. Just as the author establishes the story's setting in the first pages of the text, so does the adolescent or young adult consolidate his or her most fundamental beliefs early in the course of constructing the life story. Those relatively rare transformations in the content and structure of the ideological setting that may occur in later adulthood require that the storyteller recast the narrative in new terms. I suspect that transformations of ideological setting, therefore, are the most profound and unsettling transformations in identity, and indeed often qualify as full-blown *identity crises*. Such transformations in ideology, however, should be distinguished from the crises of action—periods in one's life when one is uncertain as to what to *do* rather than what to believe. These crises in *doing* rather than *believing*, to which men and women may be especially susceptible at midlife, do *not* generally call for a thoroughgoing reevaluation of one's most basic ontological, epistemological, and ethical beliefs. Instead, they may call for a change in generative action—a reworking of the generativity script. The generativity script is the topic of the next and last chapter.

NOTES

[1] Plamenatz (1970) writes that the word *ideology* was invented in France. Translated as "the study of ideas," the term was first used at the turn of the 18th and 19th centuries to refer to a particular kind of philosophy which argued for the primacy of sensation in the derivation of ideas. Its most famous proponent was Condillac. Since then, the term has come in and out of vogue in intellectual circles, most often referring to political views and theories such as dialectical materialism, Jeffersonian democracy, fascism, the New Left, and the New Right.

I am using the term, as does Erikson, in its most general sense as a systematic body of ideas about humankind and the world. Like Erikson, furthermore, I am focusing upon personal ideologies rather than those espoused by corporate groups, though I realize that the relationships between the two are fairly complex in some cases. In his identity interviews, Marcia (1980) breaks ideology down into politics and religion. In the text, I divide it up into three abstract categories: ontology, epistemology, and ethics. There are indeed ontological, epistemological, and ethical dimensions of religious and political ideologies. The research conducted with the college students in Sample A and with a group of students from St. Olaf College concentrates on religious ideology.

[2] The attainment of formal operations in adolescence and adulthood is by no means a human universal. Though the research is sketchy, many developmental psychologists argue that formal thought may be relatively rare in traditional societies that we as Westerners might consider "primitive" (Cole & Schribner, 1974). Some psychologists have suggested, further, that a surprising number of adults in American society are either unable to engage in formal operational thinking or rarely do so (Capon & Kuhn, 1979).

[3] We have not as yet collected enough data on the ideological settings of midlife men and women to warrant inclusion of Sample B in this chapter.

[4] Parts of this section appeared first in McAdams, D. P., Booth, L., & Selvik, R. Religious identity among students at a private college: Social motives, ego stage, and development. *Merrill-Palmer Quarterly*, 1981, 27, 219–239.

[5] Two independent coders, blind to all information on the subjects as well as the study's aims and hypotheses, classified each subject's response into one of the four religious ideology statuses. The two scorers agreed exactly in 47 of the 56 cases (84 percent). The nine disagreements were decided by a third independent coder. More information on scoring and methodology is included in McAdams, Booth, & Selvik (1981).

[6] Two independent coders, blind to the study's hypotheses and other information on the subjects, rated each subject's response on the six-point scale. When a response manifested examples of more than one of the six complexity levels delineated, the coders classified the response at the "highest" (most complex) point that was exemplified. Thus, a response showing signs of points 1 and 2 would be scored at point 2. The correlation between the coder's separate scorings of the same data was .78.

[7] A criticism that could be levied against this study is that it discriminates, in a sense, against students who are not particularly "religious." One could argue that those students who have not grown up in a religious family environment or who have chosen to eschew religion in their daily lives might score relatively low on the complexity scale designed for this study. Though this criticism is not completely without merit, there are at least two responses to it that, I believe, minimize the problem suggested. First, most of the students in Sample A *have* had some religious training; the majority in the Catholic Church and/or through parochial schools. Second, the question asking for a description of religious beliefs (see Appendix B) emphasizes that one need not be a churchgoer in order to have a particular religious viewpoint. Upon receipt of the questionnaire concerning religious beliefs, the students in Sample A were told that we wished them to construe religion in very broad terms—as encompassing their basic assumptions and beliefs about the meaning of the universe and the human being's place in it. Our goal as researchers was to get across the idea of religion as something that need not be part of the institutional church. In this way, we sought to convey part of Fowler's conception of faith as a human universal.

[8] Again, two independent coders did the scoring. For RLP, their scores agreed in 67 of the 78 cases (86 percent). For CCR, agreement was 69 out of 79 (88 percent). The *Kappa* values were .72 for RLP and .77 for CCR.

Chapter 8

Generativity Script

Let us develop the resources of our land, call forth its powers, build up its institutions, promote all its great interests, and see whether we also, in our day and generation, may not perform something worthy to be remembered.

(Daniel Webster)

The magnificence of identity is its binding together of past, present, and an anticipated future. In affirming an essential sameness and continuity over time, a life story is a testament to what was and is and what will be. The past and the present find their way into the narrative via nuclear episodes (Chapter 5), an ideological setting (Chapter 7), and implicit personifications of self (Chapter 6). But the anticipated future requires a fourth story forum for its adequate expression. What is needed is a way of saying *what will happen next*. The action of the story is situated within a setting of belief and value; the main characters of the story have been established as personified and idealized images of self (imagoes); and the significant story high points, low points, and turning points—the nuclear episodes—have been organized as landmark events of the past. Given all this, *what is to be done in the future?* The stories we tell ourselves in order to live address this question by including *scripts* (plans, outlines) for chapters yet to be lived. These scripts for the future frequently and ideally center on *generativity* (Erikson, 1963, 1968, 1980). Generativity scripts for the future are as much a part of identity—as much a part of who we are—as are the setting, the scenes, and the characters emerging from our narrative reconstructions of the past and understandings of the present.

The conventional reading of Erikson is to separate neatly identity and generativity. Identity is typically understood as the central psychosocial issue of the adolescent or young adult who seeks to understand who he or she is and how he or she fits into the adult

world. Generativity, on the other hand, is the issue of middle adulthood, arising after one has achieved an identity and established intimate relationships with others and is thus ready to take on the
responsibilities of *caring for* the next generation. The simplest scenario
has it that the individual discovers an identity in young adulthood,
subsequently marries to consolidate intimacy and stave off isolation,
and then generates offspring and nurtures them through infancy,
childhood, and adolescence, so that they can repeat the cycle. Thus,
the psychosocial stages of identity versus role confusion, intimacy
versus isolation, and generativity versus stagnation—stages 5
through 7 in Erikson's scheme—unfold in a predictable sequence,
each being "resolved" in the individual's life cycle before the next, in
turn, can be confronted.

In proposing a life-story model of identity, this book holds that
the simplest scenario is too simple and that identity is too big an issue
to be confined to a discrete psychosocial stage. Though identity may
first emerge as a salient concern in adolescence, it does not go away
in adulthood, politely deferring to new and qualitatively different
issues associated with new developmental stages. Identity is a jealous
god. Once the individual becomes a biographer of self, an evolving
life story expands to encompass as much as it can. New experiences
and concerns feed into the story, influencing and being influenced by
the narrative. The process is very Piagetian. In Piaget's terms, the life
story is a large *schema*—a pattern of knowing. New experiences and
concerns may be *assimilated* into the story and thus fitted cleanly to an
existing schema. On the other hand, new experiences and concerns
may not fit well, and the story, or part of the story, may be changed
in order to *accommodate* the new. Continual assimilation and accom-
modation—continuity and transformation—defines the relationship
between identity and experience. The relationship cannot be terminated to make way for a new stage.

Generativity, therefore, is part of identity. In order to know who
I am, I must have some inkling of what I am going to *do* in the future
in order to be generative. My generativity script for the future must
make sense in terms of an established setting of belief and value, my
idealized and personified images of self, and the landmark events of
my biography. This chapter explores the ways in which men and
women envision their futures—the kinds of scripts for generativity
they incorporate into their life stories. I will begin with a recon-
sideration of Erikson's concept of generativity, drawing heavily upon
the writings of Ernest Becker. Next, I will attempt to situate generativity in the human life cycle, focusing upon the midlife crisis as a
crisis in generativity rather than ideology. I will argue that the part of
the life story that gets rewritten in the midlife crisis is usually the
generativity script and that this crisis is qualitatively different from

the "identity crisis" of the adolescent or young adult, which typically involves dimensions of an ideological setting. I will then present data on generativity scripts collected from the midlife men and women in Sample B. Relationships between structural dimensions of generativity scripts and ego development and between content dimensions of the scripts and social motives will be examined. I will also present findings supporting the proposition that generativity draws vitality from both power and intimacy motivation, reflecting the blending of agency and communion in healthy generativity. I will close with some speculative comments concerning our adult mandate to be generative.

A Closer Look at Generativity

Next to identity, generativity is the most trenchant of Erikson's ideas. Erikson's elaborations upon the term, however, are surprisingly few. In *Childhood and Society,* Erikson introduces generativity as "primarily the concern in establishing and guiding the next generation" (1963, p. 267). Generativity is most obviously actualized, therefore, in the raising of one's own children. Yet,

> the mere fact of having or even wanting children . . . does not "achieve" generativity. In fact, some young parents suffer, it seems, from the retardation of the ability to develop this stage. (p. 267)

Thus, raising children does not necessarily assure one that he or she is being generative. Moreover, raising children is not the only road to generativity. Some individuals, "through misfortune or because of special and genuine gifts in other directions, do not apply this drive to their own offspring" (p. 267). Indeed, "the concept of generativity is meant to include such more popular synonyms as *productivity* and *creativity,* which, however, cannot replace it" (p. 267).

In generativity, one *generates* (creates, produces) something. The something may be offspring, though certain other products (creations, generations) apparently qualify as well. In generativity, one is involved with the next *generation.* Those who will live after we die are literally generated (given birth to), succored, and supported by an older generation who once benefited from the same. Whereas children and adolescents are guided, adults guide, Erikson points out. Generativity makes the human being the "teaching and instituting as well as the learning animal" (p. 266).

For Erikson, generativity is a fundamental human tendency— what he understands to be a "drive" or "need." Though psychologists are wont to dramatize the dependence of the infant and child upon the adult, few recognize, argues Erikson, that mature men and women "need to be needed," that they are dependent upon the presence of other persons and things that "need" them. Part of generativity, therefore, is the realization that other people and things are worthy of one's care and that one's care is worthy of them. Erikson describes this realization as a "faith" in a community of care. Generativity requires "some faith, some 'belief in the species,' which would make a child appear to be a welcome trust of the community" (p. 267). The object of one's care, furthermore, may be larger than one's own progeny. Erikson writes that Gandhi's generativity script outlined his mission of care for an entire nation. India needed Gandhi, and Gandhi needed to be needed by India. In some of the most extraordinary sagas of generativity, the *life history* meets the *historical moment* (Erikson, 1975), and the individual and his or her world are transformed together through bold and *caring action:*

> From the moment in January of 1915 when Gandhi set foot on a pier reserved for important arrivals in Bombay, he behaved like a man who knew the nature and the extent of India's calamity and that of his own fundamental mission. A mature man of middle age has not only made up his mind as to what, in the various compartments of his life, he does and does not *care for,* he is also firm in his vision of what he *will* and *can* take *care of.* He takes as his baseline what he irreducibly is and reaches out for what only he can, and therefore, *must do.* (Erikson, 1969, p. 255, italics in original)

Our reading of Erikson suggests that generativity is a fundamental human need which involves being productive or creative as an adult and caring for others, especially the younger generation. It includes a faith that one's care is needed and that one needs to care. Caring for one's offspring is one way that generativity manifests itself. Taking bold and caring action for one's people is another, as we see in the life of Gandhi. One might assume that certain other human endeavors provide opportunities for expressing generativity: teaching, counseling, altruism. But what about painting a picture or writing a book? What about being a police officer, working in a laboratory, laboring on the assembly line, or typing a manuscript? Do these activities offer opportunities for generativity? If yes, in what way? If no, why not? Erikson maintains that "creativity" and "productivity" are popular "synonyms" for generativity but that these terms cannot replace generativity (1963, p. 267). In other words, being creative or productive as an adult is not necessarily the same thing as being generative. Something more is needed, and it seems that that something more is in some way related to "care." The relationship between creativity and care is at the heart of generativity, but this relationship cannot be clearly articulated until we move from Erikson's scattered, though provocative, notes on the topic to the writings of the late Ernest Becker.

Becker's (1973) last book, *The Denial of Death*, is a brilliant treatise on generativity, even though the term *generativity* is never used, and Erikson's name does not even appear in the index. Becker's argument is a synthesis of Kierkegaard, Freud, and Rank, and his central thesis is quite straightforward:

> The prospect of death, Dr. Johnson said, wonderfully concentrates the mind. The main thesis of this book is that it does much more than that: the idea of death, the fear of it, haunts the human animal like nothing else; it is a mainspring of human activity—activity designed largely to avoid the fatality of death, to overcome it by denying in some way that it is the final destiny for man. (p. ix)

The ultimate human motive, for Becker, is the fear of death. It is far more basic than any of Murray's needs, James's instincts, or Bakan's fundamental modes of human existence. At a much deeper level of analysis than power and intimacy motivation, and even beneath Freud's Eros and Thanatos, lies a solitary human fear. The fear of death is the mainspring of human activity, the prime mover which activates from below all other motives which are in some way derivatives of it.

As the only animal who anticipates and dreads its own demise, the human being is beset with the paradox of being within and outside of nature. On the one hand, humans are symbolic creatures who soar above the natural world, who can place themselves "imaginatively at a point in space and contemplate bemusedly" their own planet. "This immense expansion, this dexterity, this ethereality, this self-consciousness gives to man literally the status of a small god in nature, as the Renaissance thinkers knew" (p. 26). Yet at the same time,

> as the Eastern sages also knew, man is a worm, and food for worms. This is the paradox: he is out of nature and hopelessly in it; he is dual, up in the stars and yet housed in a heart-pumping, breath-gasping body that once belonged to a fish and still carries the gill marks to prove it. His body is a material fleshy casing that is alien to him in many ways—the strangest and most repugnant way being that it aches and bleeds and will decay and die. Man is literally split in two: he has an awareness of his own splendid uniqueness in that he sticks out of nature with a towering majesty, and yet he goes back into the ground a few feet in order blindly and dumbly to rot and disappear forever. It is a terrifying dilemma to be in and to have to live with. (p. 26)

Becker views the ancient duality of mind and body from a psychoanalytic perspective. In our dreams and in our myths—that is, in the unconscious—the mind is associated with the immortality of the spirit, with soaring above nature, and with escaping clean away from the earth. The body connects to the mortality of the flesh, being bound to the earth and encased within our dirty corporeality. The mind is reason, and the body is emotion; the mind is abstract, and the body is concrete; the mind is represented by the Sky God, a masculine principle of sorts, and the body is the Earth Mother, a feminine principle (deRiencourt, 1974). The paradox of seeming transcendence but ultimate corporeality is at the root of our human anxieties and the defense mechanisms we construct in order to deal with them. Indeed, the paradox was enough to drive the hero of one of Swift's poems to the brink of madness when contemplating his beautiful lover, Caelia:

> *Nor wonder how I lost my wits;*
> *Oh! Caelia, Caelia, Caelia shits!*
>
> (Becker, 1973, p. 33)

The universal response of human beings to the essential duality that defines them and to the fundamental fear which motivates all their behavior is *heroism*. Heroism is "first and foremost a reflex of the terror of death" (p. 11). In order to deny the inevitable death of the body, the human mind invents ways to be a hero and thereby attain a kind of immortality. For Becker, human societies have always existed as symbolic action systems designed to cultivate and condone human heroism. Individuals "serve" society in order to earn "a feeling of primary value, of cosmic specialness, of ultimate usefulness to creation, of unshakable meaning" (p. 5). In other words, to be a hero is to do something that matters in the larger scheme of things—to do something that lasts and lives on after the body is eaten by worms:

> They (human beings) earn this feeling by carving out a place in nature, by building an edifice that reflects human value: a temple, a cathedral, a totem pole, a sky-scraper, a family that spans three generations. The hope and the belief is that the things that man creates in society are of lasting worth and meaning, that they outlive or outshine death and decay, that man and his products count. (p. 5)

Like Erikson, Becker asserts that adults are compelled to generate products that outlive them—to "perform something worthy to be remembered," as Daniel Webster writes in the chapter's opening quotation. Generativity is heroism in that it is a way of attaining immortality through one's generations (creations, productions). As generative heroes and heroines, adults "construct" tangible or intangible "legacies" which survive them. But there is more to generativity, and to heroism, than generating something. Note the awkward sound of the phrase "to construct a legacy." We would typically say "to leave a legacy," taking for granted that the legacy represents our own creative or productive efforts. Indeed, this is the key to our closer examination of generativity, for Becker makes clear to us, whereas Erikson only hints, that generativity or heroism is twofold. First, it involves creating, producing, or generating something. Second, it involves *offering (leaving) that something as a gift.* Becker puts it this way:

> The whole thing boils down to this paradox: if you are going to be a hero, then you must give a gift. If you are the average man, you give your heroic gift to the society in which you live, and you give the gift the society specifies in advance. If you are an artist, you fashion a peculiarly personal gift, the justification of your own heroic identity, which means that it is always aimed at least partly over the heads of your fellow men. . . . The artist's gift is always to creation itself, to the ultimate meaning of life, to God. We should not be surprised that Rank was brought to exactly the same conclusion as Kierkegaard: the only way out of human conflict is full renunciation, to give one's life as a gift to the highest powers. (p. 173)

Though the fruits of our generativity can be understood as parts of us that live on after we die, once generated they no longer belong solely to us. To generate gifts but then fail to give them, fail to grant them autonomy and lives of their own, is a desperate kind of narcissism. Whether the gifts derive from one's work, play, family, or friends, one must grapple with the seeming paradox that these gifts are *me* and *not me:* They are carefully fashioned legacies of the self which must be surrendered, selflessly, as offerings to a larger community. In Erikson's sense, we are asked as adults to fashion products and then to *care* for them as precious gifts, autonomous and yet dependent upon our care. Erikson's caring attitude is Becker's giving attitude—a second step in generativity, and the feature which distinguishes it from the concepts of "productivity" and "creativity." It is an attitude we should assume vis-à-vis all our "children," all our offerings fashioned to assure some semblance of our own immortality.

Generativity's Place in the Human Life Cycle

A Plan for the Future

Our folklore is filled with standard scripts for generativity. There is the Jewish mother who devotes her energies to coddling, feeding, and educating her "son the doctor." There is the rags-to-riches entrepreneur who bequeaths the family business to the firstborn. There are the first-generation immigrants who work the steel mills and clip the coupons to save money for their children's education. There are the scientists, artists, teachers, missionaries, nurses, and philanthropists whose gifts reach a larger audience. Many of the greatest stories in the Judeo-Christian heritage are tales of generativity: God promises Abraham and Sarah a son who will become a nation; Isaac blesses

Esau with the birthright (and Jacob swindles it away); Moses leads the
Israelites out of the land of Egypt; Christ dies on a cross to save
sinners; the New Testament martyrs give their lives to spread a message to the four corners of the earth. And many of the least legendary,
most commonplace tales of daily living say the same thing. In Studs
Terkel's *Working* (1972), Mike Lefevre, a steelworker, explains what
justifies his daily labors:

> This is gonna sound square, but my kid is my imprint. He's my free-
> dom. There's a line in one of Hemingway's books. I think it's from
> *For Whom the Bell Tolls.* They're behind the enemy lines, somewhere
> in Spain, and she's pregnant. She wants to stay with him. He tells
> her no. He says, "If you die, I die," knowing he's gonna die. "But
> if you go, I go." Know what I mean? The mystics call it the brass
> bowl. *Continuum.* You know what I mean? This is why I work. Every
> time I see a young guy walk by with a shirt and tie dressed up real
> sharp, I'm lookin' at my kid, you know? That's it. (Terkel, 1972, p. 10,
> italics added)

Mike Lefevre understands his own work in terms of generativity—in terms of fashioning a gift for the next generation, a generation
personified in "my kid." Generativity may be expressed through
one's family life, friendships, work life, church or community activities, and even pastimes and hobbies. In her studies of middle- and
lower-middle-class American adults, Marjorie Fiske (1980; Lowenthal, Thurnher, & Chiriboga, 1975) has identified four clusters of
commitment, each of which, I would argue, may afford opportunities
for the expression of generativity. Fiske describes commitments in the
areas of (*a*) the interpersonal, (*b*) the altruistic (including ethical,
philosophical, and religious allegiances), (*c*) mastery/competence,
and (*d*) self-protection. According to Fiske, adult development is best
conceived in terms of shifting priorities of commitments over time.

Palys and Little (1983) have examined adult commitment areas
which may afford the expression of generativity through what they
term *personal projects.* Personal projects are action plans designed to
achieve specific personal goals. These projects vary with respect to
their difficulty, enjoyableness, and the degree to which they are oriented toward short-term versus long-term aims. Employing a Personal Projects Matrix (PPM) in which the person lists up to 10 of his
or her own personal projects and discusses the significance of each,
Palys and Little have found that individuals who report involvement
in enjoyable and moderately difficult projects oriented toward relatively short-term goals tend to be highly satisfied with their lives.
Individuals reporting less enjoyable and highly difficult projects oriented toward longer-term goals tend to score lower in life satisfaction.
Life satisfaction was also associated with the presence of a supportive
social network with which the individual shared project involvement.

In his biographical studies of midlife men, Daniel Levinson (1978) has focused on more global action plans that adults formulate for the future. A vitalizing force in the lives of many of Levinson's men is an articulated *dream* for the future—an overall script or plan concerning what is to be done. Serving as a general and multifaceted personal project for one's life as a whole, the dream propels the action line of the individual's life story into the future and thus affirms the temporal continuity which is at the heart of identity. Levinson argues that major transitions in the adult life course are occasioned by transformations in the dream. Furthermore, men who find it difficult to formulate a dream may find that stagnation frequently wins out over generativity during their adult years.

Though not explicitly couched in terms of "generativity," the studies of Fiske (1980), Levinson (1978), and Palys and Little (1983) converge on the idea that adult lives can be meaningfully conceived according to the scripts or plans for future action that men and women formulate in areas of personal commitment. For most adults, generativity involves some kind of plan for the future. Indeed, generativity's relationship to the future can be understood in two ways. In that generativity concerns guiding the next generation, it is oriented toward the future of humankind, the succession of generations, and the continuity of the species. (Recall Erikson's "belief in the species.") In that generativity may be framed in the context of an adult's overall script or plan concerning what is to be done, it is oriented toward the particular future each individual envisions for his or her own life.

Midlife Crisis

Recent years have witnessed a good deal of talk among some psychologists, journalists, and laypersons about the *midlife crisis*. Gail Sheehy's (1976) book, *Passages*, has probably done more to popularize the term than has anything else. Sheehy describes passages as predictable crises in adult lives and suggests that men and women are especially vulnerable to these crises during the "midlife years," typically between the ages of 35 and 50. During a midlife crisis, the individual may become disillusioned with the present direction of his or her life and thus come to rethink priorities and goals so as to formulate a new plan for the future. The crisis may play itself out in a variety of commitment areas: family, job, friendships, community involvement, interests, and hobbies. Though some have described these crises as thoroughgoing transformations of identity per se (Gould, 1980), I submit that they are usually crises in generativity in which the individual is compelled, often by such external circumstances as children leaving home, to rewrite the script outlining his or her envisioned contribution to future generations. Let us look more closely at how psychologists have viewed midlife.

A number of scholars have depicted the midlife period as a time in the human life cycle in which hitherto suppressed parts of the psyche become revealed and eventually reintegrated into the self. Jung was one of the first to make this point. At midlife, the man encounters his hidden anima—the suppressed feminine side of his personality. Likewise, the woman at midlife confronts her suppressed masculinity, her anim*us*. As the individual comes to accept what was hitherto latent but now made manifest, the center of the personality moves from the conscious ego, in Jung's theory, to a point halfway between the conscious and the unconscious, a place termed the *self*. In this way, the self becomes the constellating figure, at midlife, within the Jungian psychic apparatus, and the midlife man or woman becomes, in Jung's terms, more *individuated* and more whole. This is the ideal life-cycle scenario in Jung's theory: the prescription for health and maturity in the adult years. That this general scenario has been assimilated into our contemporary Western understanding of adaptation in adulthood becomes quite evident in reading the following quotation from Giele (1980):

> In America recent discussion of the middle years has given rise to a new concept of adulthood. The mature person today is one who keeps alive the energy and adaptability of youth while cultivating the wisdom of age. In similar fashion, the ideal adult also combines both masculine and feminine traits—women becoming more assertive and independent, men tending toward greater nurturance, passivity, dependence, and contemplativeness. (p. 166)

The cross-cultural work of David Gutmann (1980) supports the Jungian view. Gutmann's observations of adult development among the Navaho and Mayan and in the Middle East have led him to the conclusion that a common tendency prevails on the part of older men to abandon the vigorous and aggressive manner of young adulthood in favor of more passive and contemplative roles at midlife. Women, on the other hand, are more likely to become more powerful as they grow older, eschewing the more dependent and self-effacing ways of their youth. Whereas younger men "see energy as a feature of the self" and as "a potential threat that has to be contained and deployed to productive service," older men "see energy outside of themselves, lodged in capricious secular or supernatural authority" (Gutmann, 1980, p. 41). Furthermore, older men are more "diffusely sensual," taking pleasure in the "pregenital" delights of good food, pleasant sights and sounds, and simple talk among friends. Women, on the other hand, move with age toward a more agentic orientation. According to Gutmann, their roles become more political and managerial and they may come to exert substantial influence over many different sectors of the community, especially over the younger men.

The conclusions of Jung and Gutmann are echoed in the theory of adult development proposed by Levinson (1977, 1978, 1980, 1981). The primary concept in Levinson's theory is the *individual life structure*. The life structure "refers to the patterning or design of the individual life at a given time" (1977, p. 99). One of the more encompassing concepts in psychological theory, the life structure includes the individual's sociocultural world (class, religion, family, political systems, sociohistorical context), participation in this world (relationships and roles vis-à-vis significant others and groups), and "aspects of the self." Adult development is thereby conceived as evolution in the life structure, and it is at midlife that the structure may undergo its most comprehensive transformations.

Based on an intensive study of 40 adult men residing in the United States, Levinson proposes that life structures in men pass through periods of marked stability and marked change. After an *Early Adult Transition* (ages 17–22), the man enters a relatively stable period in which his life structure is centered on *Entering the Adult World* (ages 22–28). This is a period of exploration, a time of provisional commitments to adult roles and responsibilities. Following the *Age 30 Transition*, the man typically begins a second period of relative stability as he becomes immersed within a second life structure centered on *Settling Down* (the early 30s). During Settling Down, the man is trying to build a niche in the world and establish a position and timetable for advancement in his occupational world, while putting down roots in the sphere of his family. The man in his early 30s, preoccupied with "making it" and "building a nest," invests heavily in issues of order, stability, security, and control. His concerns are reminiscent of Erikson's picture of the second stage of psychosocial development: the anal stage of autonomy versus shame and doubt in which the toddler makes major advances in mastering and controlling self and environment as an independent agent. For the toddler, the next phase is Oedipal: Freud's universal ontogenetic tragedy of becoming the conquering king and then falling from power. Levinson's next phase of the life structure—the period of BOOM (*Becoming One's Own Man*)—likewise has a certain Oedipal ring to it:

> BOOM tends to occur in the middle to late 30s, typically in our sample around 35–39. It represents the high point of early adulthood and the beginning of what lies beyond. A key element in this period is the man's feeling that, no matter what he has accomplished to date, he is not sufficiently his own man. He feels overly dependent upon and constrained by persons or groups who have authority over him or who, for various reasons, exert great influence upon him.

The writer comes to recognize that he is unduly intimidated by his publisher or too vulnerable to the evaluation of certain critics. The man who has successfully risen through the managerial ranks with the support and encouragement of his superiors now finds that they control too much and delegate too little, and he impatiently awaits the time when he will have the authority to make his own decisions and to get the enterprise really going. The untenured faculty member imagines that once he has tenure he will be free of all the restraints and demands he's been acquiescing to since graduate school days. (The illusions die hard!) (Levinson, Darrow, Klein, Levinson & McKee, 1974, pp. 250–251)

BOOM sets the stage for the *Midlife Transition*. During this period (ages 40–45 years), 80 percent of Levinson's sample encountered serious doubts concerning the direction of their lives.[1] Taking stock of the various areas of commitment making up their life structures, many men came to question the validity and worth of their hitherto most cherished interpersonal and instrumental goals and their envisioned plans for attaining them. For many, the Midlife Transition represented the BUST following BOOM. Marital satisfaction, job performance, and enjoyment of outside pursuits declined. Confusion and despair became common as the sense of having established a home and a niche in the adult world, consolidated during Settling Down, gradually disintegrated, replaced by the nagging apprehension that one's life has been directed by and for the sake of illusions.

Much of what makes the Midlife Transition so emotionally trying is a result of the painful work of "de-illusionment." Some of the men in Levinson's sample emerged from the Midlife Transition "cynical, estranged, unable to believe in anything" (Levinson, 1977, p. 108). Many others, however, benefited from the reevaluation. The latter group fashioned new life structures which opened up new opportunities and outlets for fulfillment in family, work, and friendship. Thus, the Midlife Transition may eventuate in a rejuvenated life structure in the second half of life—a restabilization around new plans and goals designed to maximize the individual's potential for fulfillment and, indeed, generativity. Though the de-illusionment of midlife entails substantial personal risk, it portends profound personal growth as well. In Levinson's view, men who fail to question their lives in these middle years forfeit a precious opportunity for positive change.

Crises at midlife typically concern at least three fundamental issues: (*a*) the polarity of masculinity and femininity, (*b*) the sense of aging and bodily decline, and (*c*) the recognition of one's mortality (Levinson and others, 1974). The first of these has been discussed in the context of Jung's and Gutmann's theories of gender crossover at midlife—males becoming more communal and females more agentic.

The latter two take us back to Becker and forward to the intriguing work of Elliott Jacques (1965) on death and the midlife crisis. Though Becker argues that the denial of death lies at the source of most all of our meaningful life striving, Jacques suggests that denial typically breaks down at midlife as one is faced with grappling, on a conscious level, with the prospect of one's own imminent demise. In the midlife crisis, the individual becomes painfully aware of the fact that he or she "has stopped growing up, and has begun to grow old" (Jacques, 1965, p. 506). He or she has entered the second half of life; more of life now lies behind than in front. Time is running out, and one must *do something* significant before it is too late.

Jacques has explored how the midlife crisis has played itself out in the lives of some of history's greatest creative geniuses.[2] Studying a sample of 310 painters, composers, poets, writers, and sculptors "of undoubted greatness or of genius" (p. 502), Jacques concludes that the crisis may manifest itself in one of three ways: (1) the creative career may simply come to an end, either through a cessation of creative output or death; (2) the creative capacity may show itself for the first time; or (3) a decisive change in the quality of creative work and the content of the creative product may take place. With reference to the first possibility, Jacques found that the death rate among his 310 geniuses showed a sudden increase between 35 and 39, followed by an equally sudden drop in the years 40 to 44 and a return to a normal death rate after that. Dying between the years of 35 and 39 were Mozart, Raphael, Chopin, Rimbaud, Purcell, Baudelaire, and Watteau. Those whose creative output either stopped abruptly or underwent a serious decline at midlife include Michelangelo, Rossini, Racine, and Ben Johnson. In contrast, many geniuses manifested their first creative flowering during the midlife years, such as Gauguin, Goya, Constable, and Bach.

Among those geniuses who were productive before, during, and after midlife, Jacques observed a common and quite remarkable transformation in the mode and content of their creativity. For many, the creative process was transformed at midlife from a passionate and spontaneous creativity to something more tempered and refined:

> The creativity of the 20s and early 30s tends to be a hot-from-the-fire creativity. It is intense and spontaneous, and comes out ready-made. The spontaneous effusions of Mozart, Keats, Shelley, Rimbaud, are the protoype. Most of the work seems to go on unconsciously. The conscious production is rapid, the pace of creation often being dictated by the limits of the artist's capacity physically to record the words or music he is expressing. . . .
>
> By contrast, the creativity of the late 30s and after is a sculpted creativity. The inspiration may be hot and intense. The unconscious

work is no less than before. But there is a big step between the first effusion of inspiration and the finished created product. The inspiration itself may come more slowly. Even if there are sudden bursts of inspiration, they are only the beginning of the work process. The initial inspiration must first be externalized in its elemental state. Then begins the process of forming and fashioning the external product, by means of working and reworking the externalized material. (p. 503)

Paralleling the movement from a spontaneous to a sculpted creativity at midlife is an equally radical transformation in the content of the created product. The work of the younger artist may be highly idealistic and optimistic, laden with themes of pure desire and glorious romance. With the emergence of a profound anxiety about the passing of time and imminent death at midlife, the idealism may give way to a more contemplative pessimism and a "recognition and acceptance that inherent goodness is accompanied by hate and destructive force within" (p. 505). Creative products speak a more philosophical and somber language after midlife, and this is a result of the artist's own confrontation with the prospect of death. Whereas Shakespeare produced most of his lyrical comedies before he was 35, the great series of tragedies and Roman plays—*Julius Caesar, Hamlet, Othello, King Lear,* and *Macbeth*—was begun later, between the ages of 35 and 40. A similar change is observed in the writing of Dickens, whose novels become much more tragic and realistic with the publication of *David Copperfield* at age 37.

In exploring the relationships between creativity and the fear of death at midlife, Jacques recalls our synthesis of Erikson's generativity (read: creativity, productivity) and Becker's concept of heroism in the face of impending death. Like Jacques' artists and poets, I submit, contemporary men and women undergoing the so-called midlife crisis may frequently be experiencing an identity upheaval with respect to a generativity script. Like Shakespeare and Dickens, their struggles and questions may arise from an unprecedented urgency about how much time is left and the concomitant desire *to do something that lasts before it is too late.* Unlike the 18-year-old whose identity crisis typically involves a rethinking of basic ideological values concerning what is good, what is true, what to believe, and what to value, the crisis of the 40-year-old described by Gutmann, Jung, Levinson, and Jacques is more often a crisis in *generative action.* The midlife adult may ask, "How can I attain a kind of immortality through the creation or generation of my gifts?" The question may motivate the man or woman at midlife to rewrite his or her script for the future, outlining new modes and innovative plans for the generation of meaningful and long-lasting life products.

Generativity Scripts in Midlife Adults

The Complexity of the Script

> Now that you have told me a little bit about your past, I would like you to tell me about your overall dream, plan, or vision for the future. Most of us have dreams or plans which concern what we would like to get out of life and what we would like to put into it. These dreams or plans may provide our lives with goals, interests, hopes, aspirations, and wishes. Furthermore, our dreams or plans for the future may change over time, reflecting growth and changing experiences.

With these words, the interviewer introduced to each of the midlife men and women in Sample B the topic of generativity script. Follow-up questions asked them to consider in what way their overall plan for the future enabled them (a) to be *creative* and (b) to make a *contribution* to others. (See Appendix B for the entire interview.)[3] The responses to these questions varied widely with respect to both structure and content. I will first consider variations in structure.

Hypothesis 8, presented first in Chapter 2, states that persons with higher ego development should manifest greater complexity in the structure of their scripts or plans for the future. More specifically, high ego development should be associated with greater differentiation in scripts, evidenced by a greater variety of specific goals for the future. Leaving aside for the moment the degree to which a given script for the future is indeed "generative," I have predicted that midlife men and women at higher stages of ego development should construct more differentiated future scenarios embodying detailed plans for the achievement of a relatively extensive variety of action goals. Whether or not these action goals afford opportunities for generativity is another question to be considered a bit later.

As a first step in analyzing the data, my associates and I condensed the section of each interview devoted to the individual's description of his or her script for the future to a written paragraph stating in a clear and nonredundant way the main points of his or her response.[4] Focusing on concrete action goals for the future, we broke down each response into four goal categories: instrumental/occupational, interpersonal, recreational, and material. Instrumental/occupational goals are specific plans about accomplishing tasks and achieving ends in the worlds of work and education. Interpersonal goals concern hopes and plans for one's most significant relationships, such as those with family, friends, and lovers. Recreational goals concern the use of leisure time—finding enjoyment or satisfaction in extracurricular, playful pursuits lying outside the realms of work and love. Material goals include basic daily needs to balance budgets and make ends meet as well as more grandiose aspirations about accumulating massive amounts of money and surrounding oneself with the material accoutrements of the good life.

For each of the four goal categories, we identified up to two explicit and nonoverlapping goals. Thus, for each of the four categories, the individual received a score of 0, 1, or 2, indicating the number of goals identified. To determine the degree of differentiation in future scripts, then, we merely summed scores from each of the four goals categories, arriving at a total score (hypothetically ranging from 0 to 8) for variety of goals presented in the script.[5] In Sample B, these total scores ranged from 0 to 5. The mean score was 2.37 (standard deviation = 1.13).

As in the previous chapters, the analysis of ego development involved comparing individuals scoring high and low on Loevinger's (1976) scale, high being at stage I-4 or above and low being at I-3/4 or below. Supporting Hypothesis 8, we found that men and women scoring high in ego development had significantly higher scores on variety in goals than did men and women scoring low in ego development. For the former group, the mean score on variety in goals was 2.74. For the latter group, the mean was 2.04, F (1,46) = 5.02, $p < .05$. Gender appeared to make little difference in these results. The mean score on variety in goals was 2.40 for men and 2.34 for women, a nonsignificant difference. Sex differences did appear, however, within certain goal categories. Although the results were on the border between statistical significance and nonsignificance, women tended to score higher on interpersonal goals than did men (means = 1.03 versus 0.60, F (1,46) = 3.93, $p = .05$), whereas men tended to score higher than women on material goals (means = 0.60 versus 0.31, F (1,46) = 3.47, $p = .07$).

It appears, therefore, that midlife adults high in ego development bring their relatively complex frameworks of meaning to the enterprise of apprehending their own futures. The anticipated future chapters in their life stories contain a greater variety of action goals than do those chapters envisioned by their counterparts scoring low in ego development. Men and women high in ego development combine in their scripts for the future goals from diverse commitment areas, whereas those men and women scoring low in ego development appear more likely to focus on one or two areas exclusively, framing scripts significantly less differentiated and more global. Although gender does not appear to affect this relationship between ego development and the variety of future goals, some evidence does suggest that women are more likely to focus on interpersonal goals for the future and men on goals concerned with their material well-being.[6]

The Content of Generativity Scripts

The procedure for analyzing the content of future scripts is similar to that followed in previous chapters of this book. We employed again the fundamental thematic distinction between power/agency and intimacy/communion. Hypothesis 7 states that high power motivation, assessed via the TAT, should be positively associated with agentic future scripts, whereas intimacy motivation should be positively related to scripts of communion. Thus, future scripts of midlife men and women high in power motivation should reflect a predominantly agentic content—visions of the future in which the individual expands self and exerts an impact upon the world. Scripts developed by midlife adults high in intimacy motivation, on the other hand, should reveal communal motifs—visions of the future in which the person surrenders self in the context of caring relationships with others.

We rated each of the script paragraphs on a three-point scale for agency and another three-point scale for communion. On the agency scale, a rating of 3 indicated a detailed plan strongly emphasizing expanding the self, having impact on the environment, and/or exerting force and control; a 2 indicated a somewhat vague plan emphasizing the above or a detailed plan with a moderate emphasis upon self-expansion, impact, and control; a 1 indicated no such plan. On the communion scale, a 3 indicated a detailed plan strongly emphasizing the cultivation or maintenance of warm, interpersonal relationships embodying care, dialogue, and/or helping; a 2 indicated a less detailed plan of the above or a detailed plan with a moderate emphasis upon warm relations, care, dialogue, and helping; a 1 indicated no such plan.[7] Below is a script paragraph which was scored a 3 for agency and a 2 for communion:

> To obtain a master's degree in social work or a Ph.D.; to continue in social work; to keep adapting to change; to keep growing and expanding horizons; to keep moving, never stop; to get married and have kids. (Subject sees script as offering opportunities for creativity and making a contribution to others through helping others in need. Subject does not see self as making a general contribution to humankind but believes that the case-by-case help he/she offers is important in that he/she directly affects others' lives.)

Supporting Hypothesis 7, power motivation was strongly correlated with agency themes in future scripts, r (48) = .58, p < .001. Similarly, intimacy motivation and communion themes in scripts were highly correlated, r (48) = .41 p < .01. These relationships were reflected within both sex subsamples. Although women scored slightly higher than men on communion themes in future scripts (means = 1.93 versus 1.60) and lower on agency (means = 1.60 versus

1.80), these sex differences were not statistically significant. Ego development likewise was statistically unrelated to content themes of agency and communion.

The results on the content of future scripts neatly parallel those from Chapter 5 concerning the content of nuclear episodes. Whereas Chapter 5 documents thematic continuities in identity as we move back biographically to the most significant episodes in the person's life story, this chapter extends the continuities forward into anticipated biographical scripts for the life story's chapters to be lived. Table 8.1 displays the correlations between a number of key variables for nuclear episodes and future scripts. Suggesting a strong continuity in power themes across nuclear episodes of the past and envisioned action scripts for the future are the significantly positive correlations between power/agency themes in future scripts and power theme scores in a number of nuclear episodes: peak experiences, nadir experiences, and positive childhood experiences. Continuity in intimacy themes is less striking but a significantly positive correlation is revealed between intimacy/communion themes in future scripts and intimacy theme scores in nadir experiences.

Individual Differences in Generativity

But what about *generativity*? So far I have discussed dimensions of structure and content in the midlife adults' action scripts for the future, but I have not as yet addressed the question of how these action scripts afford generativity. After listening to only a few of the interview tapes, I became convinced that future scripts vary widely on this score. Some scripts appear to be much more generative than others. Indeed, the label *generativity script* may be somewhat of a misnomer for life stories in which the future puts very little emphasis upon generating a gift to be offered to the next generation. In these cases, we may be more accurate in describing the action script for the future as just that—an "action script for the future"—rather than adding the modifier "generativity." In referring to the entire sample of scripts in this chapter, however, I am sticking with the term *generativity script* to remind the reader that these outlines for the future *frequently* and *ideally* are framed in terms of generative action and that identity cannot be neatly divorced from generativity.[8]

To code the relative prominence of generativity in generativity scripts, therefore, I adopted a generativity scale developed by Ryff and Heincke (1983). Each script paragraph was given a rating from 1 to 3. A high score (3) was given to scripts which evidenced a strong concern for establishing and guiding the next generation either directly (via caregiving, teaching, leading, mentoring, etc.) or indirectly (via contributing something that one has created to others or to a

TABLE 8.1. Correlations between Dimensions of Nuclear Episodes and Future Scripts in Sample B

| | Future Scripts | | | | | | |
| | | | Goals | | | | |
Nuclear Episodes	Agency	Communion	Instrumental/ Occupational	Interpersonal	Recreational	Material	Variety in Goals (Total)
Peak experience							
Power	.31*	-.02	.21	-.09	-.07	-.10	.00
Intimacy	-.06	.12	-.07	.12	-.25	-.07	-.10
Positive child- hood experience							
Power	.34*	-.14	.17	-.03	.15	-.17	.07
Intimacy	-.20	.25	.03	.24	-.21	-.22	.00
Peak and positive childhood experience							
Power	.40†	-.16	.24	-.10	.01	.02	-.00
Intimacy	-.16	.26	-.05	.28	-.31*	-.23	-.07
Nadir experience							
Power	.40†	-.04	.18	.06	-.30*	.00	.04
Intimacy	.19	.32*	.09	.13	-.09	.01	.12

Negative childhood experience							
Power	.12	-.15	-.26	-.01	-.07	-.02	-.22
Intimacy	-.12	.15	.06	.14	.07	.21	.27
Nadir and negative childhood experience							
Power	.41†	-.09	.08	.02	-.29	-.03	-.17
Intimacy	.12	.36*	.16	.23	-.13	.08	.26
All four experiences total							
Power	.48†	-.16	.10	-.07	.14	-.14	-.11
Intimacy	-.04	.40*	.06	.33*	.29	-.11	.11
Number of nuclear episodes in interview	.02	.25	.18	.13	-.27	-.22	-.00
Number of nuclear episodes in interview classified as "turning points"	.07	.30*	.13	.20	-.01	-.30*	.08

Note: N = 50
a Dimensions of nuclear episodes are described in Chapter 5.
* p < .05
† p < .01

community at large, as in the case of literary, scientific, artistic, or altruistic contributions). In scripts scoring high in generativity, the individual appears to possess an awareness of responsibilities to others, be they responsibilities to specific loved ones or to a larger community of others. The individual may view himself or herself as a "norm bearer" or "destiny shaper" with a "sense of maximal influence capacity" (Ryff & Heincke, 1983, p. 809). A low score (1) on generativity indicates none of the above. In this case, the individual shows little interest in establishing or guiding the next generation through contributing something, sharing knowledge, and so on. The individual may even manifest excessive self-preoccupation or narcissism. An intermediate score (2) was given to scripts which manifest a "moderate" degree of generativity concern.[9]

Approximately two thirds of the midlife adults manifested at least moderate levels of generativity in the scripts (33 out of 50). Receiving the highest rating of 3 were 10 (20 percent) of the adults, and 23 (46 percent) received ratings of 2. Seventeen (34 percent) of the adults showed no evidence of generativity concerns in their future scripts. The average generativity score was 1.93 for women and 1.75 for men, a nonsignificant difference.

Relationships between generativity ratings and a number of other variables are shown in Table 8.2. Intimacy motivation was positively associated with generativity ratings, but the correlation was quite small and barely significant ($r = .29, p < .05$). Power motivation was positively but nonsignificantly related to generativity ($r = .18$).

TABLE 8.2. Correlations between Generativity Ratings and Selected Other Variables

Variable	Entire Sample (N = 50)	Women (N = 30)	Men (N = 20)
Power motivation	.18	.14	.26
Intimacy motivation	.29*	.28	.28
Power plus intimacy motivation	.40†	.34	.48*
Career satisfaction	.11	.19	−.08
Relationship satisfaction	.20	.15	.29
Overall life satisfaction	.05	.09	−.08
Agency content in scripts	.15	.01	.48*
Communion content in scripts	.57††	.53†	.62†
Occupational/instrumental goals	.41†	.27	.64†
Interpersonal goals	.53†	.40*	−.68††
Recreational goals	−.09	.12	−.45*
Material goals	−.39†	−.38*	−.37
Complexity of script (total goals)	.41†	.31	.58†

*$p < .05$
†$p < .01$
††$p < .001$

Strong positive correlations were obtained between generativity ratings and (*a*) complexity in the generativity script ($r = .41, p < .01$)
and (*b*) communion content in the script ($r = .57, p < .001$).[10] Generativity was positively correlated, furthermore, with occupational/
instrumental and interpersonal goals and negatively associated with
material goals. Finally, generativity ratings were unrelated to ego
development ($F (1,46) = 2.19, p = .145$).

The most interesting finding, however, may seem surprising at
first glance. Observing that the two motives were each positively
though not strongly related to generativity ratings, I combined standardized scores on power and intimacy motivation into one total
motivational score for each adult in Sample B and correlated these
combination power plus intimacy scores with generativity.[11] As Table
8.2 shows, the correlation between power plus intimacy motivation
and generativity was positive and highly significant ($r = .40$,
$p < .01$), and the relationship was reflected within both sex subsamples. This means that whereas power and intimacy motivation by
themselves are each relatively weak though positive predictors of
generativity in action scripts for the future, power and intimacy motivation added together predicts generativity remarkably well. Thus,
men and women in their 30s and 40s whose life stories evidenced the
greatest concern for generative action in the future tended *to score high
on power and intimacy combined*. If power and intimacy are seen as two
fundamental motives in human lives, then we can say that highly
generative adults bring forth more raw motivational material in their
fantasy productions—their TAT stories—than do those adults whose
scripts for the future neglect generativity. In the language of Chapter
3, the most generative of identities may be those through which the
thematic lines of power *and* intimacy run most deeply.

Though surprising at first glance, the positive relationship between generativity and power plus intimacy motivation makes a good
deal of sense in light of our earlier discussion of Erikson's and
Becker's writings on generating gifts in adulthood. Remember that
generativity, as I have conceptualized it in this chapter, involves both
creating and *giving up*. In generativity, one creates a product which
represents an extension of the self and a claim to immortality. Then,
one renounces ownership of the product, granting it a certain degree
of autonomy and offering it to the world. The first step represents a
powerful expansion of the self—an agentic act *par excellence*. The
ultimate example: God creates Adam. The second step represents a
surrender of the self, a renunciation of control. Offering a gift involves
an intimate exchange with a community: God grants Adam free will
(and offers him up to the universe). Our generative gifts may be
creations in our own image, but the creations must be offered up to
others if we are to meet generativity's double demand. As religious

men and women the world over have traditionally attributed to their gods both powerful and loving qualities, so do generative adults in the act of creating and then giving their gifts experience agency and communion, power and love. This chapter's finding that power plus intimacy motivation is positively associated with generativity in action scripts for the future is the first piece of empirical evidence with which I am familiar—albeit a small piece—that generativity challenges us as adults to be both powerful and intimate, expanding the self and surrendering to others in the same generative act.

A Postscript

I have twice suggested that the action scripts adults compose to outline the future chapters in their life stories should be called *generativity scripts* because these scripts *frequently* and *ideally* concern generativity (as I have characterized it in this chapter). That adults' future life scripts *frequently* center on generativity is an empirical claim, and the fact that about two thirds of the midlife men and women in Sample B underscored generativity when describing their overall plan or vision for the future provides some support for this claim. That adults' future life scripts should *ideally* concern generativity, on the other hand, is a philosophical statement, and here I am revealing my own prescriptive bias concerning psychosocial maturity in the adult years. It is a bias shared with Erikson, Becker, and Freud.

For Erikson, generativity is the hallmark of maturity during the adult years. The contrasting phenomenon is *stagnation*—the sense that one's life is going nowhere, that one cannot create and cannot give to the next generation. For Becker, the best that men and women can do during their adult years is to strive to be heroes and heroines through their gifts. For Freud, maturity in adulthood is captured in his pithy phrase *Lieben und Arbeiten*. Human beings in their adult years minimize their anxiety and maximize their instinctual pleasure through productive love and work. Hale (1980) describes Freud's view:

> Reduced to the simplest level, both work and love are governed by the search for the same goal: more lasting, realistic, and socially responsible pleasure. Artistic creation and scientific discovery are the highest and most intensely enjoyable kinds of work because in them sublimated energies of sexuality and aggression play a major role. Work not only attaches the individual to reality but "gives him a secure place in the human community" [Freud, 1964d, 79–80]. Optimal love includes the working through of ambivalence, fantasy, disgust, and narcissism. Optimal love also includes the adult union of sexuality and affection in marriage and caring of the young, the functions Erik Erikson has developed into the concept of generativity.

Work and love can function optimally only in the context of civilization, which jointly they make possible. (p. 30)

Generativity may be our most solemn mandate and our greatest challenge in the adult years. To achieve generativity is to help assure one's own continuity through one's self-generated products and, more important, the continuity of the human community via the next generation. In this sense, the concept of generativity bears a striking resemblance to what sociobiologists describe as our biological mission to facilitate the passing on of our genes to the next generation—a biological mandate we share with all other species in the animal kingdom (Wilson, 1978). Whereas the failure to fulfill one's biological mandate may threaten the continuation of a particular genetic strain, failure in generativity—what Erikson terms stagnation—takes many forms, from the neurosis of failing to create meaningful life products to the narcissism of failing to offer those products to the world around us. As researchers, clinicians, and laypersons, we are repeatedly confronted in our personal lives and in the lives of our subjects, clients, and friends with examples of failure in generativity. Yet, there are also those heroic moments in which we or those around us, in Daniel Webster's words, "perform something worthy to be remembered." It is in those moments that adults fulfill their psychosocial mandate to be generative.

In an unforgettable passage from Terkel's (1972) *Working*, a Brooklyn firefighter named Tom Patrick describes his perspective on generativity:

The fuckin' world's so fucked up; the country's fucked up. But the firemen, you actually see them produce. You see them put out a fire. You see them come out with babies in their hands. You see them give mouth-to-mouth when a guy's dying. You can't get around that shit. That's real. To me, that's what I want to be.

I worked in a bank. You know, it's just paper. It's not real. Nine to five and its shit. You're looking at numbers. But I can look back and say, "I helped put out a fire. I helped save somebody." It shows something I did on this earth. (p. xxx)

The same sentiment is expressed in the final passage of Becker's *The Denial of Death*. I close this chapter with that passage:

We can conclude that a project as grand as the scientific-mythical construction of victory over human limitation is not something that can be programmed by science. Even more, it comes from the vital energies of masses of men sweating within the nightmare of creation—and it is not even in man's hands to program. Who knows what form the forward momentum of life will take in the time ahead or what use it will make of our anguished searching. The most that any one of us can seem to do is to fashion something—an object or ourselves—and drop it into the confusion, make an offering of it, so to speak, to the life force. (1973, p. 285)

Summary

The *generativity script* is an *action* outline for the future which specifies what an individual plans to *do* in order to leave a legacy of self to the next generation. Synthesizing Erikson's scattered offerings on generativity and the writings of Ernest Becker on "heroism," I argued that generativity is a two-step process. The first step involves creating a product: a child, painting, book, business, following, idea—the list of products, tangible and intangible, is virtually infinite. The product can arise out of any one of a number of different commitment areas in an adult's life: one's family life, friendships, occupational life, hobbies, interests, community involvements, etc. The second step involves giving the product up, that is, offering the product to a community that will, in some way, benefit from the product. Erikson describes the second step in terms of caring for the product, granting the generated extension of the self an autonomy of its own such that the product, which becomes a gift, is both *me* and *not me*. In generativity, the adult acts to assure two kinds of continuity. In the sense that the generated product lives on as an extension of the self, generativity makes for a kind of personal immortality—a continuity of the self into future generations. In the sense that the generated product is offered as a gift to a larger community, generativity makes for the continuity, and perhaps even the progressive development, of some aspect of the human enterprise.

The life-story model of identity implies that the conventional demarcation in Erikson's theory between identity as an issue of adolescence and generativity as an issue of middle adulthood is highly misleading. In the life-story model of identity, a future script for generative action is as much a part of the life story as are the ideological setting, nuclear episodes, and personified images of self. Thus, in order to understand well who I am as an adult, I must also know what I plan to do in the future in order to fulfill the developmental mandate of generating a life-justifying legacy. The generativity script, therefore, extends the life story into an anticipated future. Generativity is part of identity.

Other psychologists have described adult development in terms of striving for the accomplishment of a *dream* (Levinson), working on *personal projects* (Palys and Little), and fulfilling areas of *commitment* (Fiske). These ideas bear some similarity to the proposition that a script for future generative action is a major component of adult identity. I also argued that the so-called midlife crisis is often a crisis in generativity rather than ideology. Unlike the 18-year-old whose "identity crisis" typically involves a rethinking of basic ideological values concerning what is good, what is true, what to believe, and what to value, the crisis of the 40-year-old described by psychologists such as Jung, Levinson, Gutmann, and Jacques is more often a crisis in generative action. The midlife adult may ask, "How can I attain a kind of immortality through the creation or generation of my gifts?" The question may motivate the man or woman at midlife to rewrite his or her script for the future, outlining new modes and innovative plans for the generation of meaningful and long-lasting life products.

In the second half of this chapter, I presented personological data on generativity scripts obtained from the 50 midlife men and women in Sample B. Their responses to interview questions concerning what they planned to do in the future were analyzed in a number of different ways. Supporting Hypothesis 7 of Chapter 2, power motivation was positively associated with agentic content themes in adults' scripts for the future, and intimacy motivation was positively associated with communal themes. Relationships between thematic categories of nuclear episodes (Chapter 5) and generativity scripts were also examined, and the evidence suggested considerable thematic continuity in life stories across reconstructions of the past and anticipations for the future. In accordance with Hypothesis 8, I found that higher stages of ego development were associated with a greater variety of action goals for the future. Thus, adults who had reached the more complex frameworks of meaning associated with higher ego stages were more likely to construct action scripts for the future which were more differentiated, whereas their counterparts low in ego development manifested scripts with less variety in future action goals.

The adults' future life plans were also coded for the degree of generativity expressed. Intimacy motivation was positively associated with generativity ratings for these responses, but the correlation was just barely significant. A much more robust, and theoretically interesting, relationship was obtained between generativity ratings and the combination of power and intimacy motivation. In other words, adults who scored high on power plus intimacy motivation tended to construct action scripts for the future that were especially generative. Though surprising at first glance, this finding makes a good deal of sense in light of an understanding of generativity as a two-step process. In the first step, the individual creates a product which represents an extension of the self and a claim on immortality. This first step, thus, represents a *powerful* (agentic) expansion of the self. In the second step, the individual renounces "ownership" of the product and offers it up as a gift, what Erikson describes as an act of *caring* for the product and for the community which is to receive it. The second step, therefore, represents a surrender of the self, a renunciation of control via an intimate exchange with a community. The positive correlation between power plus intimacy motivation and generativity in action scripts for the future suggests that generativity draws upon our desires to be strong and our desires to be close vis-à-vis others. Generativity may challenge us as adults to be both powerful and intimate, agentic and communal, expanding the self and surrendering it to others in the same self-defining act.

NOTES

[1] The relevance of midlife crisis in the lives of most normal American adults is a matter of considerable controversy among life-span developmental psychologists. Although Levinson claims that as many as 80 percent of the adult men in his study experienced something akin to a crisis at midlife, many other psychologists suspect that these crises are much less frequent in the population at large, especially among women of all socioeconomic classes and among men in the working class. Fiske (1980) and Neugarten (1979) have expressed a great deal of skepticism about the usefulness of conceptualizing adult development in terms of predictable psychosocial crises corresponding to a sequence of progressive stages. Thus, they have been very critical of the theories and views put forth by Levinson, Gould, and Sheehy. This chapter reserves judgment on the controversy, merely asserting that the midlife crisis as described by Levinson and others reads like a crisis in generativity rather than a full-blown identity crisis per se. The latter would ideally involve a thoroughgoing revision of the life story with major changes in ideological setting, imagoes, and nuclear episodes, as well as in generativity script.

[2] Jacques reports that he took "a random sample of some 310 painters, composers, poets, writers, and sculptors, of undoubted greatness or of genius" (1965, p. 502). Further information on the selection of the sample was not forthcoming in the 1965 report. It is not clear from what sort of "list" Jacques chose his subjects nor according to what sort of criteria their greatness was assessed. All of the particular geniuses mentioned in the paper are men. It is not clear whether any women were included within the 310 subjects.

[3] Reflecting this chapter's theoretical synthesis of Erikson and Becker, our questions concerning how the subject's future script enabled him or her to be *creative* and to make a *contribution* were designed to probe for sources of generative satisfaction underneath the surface plans.

[4] Two independent coders listened to the 50 interview tapes and for each subject composed a short paragraph summarizing his or her overall response to our questions on the generativity script (see Appendix B). Next, I met with the two coders to combine the two paragraphs for each subject into one clear and nonredundant paragraph depicting the essence of the person's action script for the future.

[5] Scoring reliability here was quite high. Two independent coders scored the scripts for differentiation (variety in goals). The correlation between their two sets of scores was $r = .92$.

[6] Power and intimacy motivation were unrelated to variety of goals in the scripts. Intimacy motivation was significantly correlated, however, with scores on interpersonal goals ($r = .35$, $p < .05$).

[7] The correlation between the two independent coders' sets of ratings was $r = .92$ for agency content in the scripts and $r = .89$ for communion content.

[8] In reading an earlier draft of this chapter, Dave McClelland wondered why I had chosen to call the individual's plan for future action a generativity script. He pointed out that future scripts could accommodate a host of diverse themes and that the modifier of "generativity" appeared somewhat arbitrary. Indeed, the term *generativity script*, unlike the terms used for other components of the life-story model of identity (e.g., imagoes, ideological setting), is as much a prescriptive as a descriptive term. It prescribes a particular quality of identity—a focus on future generative action—which I believe to be a prerequisite for mature identity in the adult years. In this sense, I agree with Erikson, Freud, and Becker when they suggest that generativity is a key to adult maturity, and I will elaborate on this point a bit later. Yet McClelland is definitely right in pointing out that future action scripts in adult life stories need not have much to do with generativity. Thus, a more straightforward and purely descriptive term for the phenomenon in question might be *future script* or *future-action script*. I have no qualms about using this generic term. I would submit, however, that (*a*) most adults' action scripts for the future include generativity in one form or another and (*b*) *mature* identity *requires* a future script of generative action.

[9] Two independent coders scored the script paragraphs for generativity. The correlation between their two sets of scores was $r = .81$. When they did not agree exactly on a given score, a third coder decided between the two scores.

[10] The high correlation between generativity and communion in future scripts is in part a result of scoring overlap between the two scales. Try as we might, we could not separate any more neatly than we did the distinction between communion themes in the scripts and themes of generativity. Thus, those scripts which emphasized warm and close interpersonal relationships tended to be the same ones that emphasized the creation and offering up of a self-justifying life product to others ($r = .57$). It will be interesting to note later, however, that these two highly correlated categories— communion and generativity in future scripts —relate in very different ways to motive scores determined from the TAT. I will argue that generativity has both communal and agentic aspects to it, and I will present some empirical data backing up the claim.

[11] This was simply a matter of summing the standardized scores for each of the two motives per subject. Standardized scores for each of the two motives were *t* scores (mean = 50, standard deviation = 10). Combining the two motive scores into one gave us 50 "power plus intimacy" scores, ranging from 78 to 133, mean = 100.3, standard deviation = 14.7.

Appendix *A*
*D*emographic Information

Sample A

Sample A was made up of 90 undergraduate students attending a moderately large private university in the midwestern United States. All of the students were enrolled in developmental psychology courses taught by the author during the years 1981–82. As part of the course requirements, each student completed parts of an "identity journal" (Appendix B) and was administered a number of personality tests, including the Thematic Apperception Test (TAT) and the Washington University Sentence-Completion Test (WUSCT). These procedures are described in Chapters 2 through 4 and in Appendixes B, C, and D.

Below is demographic information for Sample A:

Number: 90 students
Sex: 57 female
    33 males
Age range: 17 to 28 years
Mean age: 20.03
Median age: 20
Modal age: 19
Undergraduate class: 2 (2.2%) freshmen
                      53 (58.9%) sophomores
                      20 (22.2%) juniors
                      15 (16.7%) seniors
Religious affiliation: 68 (75.5%) Catholic
                       15 (16.7%) Protestant
                        5 (5.6%) other
                        2 (2.2%) none
Ethnic background: 72 (80.0%) Caucasian
                      7 (7.8%) Hispanic
                      6 (6.7%) Asian
                      5 (5.6%) Black

Sample B

Sample B consisted of 50 adults between the ages of 35 and 50 years. Most of these subjects were recruited through evening classes being taught at a university in Chicago, Illinois. A minority were employed at the same university. All were volunteers who participated in two separate sessions during 1981–82. In the first session, the subjects were administered the TAT, WUSCT, and a number of other paper-and-pencil measures. In the second session, each subject was individually interviewed by a female gradute student (see Appendix B).

Below is demographic information for Sample B:

Number: 50 midlife adults
Sex: 30 female
          20 male
Age range: 35 to 50 years
Mean age: 39.6
Median age: 39
Religious affiliation: 26 (52%) Catholic
                                    16 (32%) Protestant
                                     4 (8%) Jewish
                                     3 (6%) other
                                     1 (2%) none
Ethnic background: 46 (92%) Caucasian
                                 4 (8%) Black
Marital status: 26 (52%) married
                           16 (32%) single
                            7 (14%) separated or divorced
                            1 (2%) widowed
Highest level of education: 7 (14%) post-master's degree (PhD, J.D., M.D.)
                                        7 (14%) master's degree
                                       21 (42%) bachelor's degree
                                       15 (30%) high school

Family income (1981–82):   2 (4%) $0 to $9,999
                                        10 (20%) $10,000 to $19,999
                                          8 (16%) $20,000 to $29,999
                                        12 (24%) $30,000 to $39,999
                                          7 (14%) $40,000 to $49,999
                                          6 (12%) $50,000 to $59,999
                                          3 (6%) $60,000 to $69,999
                                          2 (4%) over $70,000
Occupation: 15 (30%) business (sales, consulting, management, etc.)
                       7 (14%) clerical
                       7 (14%) primary or secondary school education
                       5 (10%) college education
                       5 (10%) homemaking
                       4 (8%) full-time student
                       2 (4%) social work
                       2 (4%) nursing
                       1 (2%) military
                       1 (2%) law
                       1 (2%) engineering

Appendix *B*

*L*ife-Story Questionnaires and Interviews

Questionnaires

Life-story questionnaires administered to the undergraduates in Sample A were included in a lengthy set of instruments composing an "identity journal." During the years 1981 and 1982, students enrolled in developmental psychology courses taught by the author completed these identity journals as part of a course requirement. The exercises and questions in the journal were designed to reflect salient developmental issues which were being discussed in class. Thus, questions concerning ideology were included in the journal while the students were learning Piaget's stage of formal operations, which assumedly paves the way to ideological thought. Similarly, questions on early memories were included at the time the students were learning about child cognition and memory. The journals, therefore, were designed for both pedagogical and research purposes. All subjects were aware that their responses would be analyzed for research. All data were strictly confidential and identified only by number and not name.

Over the course of the semester, students handed in journal assignments about every other week. Because the students were required to hand in at minimum about 80 percent of the journal assignments, responses to most questions were completed by fewer than the 90 subjects in Sample A. Nonetheless, most questions received answers from at least 80 percent of the subjects. Following are most of the open-ended questions which made up the identity journals.

1. Think back to when you were a very young child, as far back as your memory is able to go. Try to recall your *earliest memory* in some detail. Below please describe this memory in a paragraph. Please include in your description what you were doing in this early memory, what you were thinking, feeling, wishing, etc. Also set the

scene as you remember it, telling us where this early experience occurred and who was there.

2. This week in class we have been studying nativistic metaphors for development. When a psychologist or layperson uses nativistic metaphors in conceptualizing human development, he or she is generally implying that development unfolds in a relatively regular manner, virtually regardless of the environmental context in which the developing person is a part. One does not have to be real extreme about this. Certainly, the environment is important, the nativist would argue. But the *inborn* characteristics of the organism, coded in his/her genetic endowment, tend to provide a *blueprint* for development, conferring upon development a set of limits or boundaries. Although the forces in the environment (one's social class, family milieu, education, experiences, etc.) may markedly shape behavior and experience, such forces do so only within these inborn limits. As the sociobiologists, such as E. O. Wilson claim, all of us, by virtue of having evolved as *homo sapiens*, share certain inborn behavioral and experiential characteristics. Such behavioral traits, such as attachment and aggression, are *instinctual* in a sense. And as students of temperament (such as Thomas, Chess, and Birch) claim, each of us is born with a unique genetic endowment as well, which makes for individual differences that are present at birth and which continue to shape our development as we mature into adulthood.

Let us think about the kind of issues that the temperament scientist studies. In claiming that many intellectual and personality differences are present at birth and continue to manifest themselves over time, these psychologists adopt nativistic metaphors to explain how each of us *remains the same* over time. There is a core of continuity or consistency in development, they argue. In what essential ways have you remained the same over, say, the past 15 years or so? What continuities in your personality do you observe? Please take some time to think about this question and provide at least five–seven sentences as a response. Try to be specific and detailed in your response.

3. Now that you have tried to paint a picture of the continuity or consistency in your own development, I would like you to remember a *specific incident* in which you did something or experienced something completely "out of character." This would be an experience in which you acted, thought, or felt something in a way much different than you usually do. In looking back at this experience, you might be saying to yourself, "Gee, I can't believe I did that! It was so unlike me!" Please describe such an experience from your past in four–six sentences. Provide details: What happened? Who was there? What were you thinking, feeling, etc.? Also, explain in what ways this experience was so unusual for you or so unlike you.

4. I would like you to think about your life as if it were a book. Most books are divided into chapters. I would like you now to divide your own life into chapters in any way you see fit. Each chapter tells a kind of story; that is, it has a plot. Think about this for a while. Then, divide your life into between four and seven chapters. Give each chapter a name. Below, list the chapters by name and for each provide a short plot summary (two–four sentences). Try to capture the uniqueness of your biography in this exercise. Everybody's life "divides up" differently, so it is probably best to think about how your chapter structure is different from other people's. Try to think about the major events in your life as "turning points" leading from one chapter to the next. These turning points should be unique to you. (You may use the back of this sheet if necessary).

5. Many people report occasional "peak experiences." These are generally moments or episodes in a person's life in which he or she feels a sense of transcendence, uplifting, and inner joy or peace. Indeed, these experiences vary widely. Some people report them to be associated with religious or mystical experience. Others may find such a "high" in vigorous athletics, reading a good novel, artistic expression, making love, or simply talking with a good friend. These experiences have been characterized as ones of wholeness, perfection, completion, aliveness, richness, beauty, uniqueness, or insight.

Please describe in detail (four–five sentences) something akin to a peak experience that you have experienced. Please be specific. We would like to know what happened, who was there, how it felt, what you were thinking, and how (if at all) the experience changed you.

6. Describe in some detail an experience from your childhood (before junior high school) which was experienced as emotionally highly positive (enjoyable, exciting). Provide details.

7. Describe in some detail an experience from your childhood (before junior high school) which was experienced as emotionally negative (causing anger, sadness, disgust, guilt, or shame). Provide details.

8. A "nadir" is a low point. A nadir experience, then, is the opposite of a peak experience. Please think about your life. Try to remember a specific experience in which you felt a sense of disillusionment and/or despair. This would be one of the low points in your life of the past three–four years. Even though this memory is undoubtedly unpleasant, we would still appreciate very much an attempt on your part to be honest and straightforward here and to provide for us as much detail as you did for the peak experience. Please remember to be specific (four–five sentences).

9. This week in class we will be considering various environmentalistic metaphors for human development which are prevalent in general behaviorist theories including the modern derivative of social learning theory. For behaviorists, such as B. F. Skinner, human behavior and experience is shaped profoundly by the *environment*. While downplaying the role of heredity and internal blueprints of human structure and process (and thereby the work of Wilson and the sociobiologists, temperament researchers like Thomas and Chess, and structural linguists like Noam Chomsky), Skinner pays homage to *reinforcement* and *punishment* as prime movers in the *operant-conditioning* scenario of life. Other behaviorists have emphasized the role of *classical conditioning* in development (see text pp. 14–15), and more modern social learning theorists such as Albert Bandura and Walter Mischel have supplemented the behaviorist approach with arguments for the primacy of *observational learning* through *imitation* of *models*, sometimes mediated by cognitive control. Common to all is the placement of *learning from the environment* at the center of any theory of development. I would like you to adopt the behaviorists' metaphors for a while and think of yourself as a product of your environment. As you view your life at this point, what would you say is the single factor in your natural or social environment that has had the greatest effect on determining who you are today? Describe the way in which this factor has affected you in two–three sentences.

10. Many of us have implicit *models* for our behavior and experience. These are people whom we probably admire, and, therefore, we strive to model some aspect of our life around theirs. These may be people whom we know (parents, neighbors, friends, siblings) or others whom we do not know but who serve as heroes or heroines for us (famous authors, scientists, sports figures, diplomats, literary characters, etc.). Do you have any such models or heroes in your life? Below list as many as four of these (you do *not* have to list this many), and for each provide a sentence or two describing why this person is a model or hero for you.

11. In class, we have begun to consider the general topic of cognitive development: those changes in knowing and processing information about the world that humans experience over the course of the life span. The eminent Swiss psychologist Jean Piaget has articulated the most influential theory of cognitive development— what he terms *genetic epistemology*—which seeks to describe and explain four qualitatively different stages of knowing arranged in an invariant hierarchical sequence.

The first of these stages is what Piaget terms the *sensorimotor era*. During the first few years of the child's life, he/she comes to know the world primarily through action. Early patterns of knowing— "schemata"—are action patterns or strategies of manipulating the physical world and observing, through the perceptual systems, one's effect upon this world. Gradually, the infant's patterns of knowing progress from a relatively global and simplified structure to more complex and differentiated organization so that, by the end of the second year of life, we can observe a growing *mastery* of the physical world on the part of the child. Indeed, other psychologists of radically different theoretical persuasions than Piaget, such as Robert White, have remarked on the development of "mastery motivation" (sometimes called effectance motivation) in the latter part of the sensorimotor era as the toddler's growing expertise in exploration and manipulation of the physical surround bespeaks a budding and pervasive sense of *competence.*

Think back to your childhood. Try to recall a relatively early (before the age of six) experience in which you felt a real sense of mastery or competence in doing something. Please describe what in fact you did which led to this feeling. What were you thinking and feeling at the time? Did anybody remark on your accomplishment? If yes, who? Please be specific.

12. Piaget's second stage of cognitive development is termed the *preoperational* phase. Between the years of two and seven, the child's patterns of knowing become truly conceptual as they emancipate themselves, in part, from the limited domain of action. At this time, according to Piaget, a child's thought may have a kind of *magical* quality. Many psychologists have drawn parallels between this early and fantastical kind of thinking in young children and the kind of primitive thinking that seems to occur in dreams. Indeed, children during this time may themselves confuse reality with their dreams, attributing real-life causality to inner or mental fantasies and dreams. Think back again now to your childhood and try to recall a particular dream or set of dreams that stands out in your memory. This nighttime dream may be a happy one, a neutral kind of experience, or even a nightmare. Describe it in at least three to four sentences.

13. When one has attained what Piaget terms *formal operational thought,* one is generally able to operate upon his or her mental operations. In so doing the individual begins to appreciate the possibilities of form and function that are not directly experienced in daily life. With the attainment of formal operations, many of us as teenagers and young adults are able to construct organized systems of truth, beauty, and reality which provide a philosophical context for our behavior and experience. Indeed, both Piaget and Kohlberg speak of the adolescent and the young adult as lay philosophers, actively constructing their own systems of belief so as to make sense, in a new way, of their ethical, religious, political, and social worlds. The appreciation of the hypothetical, which is the centerpiece of formal operational thought, spurs in many of us the development of a personalized *ideology.*

At minimum, an ideology defines what is right (good) and true *for an individual*. As such, it may include the domains of religious belief, ethics, and morality, and one's understanding of what life on earth means in some ultimate sense.

Describe in as much detail as you see fit your present religious beliefs. Be sure to tell us not only about the beliefs you seem to share with others but also any particular understandings that you believe are fairly specific to you. (Note: One need not be a regular church attender to have a well-articulated religious belief system. Religious belief can refer to your most basic thoughts and feelings about the universe and the human being's place in it.)

14. In what ways have your religious beliefs and attitudes changed in the past 10 years? Please be as specific as you can. (If you have not changed much on this, please tell us. Also, if you do not believe that you have a particular religious viewpoint, then say so. Do not feel pressured to make something up in order to satisfy the reader!)

15. Become philosophical for a second. For centuries, philosophers have been puzzled about the meaning of life. Why in fact has man been placed on earth? Are we as a people supposed to accomplish something during our limited number of years here? Is there any meaning at all to human life? If yes, what is it? After thinking about this for a while, please share some of your thoughts on the issue. (Below write as much or as little as you please.)

16. Erik Erikson has argued that each individual over the course of his or her life span must eventually come to grips with each of eight crucial psychosocial issues. In most lives, the issues unfold in a regular sequence, each corresponding to a particular stage of development. Although a particular issue may not be confined to a particular stage in life, it will arise for the *first time* at its corresponding stage. For example, although the issue of initiative versus guilt which is embodied in the Oedipal child's central question of, "How can I be powerful?" becomes salient for the first time in Erikson's third stage, the issue will probably continue to be of at least moderate psychosocial importance at various later stages in living, e.g., in adulthood, perhaps. Hence, each stage's psychosocial issue has relevance for virtually the entire life span.

Your assignment this week is to choose *one* of Erikson's eight psychosocial issues (consult class notes in order to appreciate the flavor of each issue) and discuss below how that issue has been worked out in your life. Unlike many previous journal assignments, you are being asked to *analyze* your life as a particular developmental theorist might. Hence, I am asking you to apply parts of Erikson's very influential theory to your own life as a way of making sense of events developmentally. This may require a good bit of thinking and contemplation on your part as well as a rudimentary understanding of what Erik Erikson has to say to us. (You may use the back of this sheet if you wish.)

17. According to Erikson, identity implies an articulated perspective on, minimally, *ideology, occupation,* and personal *relationships.* Although we have spent some time in the journal dealing with ideology and relationships, little has been said about occupational choice.

This week I would like you to spend some time thinking about occupational choice. Many of you may have already made some kind of tentative decision concerning future occupational goals. Others may be uncertain—torn between or among a number of goals, perhaps. And some of you have probably not thought much about the whole thing.

Describe in two to three sentences what you see as your occupational goals for the future.

18. If you have tentatively chosen a particular career path (which is to say that you are relatively certain as to future occupational goals), describe in some detail (three to four sentences) how you came to this particular decision on occupations. For instance, when did you decide to pursue this occupation? Who influenced you? What were the alternatives?

19. An articulated identity developed in adolescence and young adulthood confers upon the individual a reassuring sense of sameness and continuity which enables that person to construct a rather detailed vision or picture of what he or she plans to get out of life and what he or she plans to put into it. Although your own vision of the future may be somewhat fuzzy at present, we would like you now to spend some time putting together in your mind some kind of such a vision. Below please relate this vision to us and describe in some detail exactly *what you plan to accomplish during your adult years.* Please concentrate on those aspects of the *vision of your own future* which may be *unique* to you.

20. Imagine that after a very full life, you die in the year 2050. A 70– to 100–word obituary of you appears in *The New York Times.* On the back of this sheet, please compose that obituary as you *realistically* think it might read.

Interview

Each of the 50 midlife adults in Sample B was administered a semistructured interview modeled in part after the identity journals used for Sample A. Following is a list of the questions making up the interview:

1. Please spend some time thinking about your life—its past, present, and future. In order to help you along, I would like to suggest that you imagine your life is like a book, and each of its major parts comprises a chapter of the book. Certainly the book is unfinished at this point; still it probably already contains a few interesting and well-articulated chapters. Please provide names for each of the chapters and describe the content of each in some detail. Highlight any turning points that may mark the end of one chapter and the beginning of another.

2. Now that you have told me a little bit about your past, I would like you to tell me about your overall dream, plan, or vision for the future. Most of us have dreams or plans which concern what we would like to get out of life and what we would like to put into it. These dreams or plans may provide our lives with goals, interests, hopes, aspirations, and wishes. Furthermore, our dreams or plans for the future may change over time, reflecting growth and changing experiences. What, then, is your present dream or overall plan for your future?

3. In what ways does your plan for the future enable you to be creative?

4. In what ways does your plan for the future enable you to make some kind of contribution to others?

5. Now, I would like you to break up your plan for the future into smaller pieces and look at it in more detail. Let's divide it up into your occupation, family, friends, and outside commitments. With respect to the first point, please describe your job to me. What are your responsibilities and major duties? What do you do on a typical day of work? Describe a specific incident when you felt that you had done a particularly good job at what you do—that is, an experience on the job in which you felt a sense of mastery, competence, etc. What occupational plans do you have for the future? What is the value of your job to you? (Note: Being a homemaker or a student was considered a job for the purposes of the interview.)

6. Now we can move on to your family and its relationship to your overall plan or dream for the future. (Inquire into general family situation: number of children at home, spouse, members of extended family living at home, etc.) How much time do you spend with your family in an average week? What are some of the major things you do together? Describe a specific incident in which you experienced a good deal of happiness and satisfaction with your family. What do you see as the future for your family?

7. Tell me a little bit about any very close friends you may have outside of your family. How often do you get together? What do you do? Describe a specific incident in which you and one of your friends

had a very rewarding or satisfying time together. What are your aspirations or plans for the future of your friendships?

8. Finally, some psychologists have suggested that major outside commitments can also have an important bearing on a person's
plan for the future. These outside commitments may include any
aspects of your life that we have not talked about so far but which in
your eyes are central in your general vision of what you are and where
you are going. These may include participation in organizations,
clubs, hobbies, or outside pastimes which give your life a good deal
of meaning or at least satisfaction. What are these for you? Why are
they important to you? What are your plans for the future in this area?

9. Briefly I would like you to describe in very general terms
what your overall plan or vision for the future was five years ago, at
age 30, 25, and 22.

10. Many of us have heroes or ideal models for our own lives.
Do you presently have, or have you had in the past, any significant
heroes to whom you have looked up? How have they influenced you?

11. Finally, I would like you to think again about your entire life
in terms of a book with chapters. When we read a book, we are often
able to excerpt from it some kind of message or philosophy which
summarizes the overall meaning of the text. In your life story, what
is the underlying theme of the book? What is your philosophy of life?
In general, what most provides your life with meaning, happiness,
fulfillment?

Appendix C

A Brief Summary of the Intimacy Motive Scoring System[1]

The intimacy motive is a *recurrent preference or readiness in an individual for experiences of warm, close, and communicative exchange with others*. It is manifested as a thematic clustering in imaginative thought samples such as those elicited through the Thematic Apperception Test (TAT). In coding a TAT story for intimacy motivation, the scorer assesses the quality of the interpersonal interaction manifested by the characters in the subject's story. In so doing, he or she analyzes the story for the presence or absence of 10 thematic categories described below. Scorers trained according to the full scoring manual complete with practice stories (McAdams, 1984c) have shown high agreement with expert scoring. After Winter (1973), the category agreement for the first two thematic categories of the intimacy motive system has ranged from 91 percent to 95 percent and the rank-order correlation between intimacy-motive story scores determined by trained scorers and the expert scoring of the manual has ranged between *rho* = +.86 and +.92.

The scoring system is composed of 10 thematic categories, 2 of which are labeled "Prime Tests" and 8 of which are subcategories. The task of the scorer is first to determine the presence (+1) or absence (0) of Prime Tests 1 and 2 (+A and Dlg) in the story. If either or both of the Prime Tests is/are present, then the scorer should proceed through the remaining eight subcategories, systematically detecting for each category its presence (+1) or absence (0) in the story. If neither Prime Test 1 nor Prime Test 2 is present, then all scoring of that story is terminated, and the story receives a score of zero. Each of the 10 categories receives either one point or zero. Each category can be scored only once per story. The total score for each story is simply the sum of the points for the 10 categories. Hence, the maximum score possible for each story is 10; minimum is 0.

Prime Test 1: Relationship Produces Positive Affect (+A)

A relationship is defined as any meeting or encounter between (among) two or more human characters in the story in which there is interaction. The interaction may be anything from two people talking with each other, to a group of people dancing together at a party, to one person thinking about another person. All people mentioned by the writer of the story are considered characters, regardless of whether or not they are pictured in the TAT picture, and any situation in which the characters relate to each other in even the vaguest way constitutes a relationship or interpersonal encounter. For instance, "John remembers the afternoons he spent with his family" constitutes a relationship even though John is only remembering them. On the other hand, "Two people sit on a bench; they are in separate worlds and do not notice each other" does *not* constitute a relationship, unless of course the two begin to interact in subsequent sentences in the story.

In order to be scored (+1) for Prime Test 1, a story must manifest explicit evidence that the relationship, as defined above, *precipitates, facilitates, or is decidedly connected with a positive affective experience on the part of at least one of the characters* in the story. In other words, positive affect is engendered because of the interpersonal encounter. There are five categories of phenomena that qualify as positive affect:

1. Feelings of *love* (romantic, platonic, or otherwise), warmth, closeness, affection, caring, intimacy, compassion, trust, tenderness, sympathy, fondness, and so on toward another (other) character(s) in the story.

2. Feelings of *friendship*, liking, camaraderie, brotherhood, fellowship, and so on toward another (other) character(s) in the story. This includes names of friendships or special bonds, such as "chums," "buddies," "pals," "cronies," "comrades," "dear (close, good, etc.) friends," etc. The word *friends* alone does *not* qualify.

3. Feelings of *happiness*, joy, enjoyment, good cheer, excitement, merriment, delight, gladness, good spirits, hilarity, exuberance, rejoicing, glee, geniality, ecstasy, bliss, conviviality, mirth, and so on experienced by at least one character in the story while engaged in an interpersonal encounter (generally an activity of some sort).

4. Feelings of *peace*, contentment, serenity, satisfaction, quietude experienced by at least one character while engaged in an interpersonal encounter.

5. *Tender behaviors* that generally denote positive affect in interpersonal contexts and which, in the context of the story, do in fact denote so. This includes smiling, caressing, laughing, kissing, holding hands, hugging, making love, and others. These are always nonverbal behaviors—generally touching of some sort, or gestures.

There is also a sixth category of phenomena that qualifies as a special case of negative affect that connotes previous positive affect. Here, Prime Test 1 can also be scored for a character's feelings of *mourning* or *sadness* associated with the *separation from or loss of* another (other) person(s), the implication being that the interpersonal relationship must be one associated with positive affect if its loss or suspension brings about sadness (e.g., grief, mourning, unhappiness, depression, melancholy). Only such feelings of sadness are scoreable here, and then only in the context of interpersonal loss or separation. Hence, feelings of anger, frustration, irritation, disgust, anxiety, fear, and so on do *not* qualify. A common manifestation of this special case that *is* scored for +A is found in stories in which one character "misses" another.

Examples

"the two *lovers* . . ."

"There is a true *affection* between the two, the feeling that exists between father and daughter."

"Although it is raining outside and on the whole is a very dreary day, Nancy is still in a *good mood*. There is no particular reason for her *happiness*, just that things are going well for her with her job and with her relationships with the important people in her life."

"They're just sitting there *enjoying being together.* "

"The man *loves* his family."

"It was a very *jovial* seduction."

"She is reminiscing about the *fun* they had *together* in Italy."

"They sat, *hand in hand.* "

Prime Test 2: Dialogue (Dlg)

Dialogue is defined as a particular kind of verbal (including written) or nonverbal *exchange of information* between (among) characters in the story. In order to be scored for Dlg, a story must manifest exchange of information that is at least one of three acceptable types: (*a*) reciprocal and noninstrumental communication, (*b*) discussion of an interpersonal relationship, or (c) communication for the purpose of helping another person in distress.

> *Reciprocal and Noninstrumental Communication.* This is a verbal or nonverbal exchange among (between) characters that exists in the context of the story *for its own sake,* that is, the communication does not serve the purpose of furthering a particular goal or implementing a particular task. Such "communication for communication's sake" implies rapport, reciprocity, give-and-take, listening, and exchange. It may include phenomena as diverse as chatting about the weather to sharing ideas on the problems of society.

> Note: In some stories, the dialogue may start out in a reciprocal manner and then subsequently deteriorate (e.g., a pleasant conversation turns into a heated argument). In other stories, the reverse may be true (from argument to mutual dialogue). In these cases, the scorer should evaluate and score only the quality of the communication as it is presented at the *end* of the story.

> *Discussion of an Interpersonal Relationship.* This is, in fact, instrumental dialogue, the purpose of which is to consider and work through a particular aspect of the characters' relationships with each other. No other purpose for the discussion can be scored for Dlg here. If the writer makes explicit reference to problems in this discussion, the story is not scored for Dlg.

> *Communication for the Purpose of Helping Another.* This, again, is instrumental dialogue. This time the purpose of the communication lies in one person's attempt to help another, especially when the other is in trouble, feels bad, or has suffered a setback of some kind. Again, if the writer makes explicit reference to problems in reciprocity of the communication, the story is not scored for Dlg.

> *Examples:*

> "They found a spot to sit and *talk.*"
> "He struck up a *conversation* with her."
> "They greeted each other warmly and sat by the Charles for a while *reminiscing* about old times."
> "The old farmers are *swapping stories.*"
> ". . . shooting the bull."
> "She *told* him about the fight with her mother. He *listened.*"
> "They are discussing both unimportant household matters and Aristotle's views on physics."

Category 3: Psychological Growth and Coping (Psy)

A relationship (as defined under Prime Test 1) is demonstrably *instrumental in facilitating, promoting, or affording psychological growth,* self-fulfillment, adjustment, coping with problems, self-actualization, self-realization, identity formation, self-esteem, psychological health, the search for self-knowledge, enlightenment, spiritual salvation, inspiration, creativity, maturity, or the like.

Examples:

"Bev is continually becoming better adjusted to everyday life and how to handle it because of Harry."

"He feels that she has changed his life. He has finally come to realize that he loves mankind."

"A warm relationship with another person can be very comforting when trouble comes up."

"When he is with his wife, whom he loves very much, he will think of a new design and solve the crisis." (Inspiration.)

Category 4: Commitment or Concern (CC)

A character in the story feels a sense of commitment to or concern for another (others) that is *not* rooted in guilt or reluctant and begrudging duty. Commitment includes feelings of loyalty to, and responsibility for, another. Concern generally indicates a felt responsibility for another's welfare, usually leading to some kind of helping or humanitarian behavior, and sometimes personal sacrifice.

Note: Some passages that score for Psy may also score for CC, especially those in which a character in the story purposely takes an initiative in helping another person cope with a problem.

Examples:

"She is devoted to her husband."

"He feels responsible for their well-being."

"Bob has commited himself to the relationship. He cannot back out now."

"He wants to give them his best."

"The youngest grandson has taken his ailing grandfather outside for a walk and some fresh air."

"The old man left his fortune to the poor family in Harlem."

Category 5: Time-Space (TS)

Two or more characters in the story are engaged in a relationship that *transcends the usual limitations of time and/or space.* This includes any explicit references made to the *enduring* quality of a relationship over an extended period of time or in the face of physical separation. If the writer merely reports objectively the length of time two people have known each other, then that time period should be greater than six months *if* the story is to be scored for TS. Furthermore, the category includes overt themes of "timelessness," "time standing still," "the eternal moment," and so on when employed by the writer in the context of interpersonal relations.

Examples:

"They have a kind of rapport that spans time and generations."

"These *old* friends. . . ."

"The three men in the preceding picture get together every year to hunt deer and shoot the bull."

"They part with plans to meet again. Each one is content with the other, not knowing what their future together might bring."

"They have been going together for a while now—nearly a year."

Category 6: Union (U)

In the story, the writer makes explicit reference to the physical or figurative *coming together of people who have at one time or another been apart.* The emphasis is upon unity, reunion, togetherness, oneness, reconciliation, synthesis, or integration. This category includes the coming together of people who are generally not found together by virtue of their dissimilarity (e.g., the atheist meets the priest; the *old* man confronts the *young* woman; the Republicans and the Democrats are reconciled). It also includes characters who have *recently* come together in marriage (i.e., newlyweds) or are planning to do so (becoming engaged).

Examples:

"This is a father and daughter who have come together after a long time."

"She will end up back home and proceed with a reconciliation with her parents."

"The *young woman* is sitting alone crying. While she is sitting there, an *old farmer* comes up to her as he walks through his fields and quietly asks her if it could be that bad."

"After years apart, she came back to Switzerland to be with her grandfather."

Category 7: Harmony (H)

Characters in the story find that they are in harmony with one another. They are "on the same wavelength," their actions are in "synchrony," one "understands" the other, they find something "in common," they share similar views, and so on.

Examples:

"They found that they *had much in common.*"

"She looks at him once and he *understands,* feels better, and looks out at the river."

"The two people are discovering a problem that both of them share."

"Usually she does not listen to her father. He is saying the same thing again, but somehow she sees why this time."

"These students met in section and through subsequent study sessions they became aware that they both avidly participate in crew."

Category 8: Surrender (Sr)

A character finds that interpersonal relations are subject to control that is in some way beyond him or her. He or she *surrenders to this outside force* (e.g., luck, fate, chance, society, God's will, etc.) or, minimally, does not struggle against the outside control. The absence of personal control over the vicissitudes of interpersonal relations, however, is *not* experienced with any anxiety or consternation. Rather, the character(s) may "go with the flow" of interpersonal events, acquiescing to the forces that he or she cannot control. Examples include quirks of fate, the unleashing of uncontrollable emotions, and accidental or chance meetings of people. It is essential to remember that the absence or loss of control must occur in the context of a relationship (as defined under Prime Test 1) if the story is to be scored for Sr.

Examples:

"A young couple *find themselves* deeply in love."

"They *accidentally met* on the road to Crown Point."

"These two people *happen to meet* on a bench next to a river."
"She *let herself go* and found that she enjoyed the party much
more."
"They are *helplessly* in love."

Category 9: Escape to Intimacy (Esc)

Character(s) in the story actively or mentally escape(s) from a
particular situation or state to another situation or state that affords
the experiencing of happiness, peace, liberation, fulfillment, meaning, etc., in the context of interpersonal relations. Characters may
escape together, as in the case of a family leaving the city to take a
vacation in the mountains or a group of meditators entering an altered
state of consciousness together in order to escape the strains of everyday existence. Or a character may escape by himself or herself. In the
latter case, the escape or its concomitant goal state or activity must
refer in some way to an interpersonal relationship if the story is to be
scored for Esc (e.g., a young man escapes to the forest to think about
his relationship with his lover, or a woman leaves home in order to
work out her decaying relationship with her parents in a more objective setting).

Examples:

"The two people were tired of being cooped up in the apartment
so they decided to take a walk on the beach."
"She is taking a walk to think out her problems with her boyfriend."
"He is taking a break from his busy day to think about them."
"Her father wants her to remain chaste and pure. But she will
run off with her lover, and they will become gypsies."

Category 10: Connection with the Outside World (COW)

The outside world is defined as any or all aspects of the non-
human world that exist outside the human body. Examples include all
aspects of nature; the cosmos; animals; environments of human origin, such as streets and skyscrapers; the weather; and God or other-
worldly forces. In order to be scored for COW, the story must manifest
explicit evidence of a *connection* between one of the characters and the
outside world. The connection must be one of two kinds:

1. A direct *interaction* with the outside world in which that world exerts a demonstrable effect upon the character's behavior, thought, or feelings.

2. A metaphoric *parallel* with the outside world in which the character or a relationship between (among) characters is seen by the writer as mirroring or being analogous to the outside world.

Examples:

". . . communion with nature."

". . . feel for the environment."

"Their love like the weather is warm and light."

"The heat is oppressive to him."

"They love the way the morning air feels and smells."

NOTES

[1] Appendix C is an abbreviated version of the full scoring manual (McAdams, 1984c). The full manual is designed to teach the clinician or researcher to score TAT stories for intimacy motivation in a reliable fashion. The manual contains further scoring explanations, many examples, 210 practice stories, and expert scoring of the practice stories. The full manual appears as:

McAdams, D. P. (1984c). Scoring manual for the intimacy motive. *Psychological Documents, 14* (2614).

Appendix D

Sentence-Completion Test

In both Samples A and B, the subject's stage of ego development was determined through analysis of responses to sentence-completion tests designed by Holt (1980) and based on Loevinger's (1976; Loevinger and others, 1978) Washington University Sentence-Completion Test for ego development (the WUSCT). Holt has presented one version of the test for males and one for females. These 12-item versions of the WUSCT are abbreviated forms of Loevinger's original 36-item test. Each subject is asked to complete the 12 sentence stems in any way he or she chooses. There is no time limit for the test, but subjects typically finish within 20–25 minutes.

For both Samples A and B, the responses were scored by two trained coders according to the scoring manuals published by Loevinger and her colleagues (Loevinger and Wessler, 1978, and Loevinger and others, 1978 for women; Redmore and others, 1978 for men). In Loevinger's system, each sentence response is scored for one of the stages of ego development, and then the 12 resultant scores for the 12 responses are put together according to "ogive rules" to determine the individual's overall stage of ego development. For the 12-item version of the sentence-completion test, the ogive rules are provided by Holt.

Below are reproduced the sentence stems used in the 12-item sentence-completion tests administered to Samples A and B:

Females

1. For a woman a career is
2. A girl has a right to
3. The thing I like about myself is
4. Education
5. A wife should
6. Rules are
7. When I get mad

8. Men are lucky because
9. I am
10. A woman feels good when
11. My husband and I will
12. A woman should always

Males

1. If I had more money
2. A man's job
3. The thing I like about myself is
4. Women are lucky because
5. A good father
6. A man feels good when
7. A wife should
8. A man should always
9. Rules are
10. When his wife asked him to help with the housework
11. When I am criticized
12. He felt proud that he

Appendix E

Life Satisfaction Questionnaire

All of the subjects in Sample B were administered a life-satisfaction questionnaire in which they rated satisfaction with career, relationships, and life in general on seven-point Likert scales at various ages. The questionnaire is reproduced below:

Ages	*Career*							*Relationships*							*Life in General*						
18 years old	1	2	3	4	5	6	7	1	2	3	4	5	6	7	1	2	3	4	5	6	7
22 years old	1	2	3	4	5	6	7	1	2	3	4	5	6	7	1	2	3	4	5	6	7
25 years old	1	2	3	4	5	6	7	1	2	3	4	5	6	7	1	2	3	4	5	6	7
30 years old	1	2	3	4	5	6	7	1	2	3	4	5	6	7	1	2	3	4	5	6	7
35 years old	1	2	3	4	5	6	7	1	2	3	4	5	6	7	1	2	3	4	5	6	7
40 years old	1	2	3	4	5	6	7	1	2	3	4	5	6	7	1	2	3	4	5	6	7
Now	1	2	3	4	5	6	7	1	2	3	4	5	6	7	1	2	3	4	5	6	7

Appendix F

Imago Description Sheet

Subject number ——————————

Imago type ————————————   Variant —————————————

Brief summary (including unique features): ——————————

————————————————————————————

————————————————————————————

————————————————————————————

Associated personality traits: —————————————————

————————————————————————————

Associated significant other (role model, parent, friend, etc.): ——————

————————————————————————————

Describe how the significant other(s) relate(s) to imago: ——————————

————————————————————————————

————————————————————————————

————————————————————————————

————————————————————————————

Biographical event giving birth to imago (describe): ————————————

————————————————————————————

————————————————————————————

————————————————————————————

————————————————————————————

Four events in which imago was displayed in behavior:

1. _____

2. _____

3. _____

4. _____

Associated wishes, aspirations, goals: _____

_____

_____

Biographical period in which imago was ascendent: _____

_____

_____

Associated antiimago (describe): _____

_____

_____

Personality traits associated with antiimago: _____

_____

Associated significant others: _____

Describe how significant others related to antiimago: _____

_____

_____

Biographical event giving rise to antiimago: _____

_____

_____

Four events in which antiimago was displayed in behavior: _____

1. _____

2. _____

3. _____

4. _____

Associated wishes, aspirations, goals for antiimago: _____

_____

Biographical period in which antiimago was ascendent: _____

_____

_____

Nature of conflict between antiimago and imago: _____

_____

_____

_____

Evidence for resolution of conflict, synthesis between imago and antiimago:

_____

_____

_____

_____

Secondary imagoes: Type _____   Variant _____

Description: _____

_____

_____

_____

Antiimago: _____

_____

_____

_____

Miscellaneous comments:

References

Adams, G. R., & Shea, J. A. The relationship between identity status, locus of control, and ego development. *Journal of Youth and Adolescence*, 1979, *8*, 81–89.

Adelson, J. Personality. In P. H. Mussen & M. R. Rosenzweig (Eds.), *Annual review of psychology* (Vol. 20). Palo Alto, Calif.: Annual Reviews Inc., 1969.

Adelson, J. The development of ideology in adolescence. In S. E. Dragastin & G. H. Elder (Eds.), *Adolescence in the life cycle: Psychological change and social context*. New York: John Wiley & Sons, 1975.

Adler, A. The aggression drive in life and neurosis. In H. L. Ansbacher & R. R. Ansbacher (Eds.), *The individual psychology of Alfred Adler*. New York: Harper & Row, 1956. (Originally published, 1908.)

Adler, A. *The practice and theory of individual psychology*. New York: Harcourt Brace Jovanovich, 1927.

Adler, A. Individual psychology. In C. Murchison (Ed.), *Psychologies of 1930*. Worcester, Mass.: Clark University Press, 1930.

Adler, A. *What life should mean to you*. Boston: Little, Brown, 1931.

Adler, A. The significance of early recollections. *International Journal of Individual Psychology*, 1937, *3*, 283–287.

Adorno, T. W., Frenkel-Brunswick, E., Levinson, D. J., & Sanford, R. N. *The authoritarian personality*. New York: Harper & Row, 1950.

Ainsworth, M. D. S. Object relations, dependency, and attachment: A theoretical review of the mother-infant relationship. *Child Development*, 1969, *40*, 969–1025.

Allen, R. M., Haupt, T. D., & Jones, R. W. Analysis of peak experiences reported by college students. *Journal of Clinical Psychology*, 1964, *20*, 207–212.

Allport, G. W., Vernon, P. E., & Lindzey, G. *A study of values: A scale for measuring the dominant interests in personality* (Rev. ed.). Boston: Houghton Mifflin, 1951.

Angyal, A. *Foundations for a science of personality*. New York: Viking Press, 1941.

Ansbacher, H. L. & Ansbacher, R. R. *The individual psychology of Alfred Adler: A systematic presentation in selections from his writings*. New York: Harper & Row, 1956.

Applebee, A. N. *The child's concept of story*. Chicago: University of Chicago Press, 1978.

Argyle, M., & Little, B. R. Do personality traits apply to social behavior? In N. S. Endler & D. Magnusson (Eds.), *Interactional psychology and personality*. New York: John Wiley & Sons, 1976.

Atkinson, J. W. (Ed.). *Motives in fantasy, action, and society*. New York: Van Nostrand Reinhold, 1958.

Atkinson, J. W. *An introduction to motivation*. New York: Van Nostrand Reinhold, 1964.

Atkinson, J. W. Studying personality in the context of an advanced motivational psychology. *American Psychologist*, 1981, *36*, 117–128.

Atkinson, J. W. Motivational determinants of thematic apperception. In A. J. Stewart (Ed.), *Motivation and society*. San Francisco: Jossey-Bass, 1982.

Atkinson, J. W., & Birch, D. *An introduction to motivation* (Rev. ed.). New York: Van Nostrand Reinhold, 1978.

Atkinson, J. W., Heyns, R. W., & Veroff, J. The effect of experimental arousal of the affiliation motive on thematic apperception. *Journal of Abnormal and Social Psychology*, 1954, *49*, 405–410.

Atkinson, J. W. & Raynor, J. O. (Eds.). *Motivation and achievement*. Washington, D.C.: Winston Press, 1974.

Atwood, G. E., & Tomkins, S. S. On the subjectivity of personality theory. *Journal of the History of the Behavioral Sciences*, 1976, *12*, 166–177.

Ausubel, D. P. *Ego development and the personality disorders*. New York: Grune & Stratton, 1952.

Bakan, D. *The duality of human existence: Isolation and communion in Western man*. Boston: Beacon Press, 1966.

Balint, M. *The basic fault: Therapeutic aspects of regression*. New York: Bruner/Mazel, 1979.

Bartlett, F. C. *Remembering*. Cambridge: Cambridge University Press, 1932.

Beck, A. T. Cognitive therapy: Nature and relation to behavior therapy. *Behavior Therapy*, 1970, *1*, 184–200.

Becker, E. *The denial of death*. New York: Reprinted with permission of The Free Press, a Division of MacMillan, Inc. Copyright © 1973 by the Free Press.

Bem, D. J. *Beliefs, attitudes, and human affairs*. Monterey, Calif.: Brooks/Cole Publishing, 1970.

Berne, E. *Games people play*. New York: Random House, 1964.

Berne, E. *What do you say after you say hello?* New York: Grove Press, 1972.

Bertaux, D. (Ed.). *Biography and society: The life history approach in the social sciences*. Beverly Hills, Calif.: Sage Publications, 1981.

Bettelheim, B. *The uses of enchantment: The meaning and importance of fairy tales*. New York: Alfred A. Knopf, 1976.

Bigda-Peyton, F., & Fine, G. A. The Hephaestus complex: Power themes in the life of James Thurber. *Biography*, 1978, *1*, 37–60.

Block, J. *Lives through time*. Berkeley, Calif.: Bancroft, 1971.

Block, J. Some enduring and consequential structures of personality. In A. I. Rabin, J. Aronoff, A. M. Barclay, & R. A. Zucker (Eds.), *Further explorations in personality*. New York: John Wiley & Sons, 1981.

Bob, S. *An investigation of the relationship between identity status, cognitive style, and stress*. Unpublished doctoral dissertation, State University of New York at Binghampton, 1968.

Boer, C. (trans.). [*The Homeric Hymns*] Dallas: Spring Publications, 1970.

Botvin, G. J., & Sutton-Smith, B. The development of structural complexity in children's fantasy narratives. *Developmental Psychology*, 1977, *13*, 377–388.

Bourne, E. The state of research on ego identity: A review and appraisal (Part 1). *Journal of Youth and Adolescence*, 1978, *7*, 223–251. (a)

Bourne, E. The state of research on ego identity: A review and appraisal (Part 2). *Journal of Youth and Adolescence*, 1978, *7*, 371–392. (b)

Bowlby, J. *Attachment and loss: Attachment* (Vol. 1). New York: Basic Books, 1969.

Bowlby, J. *Attachment and loss: Separation* (Vol. 2). New York: Basic Books, 1973.

Boyatzis, R. E. Affiliation motivation. In D. C. McClelland & R. S. Steele (Eds.), *Human motivation: A book of readings.* Morristown, N. J.: General Learning Corporation, 1973.

Breger, L. *From instinct to identity: The development of personality,* © 1974, pp. 330–31. Reprinted by permission of Prentice-Hall, Inc., Englewood Cliffs, N.J.

Broughton, J. M. Genetic metaphysics: The developmental psychology of mind-body concepts. In R. W. Rieber (Ed.), *Body and Mind.* New York: Academic Press, 1980.

Brown, N. O. *Hermes the thief: The evolution of a myth.* New York: Random House, 1947.

Bruner, J. S. Myth and identity. In H. A. Murray (Ed.), *Myth and mythmaking.* New York: George Braziller, 1960.

Buber, M. *Between man and man.* New York: Macmillan, 1965.

Buber, M. *I and Thou.* New York: Charles Scribner's Sons, 1970.

Bühler, C. (The human course of life as a psychological problem.) *Der menschliche lebenslauf als psychologisches problem.* Leipzig: S. Hirzel Verlag, 1933.

Buss, R. R., Yussen, S. R., Matthews, S. R., Miller, G. E., & Rembold, K. L. Development of children's use of a story schema to retrieve information. *Developmental Psychology,* 1983, *19,* 22–28.

Candee, D. Ego developmental aspects of the new left ideology. *Journal of Personality and Social Psychology,* 1974, *30,* 620–630.

Capon, N., & Kuhn, D. Logical reasoning in the supermarket: Adult females' use of a proportional reasoning strategy in an everyday context. *Developmental Psychology,* 1979, *15,* 450–452.

Carlson, R. Where is the person in personality research? *Psychological Review,* 1971, *75,* 203–219.

Carlson, R. Personality. In M. R. Rosenzweig & L. W. Porter (Eds.), *Annual review of psychology* (Vol. 26). Palo Alto, Calif.: Annual Reviews, Inc., 1975.

Carlson, R. Studies in script theory: I. Adult analogs of a childhood nuclear scene. *Journal of Personality and Social Psychology,* 1981, *40,* 501–510.

Carlson, R. Personology lives! *Contemporary Psychology,* 1982, *27,* 7–8.

Cohen, C. E. Goals and schemata in person perceptions: Making sense from the stream of behavior. In N. Cantor & J. F. Kihlstrom (Eds.), *Personality, cognition, and social interaction.* Hillsdale, N.J.: Lawrence Erlbaum Associates, 1981.

Cole, M., & Schribner, S. *Culture and thought: A psychological introduction.* New York: John Wiley & Sons, 1974.

Coles, R. *Erik Erikson: The growth of his work.* Boston: Little, Brown, 1970.

Cowley, M. Hemingway's novel has the rich simplicity of a classic. *New York Herald Tribune Book Review,* September 7, 1952, 1–17.

Cross, H., & Allen, J. Ego identity status, adjustment, and academic achievement. *Journal of Consulting and Clinical Psychology,* 1970, *34,* 288.

Csikszentmihalyi, M. *Beyond boredom and anxiety: The experience of play in work and games.* San Francisco: Jossey-Bass, 1977.

Csikszentmihalyi, M. Toward a psychology of optimal experience. In L. Wheeler (Ed.), *Review of Personality and Social Psychology: 3.* Beverly Hills, Calif.: Sage Publications, 1982.

Csikszentmihalyi, M., & Beattie, O. V. Life themes: A theoretical and empirical exploration of their origins and effects. *Journal of Humanistic Psychology,* 1979, *19* (1), 45–63.

Csikszentmihalyi, M., Larson, R., & Prescot, S. The ecology of adolescent activity and experience. *Journal of Youth and Adolescence*, 1977, 6, 281–294.

Daiches, D. *Critical approaches to literature* (2nd ed.). Essex: Longman Group, 1981.

Damon, W. *The social world of the child*. San Francisco: Jossey-Bass, 1977.

deCharms, R. *Personal causation: The internal affective determinants of behavior*. New York: Academic Press, 1968.

deCharms, R., & Muir, M. S. Motivation: Social approaches. In M. R. Rosenzweig & L. W. Porter (Eds.), *Annual review of psychology* (Vol. 29). Palo Alto, Calif.: Annual Reviews, Inc., 1978.

deRiencourt, A. *Sex and power in history*. New York: David McKay, 1974.

Didion, J. *The white album*. New York: Reprinted by permission of Simon & Schuster, Inc. © 1979.

Dilthey, W. The development of hermeneutics. In H. P. Rickman (Ed.), *W. Dilthey: Selected writings*. Cambridge: Cambridge University Press, 1976. (Originally published, 1900.)

Dollard, J. *Criteria for the life history*. New Haven, Conn.: Yale University Press, 1935.

Donovan, J. M. Identity status and interpersonal style. *Journal of Youth and Adolescence*, 1975, 4, 37–55.

Dostoyevsky, F. [*The brothers Karamazov*] (C. Garrett, trans.). New York: New American Library, 1957.

Ebersde, P. Effects of nadir experiences. *Psychological Reports*, August 1970, 27, 207–209.

Edel, L. Biography: A manifesto. *Biography*, 1978, 1, 1–3.

Eliot, T. S. *Selected poems*. New York: Harcourt Brace Jovanovich, 1930.

Elkind, D. *Children and adolescents: Interpretive essays on Jean Piaget* (3rd ed.). New York: Oxford University Press, 1981.

Ellis, A. Rational-emotive therapy. In L. Hersher (Ed.), *Four psychotherapies*. New York: Appleton-Century-Crofts, 1970.

Elsbree, L. *The rituals of life: Patterns in narratives*. Port Washington, N.Y.: Kennikat Press, 1982.

Entwistle, D. E. To dispel fantasies about fantasy-based measures of achievement motivation. *Psychological Bulletin*, 1972, 77, 377–391.

Epstein, S. The stability of behavior: 1. On predicting most of the people much of the time. *Journal of Personality and Social Psychology*, 1979, 37, 1097–1126.

Erikson, E. H. *Young man Luther: A study in psychoanalysis and history*. New York: W. W. Norton, Inc. Copyright © 1958.

Erikson, E. H. Identity and the life cycle: Selected papers. *Psychological Issues*, 1959, 1 (1), 5–165.

Erikson, E. H. *Childhood and society* (2nd ed.). New York: W. W. Norton, 1963.

Erikson, E. H. *Insight and responsibility: Lectures on the ethical implications of psychoanalytic insight*. New York: W. W. Norton, 1964.

Erikson, E. H. *Identity: Youth and crisis*. New York: W. W. Norton, 1968.

Erikson, E. H. *Gandhi's truth: On the origins of militant nonviolence*. New York: W. W. Norton, 1969.

Erikson, E. H. *Life history and the historical moment*. New York: W. W. Norton, 1975.

Erikson, E. H. Themes of adulthood in the Freud-Jung correspondence. In N. J. Smelser & E. H. Erikson (Eds.), *Themes of work and love in adulthood*. Cambridge, Mass.: Harvard University Press, 1980.

Eysenck, H. J. Biography in the service of science: A look at astrology. *Biography*, 1979, 2, 25–34.

Fairbairn, W. R. D. *Psychoanalytic studies of the personality: The object relations theory of personality*. London: Routledge & Kegan Paul, 1952.

Feather, N. T. Values in adolescence. In J. Adelson (Ed.), *Handbook of adolescent psychology*. New York: John Wiley & Sons, 1980.

Ferenczi, S. Stages in the development of the sense of reality. *Sex in psychoanalysis*. Boston: Gorham Press, 1916. (Originally published, 1913.)

Ferenczi, S. Psychoanalysis of sexual habits. *International Journal of Psychoanalysis*, 1925, 6, 372–404.

Fingarette, H. *Self-deception*. London: Routledge & Kegan Paul, 1969.

Fischer, K. W. A theory of cognitive development: The control and construction of hierarchies of skills. *Psychological Review*, 1980, 87, 477–531.

Fiske, D. W. The limits of the conventional science of personality. *Journal of Personality*, 1974, 42, 1–11.

Fiske, M. Changing hierarchies of commitment in adulthood. In N. J. Smelser & E. H. Erikson (Eds.), *Themes of work and love in adulthood*. Cambridge, Mass.: Harvard University Press, 1980.

Fiske, S. T. & Kinder, D. R. Involvement, expertise, and schema use: Evidence from political cognition. In N. Cantor & J. F. Kihlstrom (Eds.), *Personality, cognition, and social interaction*. Hillsdale, N.J.: Lawrence Erlbaum Associates, 1981.

Flavell, J. H. Structures, stages, and sequences in cognitive development. In W. A. Collins (Ed.), *The Minnesota symposium on child psychology* (Vol. 15). Hillsdale, N.J.: Lawrence Erlbaum Associates, 1982.

Fodor, E. M., & Farrow, D. L. The power motive as an influence on use of power. *Journal of Personality and Social Psychology*, 1979, 37, 2091–2097.

Fodor, E. M., & Smith, T. The power motive as an influence on group decision making. *Journal of Personality and Social Psychology*, 1982, 42, 178–185.

Forsyth, D. R. A taxonomy of ethical ideologies. *Journal of Personality and Social Psychology*, 1980, 39, 175–184.

Fowler, J. *Stages of faith: The psychology of human development and the quest for meaning*. New York: Harper & Row, 1981.

Frank, S., & Quinlain, D. Ego developmental aspects of female delinquency. *Journal of Abnormal Psychology*, 1976, 85, 505–510.

Frenkel, E. Studies in biographical psychology. *Character and Personality*, 1936, 5, 1–35.

Freud, A. *The ego and mechanisms of defense*. New York: International Universities Press, 1946. (Originally published, 1936.)

Freud, S. Screen memories. In J. Strachey (Ed.), *The standard edition of the complete psychological works of Sigmund Freud* (Vol. 3). London: Hogarth, 1962. (Originally published, 1899.)

Freud, S. The interpretation of dreams. In vols. 4–5 of *The standard edition*. London: Hogarth, 1953. (Originally published, 1900.)

Freud, S. Beyond the pleasure principle. In vol. 18 of *The standard edition*. London: Hogarth Press, 1955. (Originally published, 1920.)

Freud, S. The ego and the id. In vol. 19 of *The standard edition*. London: Hogarth, 1961. (Originally published, 1923.)

Freud, S. Civilization and its discontents. In vol. 21 of *The standard edition*. London: Hogarth, 1961. (Originally published, 1930.)

Fromm, E. *Escape from freedom*. New York: Farrar, Straus & Giroux, 1941.

Frye, N. *Anatomy of criticism*. Princeton, N.J.: Princeton University Press, 1957.

Frye, N. *Fables of identity: Studies in poetic mythology*. New York: Harcourt Brace Jovanovich, 1963.

Giele, J. Z. Adulthood as transcendence of age and sex. In N. J. Smelser & E. H. Erikson (Eds.), *Themes of work and love in adulthood*. Cambridge, Mass.: Harvard University Press, 1980.

Gilligan, C. *In a different voice*. Cambridge, Mass.: Reprinted by permission of Harvard University Press, Copyright © 1982.

Goethals, G. W. The evolution of sexual and genital intimacy: A comparison of the views of Erik H. Erikson and Harry Stack Sullivan. *Journal of the American Academy of Psychoanalysis*, 1976, 4, 529–544.

Gold, S. N. Relations between level of ego development and adjustment patterns in adolescents. *Journal of Personality Assessment*, 1980, *44*, 630–638.

Gough, H. G. *The adjective checklist.* Palo Alto, Calif.: Consulting Psychologists Press, 1952.

Gould, R. L. Transformations during early and middle adult years. In N. J. Smelser and E. H. Erikson (Eds.), *Themes of work and love in adulthood.* Cambridge, Mass.: Harvard University Press, 1980.

Graves, C. W. Deterioration of work standards. *Harvard Business Review*, 1966, *44*, 117–128.

Grotevant, H. D., & Cooper, C. R. Assessing adolescent identity in the areas of occupation, religion, politics, friendships, dating, and sex roles: Manual for administering and coding of the interview. *JSAS Catalog of Selected Documents in Psychology*, 1980, *11* (3), 52.

Grotevant, H. D., Thorbecke, W., & Meyer, M. L. An extension of Marcia's identity status interview into the interpersonal domain. *Journal of Youth and Adolescence*, 1982, *11*, 33–47.

Guntrip, H. *Psychoanalytic theory, therapy, and the self.* New York: Basic Books, 1973.

Gutmann, D. L. The postparental years: Clinical problems and developmental possibilities. In W. H. Norman & T. J. Scaramella (Eds.), *Mid-Life: Developmental and clinical issues.* New York: Bruner/Mazel, 1980.

Hale, N. Freud's reflections on work and love. In N. J. Smelser & E. H. Erikson (Eds.), *Themes of work and love in adulthood.* Cambridge, Mass.: Reprinted by permission of Harvard University Press, Copyright © 1980.

Hall, C. S., & Lindzey, G. *Theories of personality* (2nd ed.). New York: John Wiley & Sons, 1970.

Hall, E. Children and other political naifs: Joseph Adelson interviewed. *Psychology Today*, November, 1980, p. 56.

Hall, G. S. Note on early memories. *Pedagogical Seminary*, 1899, *6*, 485–512.

Hankiss, A. Ontologies of the self: On the mythological rearranging of one's life history. In D. Bertaux (Ed.), *Biography and society: The life history approach in the social sciences.* Beverly Hills, Calif.: Sage Publications, 1981.

Hartmann, H. *Ego psychology and the problem of adaptation.* New York: International Universities Press, 1958. (Originally published, 1939.)

Hartmann, H., Kris, E., & Lowenstein, R. M. Papers on psychoanalytic psychology. *Psychological Issues*, 1964, *4* (2, Whole No. 14).

Harvey, O. J., Hunt, D. E., & Schroder, H. M. *Conceptual systems and personality organization.* New York: John Wiley & Sons, 1961.

Hauser, S. T. Loevinger's model and measure of ego development: A critical review. *Psychological Bulletin*, 1976, *80*, 928–955.

Hayes, J. M. *Ego identity and moral character development in male college students.* Unpublished doctoral dissertation, The Catholic University of America, 1977.

Heckhausen, H. *The anatomy of achievement motivation.* New York: Academic Press, 1967.

Helson, R., & Mitchell, V. Personality. In M. R. Rosenzweig & L. W. Porter (Eds.), *Annual review of psychology* (Vol. 29). Palo Alto, Calif.: Annual Reviews, Inc., 1978.

Hemingway, E. *The old man and the sea.* New York: Charles Scribner's Sons, 1952.

Heyns, R. W., Veroff, J., & Atkinson, J. W. A scoring manual for the affiliation motive. In J. W. Atkinson (Ed.), *Motives in fantasy, action, and society.* New York: Van Nostrand Reinhold, 1958.

Hogan, R. Moral conduct and moral character: A psychological perspective. *Psychological Bulletin*, 1973, *79*, 217–232.

Hogan, R. *Personality theory: The personological tradition.* Englewood Cliffs, N.J.: Prentice-Hall, 1976.

Holmes, T. H., & Rahe, R. H. The Social Readjustment Rating Scale. *Journal of Psychosomatic Research*, 1967, *11*, 213–218.

Holt, R. R. Loevinger's measure of ego development: Reliability and national norms for male and female short forms. *Journal of Personality and Social Psychology*, 1980, *39*, 909–920.

Homer, [The Homeric Hymns] (C. Boer, trans.). Chicago: Swallow Press.

Hoppe, C. *Ego development and conformity behavior*. Unpublished doctoral dissertation, Washington University, 1972.

Horowitz, M. J. *States of mind: Analysis of change in psychotherapy*. New York: Plenum Publishing, 1979.

Howe, M. J. A. Biographical evidence and the development of outstanding individuals. *American Psychologist*, 1982, *37*, 1071–1081.

Hunt, M., & Hunt, B. *The divorce experience*. New York: New American Library, 1977.

Inhelder, B., & Piaget, J. *The growth of logical thinking from childhood to adolescence*. New York: Basic Books, 1958.

Isaacs, K. S. *Relatability, a proposed construct and an approach to its validation*. Unpublished doctoral dissertation, University of Chicago, 1956.

Jacobson, E. *The self and the object world*. New York: International Universities Press, 1964.

Jacques, E. Death and the midlife crisis. *International Journal of Psycho-analysis*, 1965, *46*, 502–514.

James, W. *Principles of psychology*. New York: Holt, Rinehart & Winston, 1890.

James, W. *The varieties of religious experience*. New York: New American Library of World Literature, 1958. (Lectures originally delivered, 1902.)

Janis, I. L. *Victims of groupthink*. Boston: Houghton Mifflin, 1972.

Johnson, J. A., & Hogan, R. Moral judgments and self-presentations. *Journal of Research in Personality*, 1981, *15*, 57–63.

Johnson, N. S., & Mandler, J. M. A tale of two structures: Underlying and surface forms in stories. *Poetics*, 1980, *9*, 51–86.

Jones, E. *The life and work of Sigmund Freud*. (Ed. and abridged, L. Trilling and S. Marcus). New York: Basic Books, 1961.

Jordan, D. *Parental antecedents and personality characteristics of ego identity statuses*. Unpublished doctoral dissertation, State University of New York at Binghampton, 1971.

Josselson, R. L. Psychodynamic aspects of identity formation in college women. *Journal of Youth and Adolescence*, 1973, *2*, 3–52.

Josselson, R. L. Personality structure and identity status in women as viewed through early memories. *Journal of Youth and Adolescence*, 1982, *11*, 293–299.

Jung, C. G. The psychology of the unconscious. In *Collected works* (Vol. 7). Princeton, N.J.: Princeton University Press, 1953. (First German ed., 1943.)

Kegan, R. *The evolving self*. Cambridge, Mass.: Harvard University Press. 1982.

Kelly, G. *The psychology of personal constructs*. New York: W. W. Norton, 1955.

Kernberg, O. F. *Borderline conditions and pathological narcissism*. New York: Jason Alonson, 1975.

Kihlstrom, J. F., & Harackiewicz, J. M. The earliest recollections: A new survey. *Journal of Personality*, 1982, *50*, 134–148.

Klinger, E. Fantasy need achievement as a motivational construct. *Psychological Bulletin*, 1966, *66*, 291–308.

Kluckholn, C., & Murray, H. A. Personality formation: The determinants. In C. Kluckholn and H. A. Murray (Eds.), *Personality in nature, society, and culture* (2nd ed.). New York: Alfred A. Knopf, 1953.

Kobassa, S. C. Stressful life events, personality, and health: An inquiry into hardiness. *Journal of Personality and Social Psychology*, 1979, *37*, 1–11.

Kobassa, S. C. The hardy personality: Toward a social psychology of stress and health.

In J. Suls and G. Sanders (Eds.), *Social psychology of health and illness*. Hillsdale, N.J.: Lawrence Erlbaum Associates, 1982.

Koestler, A. *Janus: A summing up*. New York: Random House, 1979.

Kohlberg, L. Stage and sequence: The cognitive-developmental approach to socialization. In D. A. Goslin (Ed.), *Handbook of socialization theory and research*. Skokie, Ill.: Rand McNally, 1969.

Kohlberg, L. *The philosophy of moral development: Moral stages and the idea of justice* (Vol. 1). *Essays on moral development*. New York: Harper & Row, 1981.

Kohlberg, L., & Gilligan, C. The adolescent as a philosopher: The discovery of the self in a post-conventional world. *Daedalus*, Fall 1971, 1051–1086.

Kohlberg, L., & Kramer, R. Continuities and discontinuities in childhood and adult development. *Human Development*, 1969, *12*, 93–120.

Kohlberg, L., & Mayer, R. Development as the aim of education. *Harvard Educational Review*, 1972, *14*, 449–496.

Kohli, M. Biography: Account, text, method. In D. Bertaux (Ed.), *Biography and society: The life history approach in the social sciences*. Beverly Hills, Calif.: Sage Publications, 1981.

Komroff, M. Forward to F. Dostoyevsky, *The brothers Karamazov*. New York: New American Library, 1957.

Kuhn, T. S. *The structure of scientific revolutions*. Chicago: University of Chicago Press, 1962.

Labov, W., & Waletsky, J. Narrative analysis: Oral versions of personal experience. In J. Helan (Ed.), *Essays on the verbal and visual arts*. Seattle, Wash.: University of Washington Press, 1967.

Langbaum, R. *The mysteries of identity: A theme in modern literature*. Chicago: University of Chicago Press, 1982.

Langer, J. *Theories of development*. New York: Holt, Rinehart & Winston, 1969.

Larson, R., & Csikszentmihalyi, M. Experiential correlates of time alone. *Journal of Personality*, 1978, *46*, 677–693.

Larson, R., & Csikszentmihalyi, M. The significance of solitude in adolescents' development. *Journal of Current Adolescent Medicine*, 1980, *8*, 33–40.

Lasch, C. *The culture of narcissism: American life in an age of diminishing expectations*. New York: W. W. Norton, 1979.

Laski, M. *Ecstasy: A study of some secular and religious experiences*. Bloomington: Indiana University Press, 1962.

Levinson, D. J. The mid-life transition: A period in adult psychosocial development. *Psychiatry*, 1977, *40*, 99–112.

Levinson, D. J. *The seasons of a man's life*. New York: Alfred A Knopf, 1978.

Levinson, D. J. Toward a conception of the adult life course. In N. J. Smelser & E. H. Erikson (Eds.), *Themes of work and love in adulthood*. Cambridge, Mass.: Harvard University Press, 1980.

Levinson, D. J. Exploration in biography: Evolution of the individual life structure in adulthood. In A. I. Rabin, J. Aronoff, A. M. Barclay, and R. A. Zucker (Eds.), *Further explorations in personality*. New York: John Wiley & Sons, 1981.

Levinson, D. J., Darrow, C. M., Klein, E. B., Levinson, M. H., & McKee, B. The psychosocial development of men in early adulthood and the mid-life transition. In D. Ricks, A. Thomas, & M. Roff (Eds.), *Life history research in psychopathology* (Vol. 3). Minneapolis, Minn.: University of Minnesota Press, 1974.

Levi-Strauss, C. *The raw and the cooked: Introduction to a science of mythology, 1*. New York: Harper & Row, 1969.

Liebert, R. M., & Spiegler, M. D. *Personality: Strategies and issues* (3rd ed.). Homewood, Ill.: Dorsey Press, 1978.

Lifton, R. J. *The broken connection: On death and the continuity of life*. New York: Simon & Schuster, 1979.

Loevinger, J. The meaning and measurement of ego development. *American Psychologist*, 1966, 21, 195–206.

Loevinger, J. Theories of ego development. In L. Breger (Ed.), *Clinical-cognitive psychology: Models and integrations.* Englewood Cliffs, N.J.: Prentice-Hall, 1969.

Loevinger, J. Ego development: Syllabus for a course. In B. Rubenstein (Ed.), *Psychoanalysis and contemporary science* (Vol. 2). New York: Macmillan, 1973.

Loevinger, J. *Ego development: Conceptions and theories.* San Francisco: Jossey-Bass, 1976.

Loevinger, J. Construct validity of the sentence-completion test of ego development. *Applied Psychological Measurement,* 1979, 3, 281–311.

Loevinger, J. On ego development and the structure of personality. *Developmental Review,* 1983, 3, 339–350.

Loevinger, J., & Wessler, R. *Measuring ego development 1. Construction and use of a sentence completion test* (2nd ed.). San Francisco: Jossey-Bass, 1978.

Loevinger, J., Wessler, R., & Redmore, C. *Measuring ego development 2. Scoring manual for women and girls* (2nd. ed.). San Francisco: Jossey-Bass, 1978.

Lowenthal, M. F., Thurnher, M., Chiriboga, D., & Associates. *Four stages of life: A comparative study of men and women facing transitions.* San Francisco: Jossey-Bass, 1975.

Lundy, A. *The validity and reliability of the thematic measures of the intimacy motive and need for affiliation.* Unpublished manuscript, Harvard University, 1980.

Maddi, S. R. *Personality theories: A comparative analysis* (4th ed.). Homewood, Ill.: Dorsey Press, 1980.

Maddi, S. R. *Personology for the 1980s.* Opening address at the Michigan State University Henry A. Murray Lectures in Personality, East Lansing, Mich.: April 16–17, 1982.

Mandler, G. *Mind and emotion.* New York: John Wiley & Sons, 1975.

Mandler, J. M., & Johnson, N. S. Remembrance of things parsed: Story structure and recall. *Cognitive Psychology,* 1977, 9, 111–151.

Marcel, G. *Creative fidelity.* New York: Farrar, Straus and Giroux, 1964.

Marcia, J. E. Development and validation of ego identity status. *Journal of Personality and Social Psychology,* 1966, 3, 551–558.

Marcia, J. E. Ego identity status: Relationships to change in self-esteem, "general maladjustment," and authoritarianism. *Journal of Personality,* 1967, 35, 119–133.

Marcia, J. E. Identity in adolescence. In J. Adelson (Ed.), *Handbook of adolescent psychology.* New York: John Wiley & Sons, 1980.

Marcia, J. E., & Friedman, M. L. Ego identity status in college women. *Journal of Personality,* 1970, 38, 249–263.

Margoshes, A., & Litt, S. Vivid experiences: Peak and nadir. *Journal of Clinical Psychology,* 1966, 22, 175.

Markus, H. Self-schemata and processing information about the self. *Journal of Personality and Social Psychology,* 1977, 35, 63–78.

Maslow, A. H. *Motivation and personality.* New York: Harper & Row, 1954.

Maslow, A. H. *Toward a psychology of being.* New York: Van Norstrand Reinhold, 1968.

Matteson, D. R. *Adolescence today: Sex role and the search for identity.* Homewood, Ill.: Dorsey Press, 1975.

May, R. *Sex and fantasy: Patterns of male and female development.* New York: W. W. Norton, 1980.

McAdams, D. P. *Validation of a thematic coding system for the intimacy motive.* Unpublished doctoral dissertation, Harvard University, 1979.

McAdams, D. P. A thematic coding system for the intimacy motive. *Journal of Research in Personality,* 1980, 14, 413–432.

McAdams, D. P. Intimacy motivation. In A. J. Stewart (Ed.), *Motivation and society.* San Francisco: Jossey-Bass, 1982. (a)

McAdams, D. P. Experiences of intimacy and power: Relationships between social motives and autobiographical memory. *Journal of Personality and Social Psychology,* 1982, *42,* 292–302. (b)

McAdams, D. P. Human motives and personal relationships. In V. Derlega (Ed.), *Communication, intimacy, and close relationships.* New York: Academic Press, 1984. (a)

McAdams, D. P. Love, power, and images of the self, pp. 184–86, 191, and 194–200 in C. Malatesta & C. Izard (Eds.), *Emotion in adult development.* Beverly Hills, Calif.: Copyright © 1984 (b) by Sage Publications, Inc.

McAdams, D. P. Scoring manual for the intimacy motive. *Psychological Documents,* 1984, *14,* 2614. (c)

McAdams, D. P., Booth, L., & Selvik, R. Religious identity among students at a private college: Social motives, ego stage, and development. *Merrill-Palmer Quarterly,* 1981, *27,* 219–239.

McAdams, D. P., & Constantian, C. A. Intimacy and affiliation motives in daily living: An experience sampling analysis. *Journal of Personality and Social Psychology,* 1983, *45,* 851–861.

McAdams, D. P., Healy, S., & Krause, S. Social motives and patterns of friendship. *Journal of Personality and Social Psychology,* in press.

McAdams, D. P., Jackson, R. J., & Kirshnit, C. Looking, laughing, and smiling in dyads as a function of intimacy motivation and reciprocity. *Journal of Personality,* in press.

McAdams, D. P., & Losoff, M. Friendship motivation in fourth and sixth graders: A thematic analysis. *Journal of Social and Personal Relationships,* 1984, *1,* 11–27.

McAdams, D. P., & Powers, J. Themes of intimacy in behavior and thought. *Journal of Personality and Social Psychology,* 1981, *40,* 573–587.

McAdams, D. P., & Vaillant, G. E. Intimacy motivation and psychosocial adjustment: A longitudinal study. *Journal of Personality Assessment,* 1982, *46,* 586–593.

McClelland, D. C. *Personality.* New York: Holt, Rinehart & Winston, 1951.

McClelland, D. C. *The achieving society.* New York: Free Press, 1961.

McClelland, D. C. *Power: The inner experience.* New York: Irvington Publishers, 1975.

McClelland, D. C. Inhibited power motivation and high blood pressure in men. *Journal of Abnormal Psychology,* 1979, *88,* 182–190.

McClelland, D. C. Motive dispositions: The merits of operant and respondent measures. In L. Wheeler (Ed.), *Review of personality and social psychology: 1.* Beverly Hills, Calif.: Sage Publications, 1980.

McClelland, D. C. Is personality consistent? In A. I. Rabin, J. Aronoff, A. M. Barclay, and R. A. Zucker (Eds.), *Further explorations in personality.* New York: John Wiley & Sons, 1981.

McClelland, D. C. *Human motivation.* Glenview, Ill.: Scott, Foresman, 1984.

McClelland, D. C., Alexander, C., & Marks, E. The need for power, stress, immune function, and illness among male prisoners. *Journal of Abnormal Psychology,* 1982, *91,* 61–70.

McClelland, D. C., & Atkinson, J. W. The projective expression of needs I.: The effect of different intensities of the hunger drive on perception. *Journal of Psychology,* 1948, *25,* 205–222.

McClelland, D. C., Atkinson, J. W., Clark, R. A., & Lowell, E. L. *The achievement motive.* New York: Appleton-Century-Crofts, 1953.

McClelland, D. C., Davis, W. N., Kalin, R., & Wanner, E. *The drinking man.* New York: Free Press, 1972.

McClelland, D. C., Floor, E., Davidson, R. J., & Saron, C. Stressed power motivation, sympathetic activation, immune function, and illness. *Journal of Human Stress,* 1980, *6* (2), 11–19.

McClelland, D. C., & Jemmott, J. B., III. Power motivation, stress, and physical illness. *Journal of Human Stress,* 1980, *6* (4), 6–15.

McClelland, D. C., & Teague, G. Predicting risk preferences among power-related tasks. *Journal of Personality*, 1975, *43*, 262–285.

McClelland, D. C., Wanner, E., & Vanneman, R. Drinking in the wider context of restrained and unrestrained assertive thoughts and acts. In D. C. McClelland, W. N. Davis, R. Kalin, & E. Wanner, *The drinking man*. New York: Free Press, 1972.

McClelland, D. C., & Watson, R. I., Jr. Power motivation and risk-taking behavior. *Journal of Personality*, 1973, *41*, 121–139.

McCrae, R. R., & Costa, P. T. Openness to experience and ego level in Loevinger's Sentence-Completion Test: Dispositional contributions to developmental models of personality. *Journal of Personality and Social Psychology*, 1980, *39*, 1179–1190.

McCrae, R. R., & Costa, P. T. Psychological maturity and subjective well-being: Toward a new sythesis. *Developmental Psychology*, 1983, *19*, 243–248.

McDougall, W. *Social psychology*. London: Methuen, 1908.

Miller, N. E., & Dollard, J. *Social learning and imitation*. New Haven, Conn.: Yale University Press, 1941.

Milrod, D. The wished-for self-image. In A. J. Solnit, R. S. Eissler, A. Freud, and P. B. Neubauer (Eds.), *The psychoanalytic study of the child* (Vol. 37). New Haven, Conn.: Yale University Press, 1982.

Mischel, W. *Personality and assessment*. New York: John Wiley & Sons, 1968.

Mischel, W. Toward a cognitive-social learning reconceptualization of personality. *Psychological Review*, 1973, *80*, 252–283.

Morgan, C. D., & Murray, H. A. A method of investigating fantasies. *Archives of Neurological Psychiatry*, 1935, *34*, 289–306.

Monte, C. F. *Beneath the mask: An introduction to theories of personality* (2nd ed.). New York: Holt, Rinehart & Winston, 1980.

Moreno, J. L. *Psychodrama* (Vol. 1). Boston, Mass.: Beacon Press, 1946.

Morris, C. W. *Varieties of human value*. Chicago: University of Chicago Press, 1956.

Murray, H. A. *Explorations in personality*. New York: Oxford University Press, 1938.

Murray, H. A. *Thematic apperception test*. Cambridge, Mass.: Harvard University Press, 1943.

Murray, H. A. Some basic psychological assumptions and conceptions. *Dialectica*, 1951, *5*, 266–292.

Murray, H. A. American Icarus. In A. Burton and R. E. Harris (Eds.), *Clinical studies in personality*. New York: Harper & Row, 1955. Also in E. S. Schneidman (Ed.), *Endeavors in psychology: Selections from the personology of Henry A. Murray*. New York: Harper & Row, 1981.

Nabokov, V. *Lectures on literature*. New York: Harcourt Brace Jovanovich, 1980.

Nardi, P., & Tsujimoto, R. N. The relationship of moral maturity and ethical attitude. *Journal of Personality*, 1979, *47*, 365–377.

Neisser, U. *Cognition and reality*. San Francisco: W. H. Freeman, 1976.

Neugarten, B. L. Time, age, and the life cycle. *American Journal of Psychiatry*, 1979, *136*, 887–894.

Nucci, L. Conceptions of personal issues: A domain distinct from moral or societal concepts. *Child Development*, 1981, *52*, 114–121.

Olney, J. *Metaphors of self: The meaning of autobiography*. Princeton, N.J.: Princeton University Press, 1972.

Orlofsky, J. L. Identity formation, achievements, and fear of success in college men and women. *Journal of Youth and Adolescence*, 1978, *7*, 49–62.

Orlofsky, J. L., Marcia, J. E., & Lesser, I. M. Ego identity status and the intimacy versus isolation crisis of young adulthood. *Journal of Personality and Social Psychology*, 1973, *27*, 211–219.

Oshman, H., & Manosevitz, M. The impact of the identity crisis on the adjustment of late adolescent males. *Journal of Youth and Adolescence*, 1974, *3*, 207–216.

Pachter, M. The biographer himself: An introduction. In M. Pachter (Ed.), *Telling lives: The biographer's art*. Washington, D.C.: New Republic Books, 1979.

Paloutzian, R. F. Purpose in life and value changes following conversion. *Journal of Personality and Social Psychology*, 1981, *41*, 1153–1160.

Palys, T. S., & Little, B. R. Perceived life satisfaction and the organization of personal project systems. *Journal of Personality and Social Psychology*, 1983, *44*, 1221–1230.

Perry, W. C. *Forms of intellectual and ethical development in the college years*. New York: Holt, Rinehart & Winston, 1970.

Plamenatz, J. *Ideology*. New York: Praeger Publishers, 1970.

Podd, M. H. Ego identity status and morality: The relationship between two developmental constructs. *Developmental Psychology*, 1972, *6*, 497–507.

Podd, M. H., Marcia, J. E., & Rubin, B. M. The effects of ego identity and partner perception on a prisoner's dilemna game. *Journal of Social Psychology*, 1970, *82*, 117–126.

Poppen, P. J. *The development of sex differences in moral judgment for college males and females*. Unpublished doctoral dissertation, Cornell University, 1974.

Prince, G. *A grammar for stories*. Gravenhage: Mouton, 1973.

Privette, G., & Landsman, T. Factor analysis of peak performance: The full use of potential. *Journal of Personality and Social Psychology*, 1983, *44*, 195–200.

Progoff, I. *At a journal workshop*. New York: Dialogue House, 1977.

Rabin, A. I., Aronoff, J., Barclay, A. M., & Zucker, R. A. (Eds.). *Further explorations in personality*. New York: John Wiley & Sons, 1981.

Radnitzky, G. *Contemporary schools of metascience*. South Bend, In.: Regnery/Gateway, 1973.

Rainer, T. *The new diary*. Los Angeles: J. P. Tarcher, 1978.

Rank, O. *Truth and reality*. New York: W. W. Norton, 1978. (Originally published, 1936.)

Redmore, C., Loevinger, J., & Tamashiro, R. *Measuring ego development: Scoring manual for men and boys*. Unpublished manuscript, 1978.

Redmore, C., & Waldman, K. Reliability of a sentence completion measure of ego development. *Journal of Personality Assessment*, 1975, *39*, 236–243.

Riegel, K. F. *Psychology mon amour: A countertext*. Boston: Houghton Mifflin, 1978.

Rizzo, R., & Vinacke, E. Self-actualization and the meaning of critical experiences. *Journal of Humanistic Psychology*, 1975, *15*, 19–30.

Rogers, C. R. *Client-centered therapy*. Boston: Houghton Mifflin, 1951.

Rokeach, M. *The nature of human values*. New York: Free Press, 1973.

Rootes, M. D., Moras, K., & Gordon, R. Ego development and sociometrically evaluated maturity: An investigation of the validity of the Washington University Sentence-Completion Test of Ego Development. *Journal of Personality Assessment*, 1980, *44*, 613–620.

Ross, J. M. Oedipus revisited: Laius and the "Laius complex." In A. J. Solnit, R. S. Eissler, A. Freud, and P. B. Neubauer (Eds.), *The psychoanalytic study of the child* (Vol. 37). New Haven, Conn.: Yale University Press, 1982.

Rowe, I. *Ego identity status, cognitive development and levels of moral reasoning*. Unpublished master's thesis, Simon Fraser University, 1978.

Rozsnafszky, J. The relationship of level of ego development to Q-sort personality rating. *Journal of Personality and Social Psychology*, 1981, *41*, 99–120.

Rubin, Z. *Liking and loving*. New York: Holt, Rinehart & Winston, 1973.

Runyan, W. M. The life course as a theoretical orientation: Sequence of person-situation interactions. *Journal of Personality*, 1978, *46*, 569–593.

Runyan, W. M. *Life histories and psychobiography: Explorations in theory and method*. New York: Oxford University Press, 1982.

Russell, B. *A history of Western philosophy*. New York: Simon & Schuster, 1972. (Originally published, 1945.)

Ryff, C. D., & Heincke, S. G. Subjective organization of personality in adulthood and aging. *Journal of Personality and Social Psychology*, 1983, 44, 807–816.

Sartre, J. P. *Being and nothingness*. New York: Washington Square Press, 1966.

Schenkel, S., & Marcia, J. E. Attitudes toward premarital intercourse in determining ego identity status in college women. *Journal of Personality*, 1972, 3, 472–482.

Schneidman, E. S., Barron, E., Sanford, N., Smith, M. B., Tomkins, S., & Tyler, L. Aspects of the personological system of Henry A. Murray. *Personality and Social Psychology Bulletin*, 1982, 8, 604–623.

Selman, R. L. *The growth of interpersonal understanding*. New York: Academic Press, 1980.

Sheehy, G. *Passages: Predictable crises of adult life*. New York: E. P. Dutton, 1976.

Shipley, T. E., & Veroff, J. A projective measure of need for affiliation. *Journal of Experimental Psychology*, 1952, 43, 349–365.

Shweder, R. A. Liberalism as destiny: Review of L. Kohlberg's *The philosophy of moral development: Moral stages and the idea of justice*. In *Contemporary Psychology*, 1982, 27, 421–424.

Siegal, M. Kohlberg vs. Piaget: To what extent has one theory eclipsed the other? *Merrill-Palmer Quarterly*, 1980, 26, 285–297.

Singer, J. L., & Singer, D. G. Personality. In P. H. Mussen & M. R. Rosenzweig (Eds.), *Annual review of psychology* (Vol. 23). Palo Alto, Calif.: Annual Reviews, Inc., 1972.

Slavin, M. O. *The theme of feminine evil: the image of women in male fantasy and its effects on atitudes and behavior*. Unpublished doctoral dissertation, Harvard University, 1972.

Spitz, R. A. *The first year of life: A psychoanalytic study of normal and deviant development of object relations*. New York: International Universities Press, 1965.

Sroufe, L. A., & Waters, E. Attachment as an organizational construct. *Child Development*, 1977, 48, 1184–1199.

Steele, R. S. Power motivation, activation, and inspirational speeches. *Journal of Personality*, 1977, 45, 53–64.

Steele, R. S. *Freud and Jung: Conflicts of interpretation*. London: Routledge & Kegan Paul, 1982.

Stein, N. L. How children understand stories: A developmental analysis. In L. Katz (Ed.), *Current topics in early childhood education* (Vol. 2). Norwood, N.J.: Albex, 1979.

Stein, N. L., & Glenn, C. G. An analysis of story comprehension in elementary-school children. In R. O. Freedle (Ed.), *New directions in discourse processing* (Vol. 2), *Advances in discourse processes*. Norwood, N.J.: Albex, 1979.

Stein, N. L., & Policastro, M. The concept of a story: A comparison between children's and teacher's viewpoints. In H. Mandl, N. L. Stein, and T. Trabasso (Eds.), *Learning and comprehension of text*. Hillsdale, N.J.: Lawrence Erlbaum Associates, 1984.

Steiner, C. M. *Scripts people live*. New York: Grove Press, 1974.

Stevens, A. *Archetypes: A natural history of the self*. New York: Quill, 1983.

Stewart, A. J. (Ed.) *Motivation and society*. San Francisco: Jossey-Bass, 1982.

Stewart, A. J., & Chester, N. L. Sex differences in human social motives: Achievement, affiliation, and power. In A. J. Stewart (Ed.), *Motivation and society*. San Francisco: Jossey-Bass, 1982.

Stewart, A. J., & Rubin, Z. Power motivation in the dating couple. *Journal of Personality and Social Psychology*, 1976, 34, 305–309.

Stewart, A. J., & Winter, D. G. Arousal of the power motive in women. *Journal of Consulting and Clinical Psychology*, 1976, 44, 495–496.

Sullivan, H. S. *The interpersonal theory of psychiatry*. New York: W. W. Norton, 1953.

Sutton-Smith, B. The importance of the storytaker: An investigation of the imaginative life. *The Urban Review*, 1976, 8, 82–95.

Terkel, S. *Working*. New York: Pantheon Books, a Division of Random House, Inc. ©
1972.

Tesch, S. A., & Whitbourne, S. K. Intimacy and identity status in young adults. *Journal
of Personality and Social Psychology*, 1982, *43*, 1041–1051.

Thorne, F. C. The clinical use of peak and nadir experiences. *Journal of Clinical Psychology*, 1963, *19*, 248–250.

Titchener, E. B. Early memories. *American Journal of Psychology*, 1900, *11*, 435–436.

Toder, N., & Marcia, J. E. Ego identity status and response to conformity pressure in
college women. *Journal of Personality and Social Psychology*, 1973, *26*, 287–294.

Tomkins, S. S. Script theory: Differential magnification of affects. In H. E. Howe and
R. A. Dienstbier (Eds.), *Nebraska symposium on motivation* (Vol. 26). Lincoln:
University of Nebraska Press, 1979.

Trabasso, T., Secco, T., & Van Den Broek, P. Causal cohesion and story coherence. In
H. Mandl, N. L. Stein, and T. Trabasso (Eds.), *Learning and comprehension of text*.
Hillsdale, N.J.: Lawrence Erlbaum Associates, 1984.

Turiel, E. Conflict and transition in adolescent moral development. *Child Development*,
1974, *45*, 14–29.

Uleman, J. S. *The new TAT measure of the need for power*. Unpublished doctoral dissertation, Harvard University, 1966.

Uleman, J. S. The need for influence: Development and validation of a measure, and
comparison with the need for power. *Genetic Psychology Monographs*, 1972, *85*,
157–214.

Updike, J. Introduction to Nabokov, V. *Lectures on literature*. New York: Harcourt Brace
Jovanovich, 1980.

Vaihinger, H. *The philosophy of "as if."* New York: Harcourt Brace Jovanovich, 1925.
(Originally published, 1911.)

Vaillant, G. E. *Adaptation to life*. Boston: Little, Brown, 1977.

Vaillant, G. E., & McArthur, C. C. Natural history of male psychologic health: 1. The
adult life cycle from 18 to 50. *Seminars in Psychiatry*, 1972, *4*, 415–427.

Veroff, J. Development and validation of a projective measure of power motivation.
Journal of Abnormal and Social Psychology, 1957, *54*, 1–8.

Veroff, J. Assertive motivations: Achievement versus power. In A. J. Stewart (Ed.),
Motivation and society. San Francisco: Jossey-Bass, 1982.

Veroff, J., & Feld, S. *Marriage and work in America: A study of motives and roles*. New York:
Van Nostrand Reinhold, 1970.

Vinokur, A., & Selzer, M. L. Desirable versus undesirable life events: Their relationship
to stress and mental distress. *Journal of Personality and Social Psychology*, 1975, *32*,
329–337.

Waterman, A. S. Identity development from adolescence to adulthood: An extension
of theory and a review of research. *Developmental Psychology*, 1982, *18*, 341–358.

Weiss-Bourd, R., & Sears, R. R. Mark Twain's exhibitionism. *Biography*, 1982, *5*, 95–117.

Welsh, G. S. Factor dimensions A and R. In G. S. Welsh and W. G. Dahlstrom (Eds.),
Basic readings on the MMPI in psychology and medicine. Minneapolis, Minn.: University of Minnesota Press, 1956.

Werner, H. The concept of development from a comparative and an organismic point
of view. In D. Harris (Ed.), *The concept of development*. Minneapolis: University of
Minnesota Press, 1957.

White, R. W. *Lives in progress* (1st ed.). New York: Holt, Rinehart & Winston, 1952.

White, R. W. *Lives in progress* (2nd ed.). New York: Holt, Rinehart & Winston, 1966.

White, R. W. *Lives in progress* (3rd. ed.). New York: Holt, Rinehart & Winston, 1975.

White, R. W. Exploring personality the long way: The study of lives. In A. I. Rabin, J.
Aronoff, A. M. Barclay, and R. A. Zucker (Eds.), *Further explorations in personality*. New York: John Wiley & Sons, 1981.

Wilson, E. O. *On human nature*. Cambridge, Mass.: Harvard University Press, 1978.

Winter, D. G. *The power motive*. New York: Free Press 1973.

Winter, D. G., McClelland, D. C., & Stewart, A. J. *A new case for the liberal arts: Assessing institutional goals and student development.* San Francisco: Jossey-Bass, 1981.

Winter, D. G., & Stewart, A. J. Power motive reliability as a function of retest instructions. *Journal of Consulting and Clinical Psychology,* 1977, *45,* 436–440.

Winter, D. G., & Stewart, A. J. The power motive. In H. London & J. E. Exner, Jr. (Eds.), *Dimensions of personality.* New York: John Wiley & Sons, 1978.

Winter, D. G., Stewart, A. J., & McClelland, D. C. Husband's motives and wife's career level. *Journal of Personality and Social Psychology,* 1977, *35,* 159–166.

Wrightsman, L. S. Personal documents as data in conceptualizing adult personality development. *Personality and Social Psychology Bulletin,* 1981, 367–385.

Yankelovich, D. *New rules: Searching for self-fulfillment in a world turned upside down.* New York: Random House, 1981.

Yankelovich, D., & Barrett, W. *Ego and instinct.* New York: Random House, 1971.

Author Index *

* See also Subject Index for names of persons not listed in References, pages 306–20.

Subject Index

CPSIA information can be obtained
at www.ICGtesting.com
Printed in the USA
FSHW010346151118
53666FS